On Speed

Nicolas Rasmussen

On Speed

The Many Lives of Amphetamine

New York University Press • *New York and London*

NEW YORK UNIVERSITY PRESS
New York and London
www.nyupress.org

First published in paperback in 2009.

Library of Congress Cataloging-in-Publication Data
Rasmussen, Nicolas, 1962–
On speed : the many lives of amphetamine / Nicolas Rasmussen.
p. ; cm.
Includes bibliographical references and index.
ISBN-13: 978-0-8147-7639-1 (pb : alk. paper)
ISBN-10: 0-8147-7639-6 (pb : alk. paper)
ISBN-13: 978-0-8147-7601-8 (cl : alk. paper)
ISBN-10: 0-8147-7601-9 (cl : alk. paper)
1. Amphetamines—United States—History. 2. Amphetamine abuse—
United States—History.   I. Title. II. Title: Many lives of amphetamine.
[DNLM: 1. Amphetamines—history—United States. 2. Amphetamine-Related
Disorders—history—United States. 3. History, 20th Century—United States.
4. History, 21st Century—United States.   QV 102 R225o 2007]
RM666.A493R37 2007
362.29'90973—dc22   2007043261

New York University Press books are printed on acid-free paper,
and their binding materials are chosen for strength and durability.

Manufactured in the United States of America

c 10 9 8 7 6 5 4 3 2 1
p 10 9 8 7 6 5 4 3 2 1

To my parents, Laura and Norman,
  for teaching me to ask questions

Contents

Illustrations appear in two groups following pages 86 and 148.

Acknowledgments

This book benefited from so much help from so many people over so many years that it is hard to know where to begin to express my gratitude. I owe special thanks to those who have sacrificed their valuable time in commenting on drafts and excerpts, notably Jackie Biro, Mark Cortiula, Larry Diller, David Healy, Chris Kearney, Iain McGregor, Kane Race, Ned Shorter, and, especially, Andy Rasmussen. Those who helped by sharing their expertise and discussing ideas include Caroline Acker, Philippe Bourgois, Joel Braslow, Elizabeth Bromley, Christopher Callahan, Iain Chalmers, Jean-Paul Gaudilliere, Jeremy Greene, Wayne Hall, Harry Marks, Peter Neushul, Scott Podolsky, Hans Pols, Jonathan Sadowski, Jonathan Simon, Peter Steinkamp, John Swann, and Jackie Taylor. Dave Smith kindly sacrificed an entire day for interviewing, for which I am grateful. The substance of the work would not have been possible without the help and forbearance of archivists at the California Institute of Technology, Harvard University, the National Academy of Sciences USA, Rockefeller Archive Center, Tufts University, the University of California at San Francisco, the University of Pennsylvania, several U.S. National Archives and Records Administration facilities, and the United Kingdom National Archives. The research assistance of Larissa Johnson was most helpful in completing the work. I also gratefully acknowledge support from the Biot Fund of the California Institute of Technology, the American Institute for the History of Pharmacy, an Arts Faculty Research Grant and Gold Star award from the University of New South Wales, and especially an Australian Research Council Discovery Project grant, number DP0449467. Last, but certainly not least, this work owes its origins to stimulating discussions with John Gregg.

Introduction

OURS IS AN age accustomed to miracle drugs. We expect new triumphs of science that, in our lifetime, will eliminate mankind's most ancient enemies: all the illnesses that bring pain, sorrow, frailty, and untimely death. We expect these triumphs, moreover, to come in pharmaceutical form. The most famous miracle drug remains penicillin, and rightly so. In the 1940s, this microbe-derived antibiotic (and its successors) made a huge difference to human well-being and life expectancy. Thanks to penicillin, death by bacterial infection changed, almost overnight, from a commonplace tragedy to a rarity. Before penicillin's introduction, there were also a few medicines one could "fairly call miracle drugs," for example, Salvarsan, the anti-syphilis medicine in the 1910s; insulin for diabetes in the 1920s; and the first "sulfa" antibacterial agents in the 1930s.[1]

Many more drugs have been hailed as miracles since the Second World War, medicines for the soul as well as the body. In the 1950s, alongside the cortical steroids that helped the crippled walk again, came the first antipsychotic drugs like chlorpromazine (Thorazine), restoring composure to the raving mad. In the 1960s, accompanying the birth control pill and the beta-blockers for heart disease, were the benzodiazepine "minor tranquilizers," such as Librium and Valium, that saved us undue suffering from anxieties born of inner conflict.[2] And the list goes on. None of our latter-day miracles for mind and body has matched the contribution of penicillin, nor has any presented so few adverse consequences. Still, new pharmaceuticals continue to enjoy hearty acclaim as "miracle drugs." Creating or at least amplifying such acclaim is now a routine function of pharmaceutical company marketing.

Just as the the first flush of enthusiasm inevitably leads to a marvelous new drug's prescription to millions, so inevitably does consumption of a new drug by millions reveal its limits and its dark side.[3] Now cortical steroids are known to cause their own set of crippling side-effects, antipsychotics like chlorpromazine cause brain damage, the benzodiazepine tranquilizers are fiercely addictive, and the original contraceptive formulas can cause deadly blood clots and probably cancer as well. To be sure, certain people did benefit overall from these drugs. Some of them are still part of medical practice, though they are used more cautiously now than when they were first welcomed as panaceas. Other drugs have fallen completely by the wayside, as their use proved more harmful than beneficial. None produced the miracles they first promised.

Yet, despite the predictability of disenchantment, we remain prepared to welcome new miracle drugs with undiminished optimism. In the 1990s Cox-2 inhibitors, such as Bextra and Celebrex, were the miraculous breakthroughs. These drugs promised to make arthritis suffering obsolete. Joining them were the selective serotonin reuptake inhibitor (SSRI) antidepressants like Prozac and Zoloft, which transformed oversensitivity and pessimism into easily treatable illnesses. The Cox-2 inhibitors are now in dramatic decline following revelations about their potential damage to the heart. The SSRIs, too, have lost some of their lustre but have not progressed as far as the Cox-2 inhibitors through the cycle that runs from tremendous promise to bitter disappointment. If past experience is any guide, they, too, in retrospect, will be seen as overprescribed to millions of unsuitable patients who could never even have benefited from the drugs but only bore the risks. The pharmaceutical industry has long understood this pattern of overzealousness, disillusionment, and rational reassessment of a drug's place in medicine—and has learned to make the most of the initial enthusiasm. Physicians seem at least partly aware, as testified by their inside joke: "Always prescribe the latest drug—while it still works!" The rest of us apparently prefer boundless hope to cynicism, trusting in the latest miracle drugs despite the repetitive lessons of the past.

Ultimately, this book is about the way age-old human fantasies of magical cures and elixirs of youth live on in the age of science-based pharmaceuticals. It is about the place drugs have come to occupy in our culture, and the role they play in medicine. It approaches these general questions through the remarkable and unique history of amphetamine, or "speed" as it has long been known colloquially. Choosing this drug as a basis for generalizing about pharmaceuticals may seem, at first, a peculiar choice. However, although we now think of recreational street drugs when we hear the name of this powerful stimulant, amphetamine was originally another miracle drug. Its fame was so great by about 1940 that it could have been included in the above list of medical breakthroughs, alongside insulin and penicillin. According to both experts and advertisements, amphetamine not only was the first antidepressant but the very first specific medicine for a mood disorder. It was also among the first generation of medicines developed through scientific research managed by drug companies. As a new chemical invention, it was protected by the patents whose limited terms create such an incentive for manufacturers to maximize the wave of early zeal around novel drugs.

During the Second World War, amphetamine and methamphetamine were adopted in the military services on all sides, in quasi-medical efforts to tune mind and body beyond normal human capabilities. Similarly, athletes welcomed the drugs as performance-enhancing panaceas in the postwar years. Around 1950, family doctors embraced amphetamines as psychiatric medications for their distressed patients, cementing the notion that depression was both commonplace and easily treatable. Moreover, amphetamines were hailed as a breakthrough in weight loss and enjoyed enormous success as diet pills, helping to transform obesity into the menacing though preventible and treatable epidemic that medicine views it as today. When scientists and drug firms began looking for improved antidepressants and diet drugs in the later 1950s, they based that search on amphetamine and the benchmarks it set in both areas of medicine. In revolutionizing the understanding and management of disease and paving the way for progress, amphetamine behaved as a model miracle drug, a pathbreaking pharmaceutical.

As with miracle drugs before and since, the imperfections of amphetamines emerged with extensive prescription use. In the late 1950s, researchers gradually learned that amphetamine and related drugs are addictive, and that heavy enough use may cause a severe psychotic condition. Psychiatrists abandoned amphetamines for newer, better antidepressants by the beginning of the 1960s. Remarkably, though, the consumption of amphetamines did not decline, as one would expect of outmoded miracle drugs. In general practice amphetamines remained the drugs of choice for lifting mood, and for aiding in weight loss. In the late 1960s, at the peak of the drug's popularity, one in twenty American adults were active users of amphetamines by prescription; at least half as many were using "speed" without prescriptions—altogether around 10 million people, equal to the entire combined populations of New York and Philadelphia at the time.[4] Amphetamine abuse was recognized, briefly, as the leading drug problem in the United States. Finally, in the early 1970s, strong government actions overcame drug industry resistance and restricted the supply of pharmaceutical amphetamines. By the late 1970s, America's speed epidemic seemed almost a concern of the past.

This one-time miracle drug still refused to retire gracefully, however. Speed remains with us today, despite relentless narcotics enforcement. Indeed, we are now suffering another epidemic of amphetamine abuse and addiction, driven by a recent surge in the popularity of crystalline methamphetamine or "ice," as well as the amphetamine derivatives known as "ecstasy." And, once again, amphetamine and its close relatives have become enormously popular pharmaceuticals, this time for Attention Deficit Disorder. The replacements for amphetamine offered up by the drug industry as diet drugs, from the 1970s to the mid-2000s, have remained closely related to amphetamines. We might also consider the antidepressant drugs which, although not amphetamines, have recently acquired the psychiatric market once belonging to amphetamine. From the perspective of user demand, more than one in ten Americans is now using drugs that, in the 1960s, would have been amphetamines. It seems that America's need for speed has doubled since 1970. So, although looking at the business of pharmaceuticals through the lens of amphetamine may seem odd initially, I believe just the opposite to be true. In one sense, there has never been a more successful pharmaceutical.

Amphetamine's triumphant career makes its history an excellent vehicle for understanding our society's routine miracle, the pharmaceutical blockbuster. Its late deviations from a breakthrough medicine's typical life cycle only help cast extra light on the place of drugs in our culture, and on what drives demand and success in the drug business. Of course, researching the history of commercial drug development, especially the action behind the experimental reports and advertisements published in the medical journals, is always challenging for the historian. Reliable documentary evidence on what occurs within corporations is rare. In the case of this particular drug, rumors and fables abound. Certainly, I have been fortunate in having the excellent work of other historians to study, as well as the work of social and medical theorists about drugs, all cited where the value of their contributions to this story is especially great. Where I have been able to go further than previous authors in finding the facts about amphetamine's history and sorting fact from fiction, I have done so largely by using evidence generated in the course of intellectual property lawsuits, where often secretive drug companies must publicly struggle to reconstruct and document the past. In certain places I have had to calculate key measures of past amphetamine consumption for comparison with recent figures, and while readily admitting that these do not meet the precision standards of current drug epidemiology, I still believe that conservative estimates based on the best available evidence are better than no quantitative knowledge of the past. The story of amphetamine encapsulates America's love affair with pharmaceuticals, and that story now needs to be told.[5]

The New Sensation

ON JUNE 3, 1929, a twenty-seven-year-old chemist in Los Angeles took an injection of a mystery chemical he had recently created. Beyond an estimate of how much it would take to kill him, and the expectation that his blood pressure would rise—both derived from guinea pig tests—he had little idea what the injection would do. He was hoping to discover a new allergy medicine that day. It took a little while for anything to happen, because his doctor friend had injected the drug subcutaneously, rather than directly into a vein. But within ten minutes his blood pressure started to go up sharply, worrying both men until it stabilized a couple of hours later at about one and a half times his normal level. Around the time that he starting feeling some small effect, the chemist sniffed and, optimistically, recorded that his nose was clear. Soon after, some eighteen minutes after the injection, he noticed something more interesting and unexpected. "Feeling of well being," reads the notebook entry dryly. The chemist was enjoying this experiment. His doctor friend, Hyman Miller, sat with him for a few hours, chatting with the unusually talkative chemist and checking his blood pressure regularly, eventually inviting him home to dinner with his wife. The chemist recalled being an especially witty guest that evening. After Miller packed him off to bed, the chemist, still in good spirits, experienced a "rather sleepless night" where his "mind seemed to race from one subject to another," according to his notebook (Figure 1). Still, he felt fairly well in the morning.[1]

As a chemist, Gordon Alles called the substance he took that day beta-phenyl-isopropylamine, better known today as amphetamine. That day Alles had taken 50 milligrams (mg), five times what would become the standard dose once the substance was medically approved eight years later. Although he had no idea what it would be used for, the chemist knew right away that he had made a significant discovery. What no one could have guessed is how irresistible this powerful drug would prove to be, holding Americans in its thrall for three generations, all the way to the present day. So began the age of speed.

Adrenalin: New Medicine for a New Century

Alles, appropriately enough, was born in 1901, the year that Parke-Davis & Company of Detroit launched its brand-name "Adrenalin" on the market. At the time the drug business was undergoing drastic change. Adapting to dramatic advances and new attitudes in medicine presented a great challenge to pharmaceutical firms accustomed to selling mostly traditional herbs and tinctures. In Europe, the past few decades had seen the triumph of a totally new approach to healing. Called "scientific medicine," it was based in part on the careful, quantitative analysis of how well different treatments worked when administered under controlled conditions, like those found in the large hospitals that had recently been linked to medical schools. This new approach was also based in the laboratory work of experimental biologists, especially in the fields of bacteriology and physiology. Bacteriologists like Louis Pasteur and Robert Koch had identified the microbes that caused many dreaded illnesses, and also invented new vaccines that could prevent some of them. In the case of a few diseases such as diphtheria, they had even invented serums that could be used to save those already ill. Meanwhile, physiologists had been probing the chemical function of the different organs and discovered that some controlled bodily function by releasing powerful biochemical signals, or "hormones." In 1894, British physiologists identified a hormone made by the adrenal gland, soon named "adrenaline,"[2] by showing that an extract of the organ raises blood pressure when injected in experimental animals (implying that the adrenal gland plays a role in regulating circulation under some circumstances). Several scientists in Germany claimed success in isolating the hormone, and drug companies working closely with them put purified adrenal hormones on the market around 1900. But the most successful was Parke, Davis "& Company's 'Adrenalin'" preparation, based on a procedure developed by the leading American pharmacologist of the day, J. J. Abel of Johns Hopkins University (although it was the Japanese biochemist Jokichi Takamine who, after working briefly with Abel in Baltimore and improving his method, patented it and sold it to Parke, Davis).

This product, arguably the first important new drug to emerge from advances in physiology, was a milestone (Figure 2).[3] The life sciences were proving that they could yield practical benefits in the form of new medicines that could aid both doctors and patients, and nowhere was the potential more exciting than in the new science of the glands.

Adrenalin was also a special landmark for American medicine since it was invented in the United States, and commercialized by an American company, at a time when that nation lagged woefully behind Europe in both medical science and pharmaceuticals. To bring the American medical profession up to French and German standards, medical leaders in the 1890s had launched an aggressive reform program to introduce much more science into the medical school curriculum.[4] The crisis in American medical education around the turn of the century coincided with a crisis in the nation's pharmaceutical industry. That Adrenalin, a scientifically credible drug, had come from an American firm in 1901 was surprising, because the American drug industry was mainly selling snake oil at that time. There had long been makers of "ethical" drugs, medicines whose mostly plant-based ingredients were accurately disclosed and which were marketed mainly to doctors for prescription. In the late nineteenth century, however, these drugs were being crowded out by junk nostrums or so-called patent remedies—in 1900, these dubious drugs represented 72 percent of pharmaceutical industry sales, more than double their share of the American drug market twenty years earlier. Hype and mystery were the leading ingredient in the "patent" medicines (a misnomer, since the formulas of these potions and pills were typically secret, and, in any case, were not patentable). Many also featured a hefty percentage of alcohol, like Doctor Hotstetter's Celebrated Stomachic Bitters (64 proof) and Peruna, the best-selling cure-all (56 proof). These sold especially well in areas under the control of Temperance forces.[5] Some patent medicines promised health based on the recent breakthroughs of medical science, like Radam's Microbe Killer, and Radol, a "marvellous radiotized fluid" that supposedly cured cancer. Fortunately for gullible users, Radol contained no actual radium; both were basically water. Such fraudulent products were still seen as a menace to public health by the scientific medicine reformers, since users, believing they were being treated, avoided seeing doctors for (marginally) more effective professional care. But, in 1901, the most sinister pharmaceuticals were the patent remedies that contained the few really powerful drugs then known to medicine, particularly morphine-based sedatives and cough syrups, and invigorating cocaine-based tonics and decongestant snuffs. Product labels often did not reveal the presence of these ingredients, so it was easy to get hooked, or to overdose.[6]

All these useless and dangerous medicines were available by mail order and over the counter at pharmacies everywhere, but the American medical profession shared responsibility for their unhealthy popularity. A study in the 1890s found that 90 percent of doctors had actually prescribed a patent remedy. Patent medicine makers disguised their products as drugs with scientific credentials, fooling physicians with technical-sounding names (like "Fellows' Syrup of Hypophosphites"), serious-looking advertisements in medical journals (Figure 3), professional "detail men" who called on doctors with samples and informational sales pitches, and commissioned research articles in reputable journals testifying to the therapeutic power of their remedies. In all of this they resembled the practices of the ethical drugmakers who, unwilling to neglect the lucrative nostrum business, were in truth not so very different.[7] For instance, for decades after its 1901 invention, one of the leading products of the Philadelphia firm Smith, Kline & French was an elixir called Eskay's Neurophospates. Like the venerable Fellows' Syrup, the only active drug in Neurophosphates was strychnine. This ingredient has some inconsistent stimulating effects, but it was included in nerve tonics mainly for psychological reasons, exploiting the common belief that powerful poisons are powerful cures. Strychnine, in combination with phosphorous, was standard in tonics designed for that popular and poorly defined epidemic of the period "neurasthenia" (depression understood as nervous depletion or chronic fatigue).[8] That a new medicine like Neurophosphates could be launched on the market by a reputable, ethical firm in the same year as Adrenalin, and then enjoy decades of success, speaks volumes about the American pharmaceutical business at the beginning of the twentieth century.

This free market pharmaceutical pandemonium outraged the more scientific-minded medical professors. The same reformers who were trying to educate doctors scientifically so they could "distinguish the rank fraud from the efficacious remedy, honestly made and sold," turned their attention to disciplining the American drug industry. Extravagant publicity and dubious company-sponsored research had too long been "debauching our medical journals" and "tainting our textbooks," thundered George Simmons, editor of the influential *Journal of the American Medical Association* (*JAMA*). In 1905, Simmons helped found the American Medical Association (AMA) Council on Pharmacy and Chemistry (later, Council on Drugs), consisting mainly of pharmacology professors and chemists, to police drug advertising in *JAMA*. Medicines that failed accurately to disclose their active ingredients could not be advertised. Ethical drugs with adequate labeling could be advertised, but only in ways that the Council considered justified. To win Council approval for an advertising claim, careful laboratory work and careful clinical trials were required. Doctors' testimonials boasting a handful of amazing "cures," commonly commissioned by drug makers, were no longer sufficient. A number of other major medical journals joined with *JAMA* by only running Council-approved ads, making this voluntary system of regulation the main guarantee of a drug's rational use for many years. (In fact, until the Second World War, this system remained much more effective than the regulation provided by federal Food and Drug law, which, from 1906, only ensured truthful labeling.) The net effect of the reforms for drug firms wishing to compete in the ethical field was to put an ever greater premium on science, as a source of new products, to justify claims of effectiveness, and also for general marketing use.[9] With its impeccable scientific pedigree, Adrenalin was an early example of what all good medicines were now supposed to look like.

The different actions of adrenaline on the body made pharmaceuticals containing the hormone medically useful in numerous ways. Adrenaline could restart the heart if injected straight into it, a procedure sometimes necessary in cases of shock, including allergic or "anaphylactic" shock—not uncommon in doctors' offices at the time because it can be caused by one too many serum injections. The hormone also constricts capillaries, making it popular with surgeons, who mixed it with a local anesthetic such as cocaine to slow bleeding during operations. All manner of elective surgery on soft tissues became safer and thus more popular. On the blood vessels of the lungs, adrenaline has an opposite effect, easing lung circulation and relaxing the air passages. This made it a very popular drug for asthma, more effective at halting an asthmatic attack than cocaine, sold at the time for asthma because of its similar effects. Sprayed into the nose, it was also a handy—if short-acting—decongestant. Adrenaline has a range of other effects, too, stimulating tear and sweat glands, causing the pupils to widen, and relaxing the intestinal muscles. Though less marketable, these actions of the hormone aroused great interest among physiologists.

Especially fascinating to scientists at the time was that each of these effects of adrenaline on various parts of the body looked exactly like the effects of electrical stimulation of certain nerves. The nervous system is divided into two main sections: the central nervous system consisting of the brain and spinal cord, and the peripheral nervous system. In the early twentieth century, the peripheral nerves were themselves usually subdivided into two groups: on the one hand, the sensory and motor nerves (grouped with the central nervous system now, and sometimes then), with which we feel and carry out voluntary movements, and, on the other, the involuntary or "autonomic" nerves that govern all the many functions over which we have little control, such as digestion, blood circulation, sexual function, pupil dilation, sweating, and salivating. Many of the muscles that perform these involuntary functions are, in fact, controlled by two sets of peripheral nerves, each with distinct structures and opposite functions: the sympathetic and the parasympathetic. Stimulate the sympathetic nerve to the eye of an anesthetized cat, and its pupil widens; stimulate the parasympathetic, and the pupil narrows. Adrenaline triggers the same effect on the eye, and indeed on most organs, that sympathetic nerve stimulation would cause. Soon after adrenaline was on the market and widely available for physiologists to use in their experiments, suspicions began to grow that nerves may actually transmit their impulses chemically, and not just electrically. Sympathetic nerves might transmit their signals with adrenaline, and the parasympathetic nerves might use another chemical, identified (in a parallel line of research) as acetylcholine. Decades would pass before physiologists stopped debating, especially about the central nervous system. But the theory that nerves transmit signals chemically gained support in medical science gradually throughout the teens and twenties, thanks partly to the availability for experiments of adrenaline, nerve juice in a jar.[10]

Commercial and medical interest in adrenaline did not wait for the neurophysiologists to solve their puzzles. Academic biochemists and drug firms in the first decade of the twentieth century sought new ways to extract adrenaline out of adrenal glands from the slaughterhouse. Nothing proved better than Takamine's and Parke, Davis's extraction method, however. Other scientists searched in plants for chemicals of similar chemistry and physiological effect, hoping to get around the Takamine patent on the best production method from animal material. Still others looked for synthetic drugs to substitute for natural adrenaline. One of these was the Cambridge University–trained physiologist Henry Dale. Working with chemist George Barger at the British drug company Burroughs-Wellcome, the young scientists created a series of chemicals similar in structure to adrenaline. The most active molecules all shared certain key structural features with adrenaline, in particular a benzene ring with a short side-chain of carbon. Surprisingly, some of these synthetic adrenaline variants had actions that mimicked sympathetic nerve stimulation—but not in exactly the same way as adrenaline. For example, one of them raised the blood pressure much longer than adrenaline did, but did not relax the lungs nearly as much. They named it "Tyramine," and Burroughs-Wellcome sold it as a treatment for shock. The 1910 paper in which Barger and Dale described these experiments quickly became a classic for pharmacologists, an example of how one could discover new remedies by systematically exploring a wide range of chemicals related to a hormone or other natural drug. As novel chemicals, these new remedies could then be patented and marketed as improved, scientific medicines, a lesson not lost on the pharmaceutical industry. Drug discovery was on its way to becoming a routine business function.[11]

The Drug Lab behind the Allergist's Office

By the 1920s Adrenalin had been joined by a number of other purified hormone medicines, as the drug business transformed itself into the science-based industry that we know today. Indeed, the advance of physiology and the thirst for new scientifically credible medicines had set off a "gold rush" in the hormone field. The 1921 appearance of insulin, the pancreas-derived hormone that turned a diabetes diagnosis from a death sentence into a manageable condition, was especially sensational. Insulin had been introduced to medicine through a collaboration between the University of Toronto physiologists who discovered how to extract the hormone, and the Eli Lilly firm of Indiana, which manufactured and marketed it. There was money in glands, without a doubt. Forward-thinking drug firms avidly sought top-notch academic scientists to help them, and every hormone researcher ambitious to be the first to purify the hormone of this or that gland wanted an industrial partner. The reason was summed up by the pharmacologist J. J. Abel, who, in 1918, lamented that a university scientist who wanted to isolate the hormone of the pituitary gland had "no chance to solve a problem of this sort without generous financial assistance."[12]

Pituitary glands, for example, cost ten times more than any part of the cow found in stores, and a biochemist would typically have to process tons of raw material, starting from great vats of bodily fluid or finely ground raw meat, only to end up with a few tiny crystals of pure hormone. The German biochemistry professor Adolf Butenandt spent the greater part of the 1920s trying to identify and purify a male sex hormone. He finally succeeded in 1931 by distilling 25,000 liters of urine—a swimming pool's worth—collected from Berlin policemen (who were considered manly and therefore a good source for the hormone). His industrial partner, the Schering drug firm, handled much of the large-scale urine extraction. Butenandt's rival in St. Louis, E. A. Doisy, had similar help from Parke, Davis in isolating an estrogen from four tons of pig ovaries. Vitamins were just as hard to get. In the teens, a ton of rice bran was required to produce five grams of vitamin B1 for study, and thirty thousand eggs were used to isolate 0.1 gram of riboflavin.[13] So collaborations between pharmaceutical firms and academic researchers made good economic sense: the university scientists would get the money, technical support, and other material resources they needed, and the sponsors would get a new drug to market, usually based on the patented procedures of their scientist partner. Gordon Alles's formation as a biochemist took place in this heady, entrepreneurial atmosphere. Brilliant, energetic, and, at 6 feet, 200 pounds, physically powerful (Figure 4), Alles majored in chemistry at the California Institute of Technology in 1922, just as this institution was starting to transform itself from a sleepy technical college into the scientific powerhouse that "Caltech" became by the Second World War. After two brief jobs as an industrial chemist, Alles returned to Caltech in 1923 for a master's degree in organic chemistry, and then continued for a doctorate in biochemistry. All his graduate school research focused on drugs. Alles's 1924 master's thesis dealt with the chemical properties of insulin, the hormone wonder drug that had just been launched on the market. Abel was visiting Caltech that year, and Alles worked with the great old man, who capped his reputation by being the first to isolate insulin in pure form.

Alles's Ph.D. thesis dealt with the physiological action of some new chemicals, particularly their effects on blood pressure, respiration, and blood sugar in rabbits. In this project, Alles appears to have been seeking a synthetic substitute for insulin, which could have made him very rich had he succeeded. Unable to find an academic job when he graduated in 1926, Alles worked for George Piness, a Los Angeles allergist with a busy practice in the genteel western outskirts of Los Angeles's old downtown district. Alles's main job there, which he had begun part-time as a graduate student, was making extracts of cat fur, pollen and so forth, to inject as desensitization treatments for allergy sufferers. He broke up the routine with his own research sideline into new allergy medicines.[14]

In late 1926 and early 1927, when Alles started working for Piness, the biggest news in the allergy business was ephedrine. Derived from the Chinese medicinal herb Ephedra, ephedrine had a molecular structure closely related to adrenaline's, and it also had many of adrenaline's effects on the body, like raising blood pressure and relieving congestion. Because ephedrine relaxes the bronchial passages as well, but unlike adrenaline could be taken by mouth, the drug became very popular with asthmatics for preventing attacks.[15] Demand quickly outstripped supply of Lilly's product, creating an incentive for chemists to develop substitute drugs. One experimental drug Alles worked with that year was phenylethanolamine (Figure 5), a chemical first created and tested by Dale and his colleagues at the Burroughs-Wellcome firm in 1910. Alles and Piness dubbed it "Alin," and they tried it as an ephedrine substitute in nose drops, finding it reasonably effective for congestion. They made plans to register their brand name for the compound and to market it. But "Alin" seemed to have no effect when taken as a pill, and Alles lost interest in it. Just another nose drop was unlikely to make anyone famous or rich, even if it could have been patented—and it could not have been, given that Barger and Dale had already created it, proved it to have adrenaline-like effects, and described it all in print. To patent an invention, it has to be new as well as useful.

After a year of postdoctoral work at Harvard Medical School, working on biochemist Edwin Cohn's collaborative project with Lilly in pursuit of a new anemia drug derived from liver, Alles returned home to Los Angeles in 1928.[16] With no immediate academic career prospects, he returned to his job producing pollen shots for Piness's allergy patients. He rededicated his spare time to the search for a cold or asthma pill better than any on the market. Like Dale and the Wellcome group over a decade earlier, Alles synthesized a series of new molecules related to ephedrine and adrenaline, trying to learn which atoms on the basic adrenaline skeleton were responsible for which of its many biological effects. His hope was to create an artificial drug superior to the natural hormone in one or two of these specific effects, especially bronchial relaxation and decongestant action. This was the pathway that would soon lead him to amphetamine.

In November and December, Alles took time off from the Piness practice and went to the San Francisco area to test his new synthetic adrenalines on dogs and rabbits at the University of California's physiology department, through a friend who was a Berkeley graduate student. Using anesthetized animals, he measured the effects on blood pressure of all these compounds both by mouth and by injection, in search of adrenaline's basic action: the boost to blood pressure, or "pressor" effect. At some point around the beginning of 1929, Alles took a special interest in beta-phenyl-isopropylamine, the chemical now known as amphetamine. In animals it raised blood pressure when taken by mouth, like ephedrine, but had a longer-lasting effect.[17] Moreover, the blood pressure effects appeared at much lower doses than those lethal to his experimental animals, suggesting that the chemical might be safe when used as a drug. When Alles had Miller inject him with 50 mg of amphetamine that June day, it was his latest effort to discover a new hybrid between adrenaline and ephedrine.

Bold self-experimentation was not unusual among medical researchers at the time, a tradition extending to Pasteur and even earlier. Medical scientists believed that trying a drug on oneself was not just scientifically crucial, since effects on humans can differ from effects on animals, but also morally necessary. Doing no harm to patients, or at least more good than harm, represents the first principle of medical ethics. In those days, taking a new treatment first was how a medical researcher proved his belief in its safety, its harmlessness; afterward, he could try it on patients. Perhaps this perspective reflects the innocence of an earlier day's trust in science, since self-testing offers no protection against bad scientific judgment—only against bad faith. Today, human experimentation remains as essential as ever, pharmacologically. However, we now recognize that a drug's inventor is particularly likely to have excessive confidence in the safety and value of his or her brainchild, so best practice calls for an independent review of risk before anyone tries a human experiment. We also now recognize that human subjects who take an experimental drug should be informed about its risks, whether or not the experimenter has taken it first, and that only those least likely to suffer harm should be exposed to significant risk. These ethical principles developed later.[18] Thus, the experiments that Alles and his colleagues would soon conduct in the Piness clinic—and, likewise, the experiments that drug companies would sponsor to test amphetamine's safety and effectiveness (discussed in chapter 2)—did not breach ethical standards of the time in a clear-cut way, although it might now seem outrageous that the patients did not know what they were getting.

So, in June 1929, Alles thought his new chemical was safe and he wanted to prove it. Furthermore, he wanted to see if amphetamine caused any unpleasant effects that might limits its commercial prospects. His self-experiment was quite promising: nobody would complain about a "feeling of well-being," and he felt nothing worse than brief "palpitation" that first time. Two days later, Alles and Piness gave 20 mg of the new drug, by mouth, to one of the allergist's patients during an asthma attack. Much like Alles, she reported "exhilaration" and "palpitation." After waiting two hours with only some minor relief, the long-suffering volunteer was finally given an adrenaline shot to stop the wheezing. A week later, the same patient was injected with 50 mg of amphetamine during another asthma attack. Her pulse went from 106 beats per minute up to 180 after the injection, and her blood pressure jumped 50 percent. "Wheezing better, violent headache, asthma almost gone, nauseated," the case notes reported. She vomited, but the nausea remained, as did a "throbbing headache" that lasted for hours. So it seemed that enough amphetamine to help at all with an asthma attack caused the same unpleasant side-effects as a heavy dose of ephedrine.[19]

Two more asthma patients were given 50 mg doses by mouth that June, and although they did not complain of severe headaches, they, too, found that the experimental drug did not relieve their asthma completely and it also caused insomnia. Alles and Piness tried it out on congested patients, in nose drops. By late 1929, the handful of trials they had done suggested that the new drug might make a decent decongestant in nasal drops or spray but was, at best, a mediocre asthma remedy. However, it was a very reliable central nervous system stimulant—and, with its exhilarating effect on the spirits, quite pleasant in moderate doses. Alles wrote up their experiments, and Piness presented them at the West Coast AMA meeting in Portland, Oregon, that autumn.[20]

In late 1929, of course, it was hard to keep spirits up. The stock market collapsed in September, sending high-flying Wall Street players out the windows of New York's skyscrapers. After a brief rally, the market resumed its downward spiral by the start of 1930. Businesses closed, and unemployment rates climbed toward 35 percent. Everywhere, soup kitchens gathered queues that stretched around the block. The Great Depression had abruptly replaced the Roaring Twenties. Alles, who had been biding his time in the hope of landing a junior professorship at Caltech or at another good university, was now lucky to have his job making pollen shots for an allergist. The twenty-eight-year-old biochemist must have realized that he had to settle in and make the best of his situation. Around this time he struck a handshake agreement with Piness: the allergist committed to support his research on new drugs, provided Alles gave him 50 percent of whatever royalties he might receive from his inventions.[21] If either man had any inkling of the huge sums that would eventually hinge on their deal, or the legal wrangling over millions they would face one day, they surely would have written something formal on paper.

On January 23, 1930, Alles and three friends began an experiment to see how taking a smaller, daily dose of amphetamine would affect them. These friends included Alles's future wife, Maxy Pope, a biologist then working for Piness as a technician. For a week, they simply recorded their pulse and blood pressure at 9:00 AM, 12:00 noon, and 5:00 PM to establish their normal rates. Then, on January 31 at about 8:00 AM, they all took a dose of amphetamine, 18 mg for Alles and proportionally smaller doses for those who weighed less, and went to work as usual. They recorded their pulse and blood pressure periodically for the rest of the day, as well as other impressions. They continued to do so for nine days, following their normal routines. During the experiment, the four friends saw little effect on their blood pressure or pulse. However, three reported having insomnia or restlessness at least one night, three claimed they felt "jumpy" or "trembly" at some point, and all four reported feeling "exhilarated" or "peppy."

Some improvements in sinus congestion were also noticed. Alles enjoyed—perhaps more than usual—his regular lunchtime handball game with Miller. Altogether, there seemed not to be much of a problem in taking the drug every day: most of amphetamine's limited effects on congestion, as well as the mind, could be felt at a dose low enough that it did not raise blood pressure or cause headaches. Alles used himself as the guinea pig in a test of the drug's influence on metabolic rate and on the electrical activity of the heart, both of which showed little to no effect. Overall prospects must have seemed promising, as he wrote up a patent application on the salts of amphetamine that could be taken by mouth, for use in the same ways as ephedrine, and submitted it in September 1930.[22]

Though he believed he had made a real discovery in amphetamine, there was no celebration in 1930, and Alles pressed on in search of a better asthma drug without so many stimulating "side-effects." He introduced oxygen atoms, three of which are found naturally in adrenaline, at various positions on his amphetamine molecule. There was some animal testing of the new derivatives for toxicity and blood pressure action. With an idea of what would be a lethal dose, Alles would then, as before, try the experimental drug on himself to learn its effects on the human circulation, on the sinuses, and also on the mental state. By now he was looking out for changes in his emotions and perceptions, but nothing could have prepared him for his experience on July 16, 1930, with 126 mg of beta-3,4-methylene-dioxyphenyl-isopropylamine hydrochloride. Under the influence that day, Alles recorded this chemical's strange effects, such as "pupils markedly dilated" and "tendency to close jaw tightly and grind rear teeth" (Figure 6). The physical symptoms were accompanied by hallucinations: "very shakey, when relaxed room seems to be filled with curling smoke." "Cannot think in long chains, thought skips rapidly but seems quite clear," he also found. Gradually, once he calmed down, he started to find the experience amusing. Though he had seen some things that were not there, Alles noticed that the drug also made him more aware of his surroundings. "Seem exceptionally aware of sound perceptions can readily pick out minor sounds accompanying louder sounds such as street cars," which, in 1930 Los Angeles, were not hallucinations but part of one of the best public transportation systems in the country. "Generalized feeling of well-being," Alles concluded, and, moreover, he felt fine the next morning.[23]

Alles had discovered ecstasy. To be precise, this is the first experience with the drug now known as methylene-dioxyamphetamine or MDA, one of two main chemicals famous today under the street name "ecstasy."[24] (It differs from methylene-dioxymethamphetamine or MDMA, the drug more commonly called ecstasy, in the same way that amphetamine differs from methamphetamine, that is, by one small methyl group. To drug users, the subjective effects are virtually indistinguishable, as with amphetamine and methamphetamine. See Figure 5) Despite its pleasant side, Alles does not seem to have seen much promise in MDA. The drug would sit in his drawer for another two decades before he finally found a use for it.

Searching for Amphetamine's Fortune

By the second half of 1931 Alles returned to his tinkering with the adrenaline and ephedrine molecules, creating a new series of amphetamine derivatives with extra oxygens in various positions on the molecule's basic skeleton. Perhaps wary of further service as a guinea pig, Alles wanted to do more thorough animal testing of this batch of chemicals than he could in the Los Angeles allergy practice. His connections led him to Chauncey Leake, the new pharmacology professor at the University of California medical school, which was just moving from Berkeley to San Francisco at the time (the institution is now known as UCSF). Leake was a young, energetic, and affable Easterner with top academic credentials—a Ph.D. from Wisconsin, then the leading pharmacology department in the country, and, before that, a Princeton bachelor's degree and a brief stint in the Army's Chemical Warfare Service during World War I. He had been hired in 1927 to teach medical students about drugs, and the next year he set up UCSF's laboratory for pharmacology and drug physiology. The lab occupied a partly renovated space at the top of an old hospital building, up 219 steps from the street, without an elevator. In Leake's words: "Facilities were poor, animal quarters were inadequate, and there was little equipment."[25]

Leake furnished the shoestring laboratory loft as best he could, doing routine testing work commissioned by local chemical companies to help pay for the equipment. But, more important than hardware, Leake provided the enthusiasm and encouragement to attract a rotating handful of keen students doing research on drugs. Photos from the early 1930s show a closely-knit gang of young men crowding the simple, high-ceilinged laboratory room, with a pile of cages in the middle hinting at the lack of space, a bookshelf of journals, and a large seminar table where they all must have talked and studied together for long hours (see Figure 4). Though literally towering above the others, Alles fit in comfortably with the informal, free-wheeling group, quickly winning Leake's deep respect for his meticulous labwork and razor-sharp reasoning, and becoming something of an older brother to Leake's students. At UCSF Alles found his second home, returning to San Francisco for visits of several weeks once or twice a year for more than a decade following his first stay in 1931–1932.[26]

Alles's experiments during his first year visiting at UCSF show that he was still mainly interested in finding the perfect asthma drug in some variant of his amphetamine molecule. Working with Myron Prinzmetal, a medical student studying with Leake, Alles applied an advanced physiological testing procedure (or "assay") to amphetamine, and to his modified amphetamines that more closely resembled adrenaline in various ways. The purpose of the assay was to test the relaxing effect of these drugs on the lungs, apart from their effect in raising blood pressure. Like many experiments in physiology, the procedure was more than a little grisly. Alles would put a dog, cat, or guinea pig under ether anesthesia, and then poke a sharp object through the eye to destroy the higher parts of its brain. This was meant to eliminate any adrenaline-like effects that acted via the central nervous system; only peripheral and direct effects on circulation and the lungs would, ideally, be observed. The animals were then kept alive with artificial respiration under constant pressure, and the amount of air the lungs took in was measured. Relaxed bronchial passages would register as increased air volume. Leake's elaborate assay for bronchial relaxation showed that Alles's oxygenated amphetamines were more effective for relaxing the lungs, as well as much more powerful for raising blood pressure, compared to amphetamine. One of these was identified as a promising heart stimulant and decongestant, because it was less toxic than amphetamine, had a much longer effect than adrenaline, was active in pill form, and (as it soon emerged through self-experimentation) gave less of a subjective lift as well. Parahydroxy-phenylisopropylamine or "hydroxyamphetamine" would ultimately become Alles's second most rewarding invention, under the trade name "Paredrine." But no perfect asthma remedy ever emerged from this line of research, although Alles continued pursuing it for another two years.[27]

During this time, Alles sought medical applications for amphetamine where the stimulating effect on the central nervous system might serve a purpose, rather than present an inconvenient side effect. He supplied the drug to several physician colleagues to use in experimenting with their patients. In 1933, Alles gave some to Prinzmetal, then a resident at Washington University Medical School in St. Louis, to try on narcoleptic patients. People suffering narcolepsy fall deeply asleep without warning, and medical journals had recently reported that ephedrine kept narcoleptics awake. Amphetamine, he thought, might be a better stimulant for these patients, as people generally found it more pleasant. That year Alles also supplied Morris Nathanson, a Californian doctor and acquaintance working at the time in Minneapolis, with amphetamine to test along with ephedrine and adrenaline as a heart stimulant. Alles supplied amphetamine to another alumnus of Leake's UCSF group, S. Anderson Peoples, who wanted to try it on mental patients during his fellowship at London's progressive Maudsley psychiatric hospital, and to Michael Leventhal, a Chicago gynecologist (and likely another friend of Alles or Leake) who wished to try the drug for "dysmenorrhea," or painful menstruation. While he waited for his informal network of clinical researchers to turn up some promising results, Alles approached the drug firm Merck, and also Smith, Kline & French, to ask if they might like to buy rights to his amphetamines. It was a wise move. Transforming a mere chemical into a medically accepted and profitable drug is no simple matter, and, even in those days, an amateur like Alles stood very little chance compared to the large drug companies that made this commercial alchemy their business.[28]

Alles's patent had been granted in 1932, making him the official inventor of the chemicals described in it, and giving him exclusive rights to his invention for the then standard term of seventeen years. To be precise, his patent claimed the invention of amphetamine sulfate and amphetamine hydrochloride and other orally active amphetamine salts as new chemicals, as well as the medicinal use of same substances for their ephedrine-like effects. This double claiming was a common strategy: if someone challenged Alles's patent in court, the claim to discovering the chemicals themselves might be rejected, but the claim for discovering that these substances could be used as medicines might still hold up. Then, in 1934, Alles must have decided that his claim to be the actual creator of amphetamine was not defensible; a German journal article, published in 1887 by a chemist named Edeleano, described the production of amphetamine and some of its salts (though the specific salts were not named). So Alles filed what is known as a "disclaimer" with the patent office, limiting his claims to the discovery that amphetamine was a medicine, which would reduce the chances of his patent being overthrown in court.[29] As with almost every successful pharmaceutical, the details of the patent would later be raked over by gangs of lawyers working for companies both attacking and defending Alles's claims, in excruciating detail and with a highly uncertain outcome. But in 1934, when he approached the big drug companies, Alles felt reasonably secure that amphetamine was his invention to sell.

At the time Alles contacted Smith, Kline & French (SKF) in 1934, the Philadelphia firm had just released a new decongestant called Benzedrine (Figure 7). Packaged in a small metal tube with a capped opening at one end, this product was the same chemical as Alles's invention (phenylisopropylamine, i.e., amphetamine), in a volatile form. When inserted in the nose, the drug vaporized out of the tube and went directly into swollen sinus tissue, where it caused capillaries to contract, thus relieving congestion in the same way that adrenaline spray did. The volatile amphetamine base in the Benzedrine Inhaler had been patented as a medicine by SKF chemist Fred Nabenhauer at almost the same time that Alles filed his own patent on amphetamine salts, the form of the chemical suitable for taking as a pill. (SKF would stick to a different story, but Alles later learned that an agent of the firm heard the talk at the 1929 AMA meeting where he and Piness first described amphetamine's effectiveness as a decongestant, convincing Alles that the firm had copied his invention.)[30] Although not exactly identical, the two patents were similar enough that SKF could not afford to ignore the independent inventor.

Moreover, in the mid-1930s, Smith, Kline & French badly needed exciting new medicines, and also long-term help in finding them. The large but old-fashioned company had been selling a huge line of some fifteen thousand specialty products, mostly grooming supplies and non-prescription remedies. If you wanted to open a drugstore, you could stock the entire shop from an SKF catalog, boasted the firm.

Their leading prescription pharmaceutical was still "Eskay Neurophosphates" nerve tonic from 1901. In the new game of drugs with solid scientific credentials, the firm lagged behind powerhouses Merck and Lilly, leaders of the U.S. industry in tapping cutting-edge life science to develop new (and preferably patented) medicines. Still partly controlled by the founding families, SKF had brought in dynamic new management to catch up, in the form of the executive vice president Frank Boyer and research chief W. Furness ("Bill") Thompson. In the 1930s, this new executive team beefed up the scientific staff and tried to foster creative and chancy projects, becoming known for tolerating "nonconformists" and "oddball" employees as a source of new ideas.[31] Perhaps this was the way they saw Alles, too, as an oddball but potentially an asset for their drive to become more science-savvy.

At first, however, rather than actively involve Alles, SKF simply tried to acquire his invention as cheaply as possible. SKF management answered Alles that, although their lawyers were sure his patent would not stand up, they would be magnanimous and offer to buy it —for $250. The offer was paltry, but Alles did not want to sell his creation for a fixed sum at all; he insisted on royalties, a percentage of sales, so that he could share directly in its success. Moreover, he demanded provisions that if the firm did not actively develop new uses of amphetamine, the patent would revert back to him. Negotiations dragged on for the better part of a year, with Alles and a lawyer friend skillfully parrying the drug company's efforts to push him into parting with his invention for a song. Finally, in December 1934, an agreement was reached. SKF would pay Alles 5 percent royalties on sales of his orally active amphetamine salts in exchange for his patent rights, and also accepted the provisions binding the firm to develop the salts commercially. Another stipulation was that the firm gained first refusal, on similar royalty terms, to his future inventions, and SKF started by acquiring Alles's hydroxyamphetamine (soon branded "Paredrine").

By the end of these negotiations SKF came to view Alles as a wellspring of new drug ideas. In addition to royalties on amphetamine sulfate—now dubbed "Benzedrine Sulfate" to match SKF's amphetamine inhaler product—the firm would pay Alles a yearly research subsidy and a consulting retainer of $3,600. This retainer alone was a science professor's salary at the time, and almost twice what Alles was paid by Piness.[32] The partnership with SKF gave Alles another way to realize his dream of a career inventing drugs, outside the academic world. He would soon break free from Piness and, within a few years, build a chemical research firm and laboratory of his own with the mounting royalties from amphetamine.

2

Benzedrine

The Making of a Modern Medicine

ALLES HAD FOUND a splendid partner to make his creation a blockbuster. Although Smith, Kline & French could not yet boast many scientifically impressive pharmaceuticals in its product line (Figure 8), the firm had the marketing skills to turn a mere chemical into a successful medicine. The period in which amphetamine underwent this transformation, 1935 through 1937, was the twilight of the age when pharmaceuticals remained largely unregulated. In the United States, federal law still required only the accurate labeling of medicines. Apart from listed narcotics, a doctor's prescription was not legally required to purchase drugs from pharmacies. However, much had changed since the turn-of-the-century crisis generated by the free market in drugs. The contents of medicines were now truthfully labeled and were "pure"—thanks to the 1906 Federal Food and Drug Law. And, as we saw, the AMA Council on Pharmacy required manufacturers to provide scientific evidence that a drug was effective as claimed, and safe in typical doses, before approving advertising in participating medical journals. Marketing plans needed to take science into account.

So, like any company with a new medicine to offer, SKF had to arrange for convincing safety studies with amphetamine. The firm also had to identify some medical conditions that the drug helped, and to gather evidence from clinical trials proving amphetamine beneficial by the scientific standards of the day. Arranging for this efficacy testing meant selecting some of the drug's many effects: perhaps the way it kept one awake, or made the mind race, or another effect on the brain like the "feeling of well-being" Alles reported—or perhaps some of the adrenaline-like effects on involuntary muscles. Through clinical studies testing these specific amphetamine actions on patients with certain conditions, a few would be defined as the drug's official, medically useful effects, and the rest as side effects. Following AMA review and approval of the evidence, the manufacturer would then market the drug to doctors using journal advertising, as well as direct mail and the sales force of "detail men."[1]

Safety studies for the AMA Council were straightforward in those days. SKF only needed to conduct animal testing to establish the drug's toxicity, that is, to determine precisely what dose levels were probably lethal and whether any obvious harms occurred from taking high doses. The firm also had to test the drug more formally on people in the relevant dose range—that is, doses well below lethal levels but high enough for medically valuable effects to be felt—to check for dangerous or unpleasant side effects. After some delays and false starts, in mid-1936 the firm commissioned a toxicity study from University of Pennsylvania pharmacology professor Edward Krumbhaar, a friend and close neighbor of SKF vice president Boyer. Krumbhaar documented no harm from massive doses in rats over several weeks, then moved on to dogs, rabbits, and guinea pigs. Eventually he published his findings, and, meanwhile, SKF prepared a summary of his results to mail to doctors already experimenting with the drug, to help allay any safety concerns.[2]

To demonstrate that amphetamine was safe for people to take orally, SKF commissioned a study by a University of Pennsylvania medical school (Penn) professor of internal medicine named Wallace Dyer. Because amphetamine was thought of as an artificial adrenaline, one of the most obvious issues was the rise in blood pressure that it caused. This effect might be beneficial for those with low blood pressure, but it might be a dangerous side-effect for patients with high blood pressure. To establish whether such people would have to be be ruled out for Benzedrine Sulfate prescriptions, whatever the drug's medical use might be, Dyer recruited subjects with normal, low, and high blood pressures from among his patients in the Penn hospital. At first he gave them all 10–20 mg of amphetamine a day, and then, after a few months, on instructions from SKF, he raised the doses to 30 mg per day. Today, Dyer's experiment would be ethically unacceptable, since his patients with high blood pressure stood a particularly good chance of being harmed and could not reasonably be expected to benefit. In those days, however, doctors had few doubts about their own beneficence, and there was nothing very unusual about such experimentation. Only after the Nazi medical atrocities of World War II were revealed did American medical researchers begin to reconsider their own ethics around human experimentation. In any case, nothing bad seems to have happened to Dyer's patients, and his study was eventually published in the high-profile *American Journal of Medical Science*.[3]

Drug Seeking Disease

In the 1930s, proof of safety was required only for AMA permission to advertise. Legally, a new drug could be used on people, and indeed sold at pharmacies, before animal studies were even done. So, while the safety studies were under way in 1935 and 1936, SKF also worked on clinical testing to solve the more difficult problem, that is, to help Benzedrine Sulfate find its place in medicine by discovering how the drug might be useful. Amphetamine, in other words, was a "drug looking for a disease," to borrow sociologist Rein Vos's memorable phrase. In 1936 almost any use was imaginable, since amphetamine had adrenaline-like effects on the circulation, respiration, and involuntary muscles, as well as the brain. So SKF took a two-pronged approach. The first consisted of providing a free drug supply to almost any interested doctor, asking, in exchange, only to be kept informed. By mid-1936 SKF already had a list of "sixty-odd men doing special work" on amphetamine, most of them freelancers following their own scientific interests. Doctors both eminent and obscure were sent samples of the drug for experiments on conditions ranging from colitis to multiple sclerosis.[4] SKF even sent some in liquid form to a Buffalo, New York, endodontist who wanted to try it instead of adrenaline as an additive with local anesthetic injections—even though laboratory tests had already shown that amphetamine was inferior to adrenaline for constricting capillaries, and therefore a poor choice for reducing surgical bleeding. SKF research managers greatly appreciated such "scientific hunches" coming from practitioners, who after all were the prescribers on whom sales ultimately depended. If these free-lance experimenters should turn up "something of interest or value" the firm wanted to know, whether or not they intended to publish, so the researchers were regularly "tickled" for updates (in the words of SKF's Assistant Director of Research, Ted Wallace).[5]

On the other hand, not everything could be left to the random hunches of the medical profession. Thus, the second prong of SKF's approach consisted of commissioning targeted studies by relevant experts to explore the most obvious and potentially lucrative possibilities for the new product. Apart from narcolepsy, which Alles's old friend Prinzmetal and several others were already pursuing, two of the most obvious potential uses of amphetamine were for asthma and allergies, and for dysmenorrhea. The dysmenhorrea idea seemed plausible based on laboratory physiology, since the drug reduced contractions in uterus muscle. The market might be huge: because dysmenorrhea was extremely common and little could be done for it, the complaint was the "bete-noir of the gynecologist," as one of them, J. M. Hundley of the University of Maryland, put it. Along with Alles's acquaintance Leventhal, Hundley was one of several gynecologists trying out Benzedrine Sulfate with funding from SKF in 1936. The first results from a study on 40 women complaining of dysmenhorrea were very encouraging; many patients were coming back to the doctor, asking for more of the new pills. So Hundley and colleagues arranged a larger trial with women working in a General Electric factory. Although 114 of 186 women treated for dysmenhorrea over six months experienced "good" results in that they reported that their menstrual pain subsided after one 10 mg tablet, SKF did not ultimately choose dysmenorrhea as its main path for bringing amphetamine to market. The reason may be that other experimenters were not finding any such benefits, or the latest physiological research suggested that dysmenorrhea was not actually caused by abnormal contraction of the uterus. The firm may also have realized that these "good" results might have come from the drug's mental side effects; many women reported that the pills made work easier and that they left the factory feeling remarkably energetic. [6] Neither did studies to test amphetamine for asthma find the drug particularly useful. Amphetamine would not find its place with the allergists or gynecologists.

Another possibility for amphetamine specially targeted by SKF was the use of the drug for mental performance enhancement. Higher intelligence test scores with the drug were reported by psychiatrist William Sargant, from London's Maudsley clinic, in the prominent journal *Lancet* in late 1936. (Recall that Alles's old San Francisco friend, Peoples, had brought amphetamine along when he went for training there). To follow up, SKF funded psychologists William Turner and George Carl at the University of Pennsylvania hospital to conduct an extensive battery of tests on normal volunteers, mostly nurses and other hospital staff. The tests were intended to show how the drug affected performance in various mental and physical tasks, and also to assess effects on a wide range of psychological factors such as imagination, optimism, and other aspects of personality. These researchers found that the drug indeed improved efficiency in simple mental tasks and tests of hand-eye ("psychomotor") problem solving, especially those requiring persistence and alertness. They concluded that the increased performance on mental tasks did not come from any actual improvement in thinking ability but from increased confidence and other mood effects of the drug. And while these researchers did not conclude that the drug caused true personality change, their psychometric tests showed evidence that amphetamine typically produces increased optimism, extroversion, initiative, and aggression.[7]

A medical market for mental performance enhancement might be found among psychiatrists specializing in the field then known as "orthopsychiatry," and today "learning disabilities" or "child psychiatry." So SKF also funded Matthew Molitch, neurology professor at Penn and resident psychiatrist at the New Jersey State Home for Boys, to assess the effect of amphetamine on standardized intelligence and school achievement test results. Molitch and colleagues similarly found improved average performance across the board, both in boys rated as having normal intelligence as well as those rated as "subnormal." As in much of the testing organized by the drug firm, both the Pennsylvania and New Jersey Home studies used "placebo" controls, sugar pills that look identical to the test drug so that patients do not know whether they are receiving the drug. (Placebos allow the biological impact of the drug to be distinguished from the psychological effects of expecting pills to work—the surprisingly dramatic "placebo effect" that often confuses medical research.) SKFs seemingly routine production and distribution of placebos in the testing phase of amphetamine suggests that, contrary to the opinions of some historians, the use of placebo controls was already commonplace by the late 1930s. Furthermore, several of the SKF-funded studies described here also used the latest statistical methods and "double-blinding" to prevent the evaluating experimenters from knowing which subjects were on drugs. This suggests that drug firms in the period liked to sponsor clinical studies with advanced clinical trial methodology, presumably to add credibility and to boost the impact of any resulting publications.[8]

Work on children similar to Molitch's was being conducted by another researcher, one of the many volunteers who approached SKF after the firm began offering experimental supplies of 10 mg Benzedrine tablets and identical placebos around the beginning of 1936. Charles Bradley, chief psychiatrist at a children's mental institution in Rhode Island, tried the new drug on thirty boys and girls with learning disabilities, many of whom were diagnosed with a neurological problem and others only emotionally disturbed. Bradley found that about half the children scored higher on tests with amphetamine, and these same children were the ones who showed a surprising, even paradoxical drug reaction. Benzedrine made them calmer and more cooperative in the classroom, suggesting an unknown biological cause behind their typically unruly behavior. However, the amphetamine made other unruly children even more agitated, thus raising the question of what the difference was in those who responded positively. Though the Rhode Island group gathered some evidence for a subtle defect in the higher functions of the brain, together with an abnormal brain wave profile that might identify children likely to respond well, Bradley was unable to pin down the factors that defined the right kind of "problem child" for medication. Because Bradley is seen today as the individual who discovered both Attention Deficit Disorder and the "paradoxical" effect of stimulant drugs in helping the condition, it is interesting to consider why SKF took a much greater interest in the parallel work by Molitch. A key may lie in market factors: where Bradley believed that the amphetamine effect depended on a brain defect, Molitch characterized his subjects as biologically normal juvenile delinquents. A large market for Benzedrine in learning enhancement would be more likely were the drug to be found effective on any children with problems in school, not just those with abnormal brain waves. A similarly large market was explored by Molitch with another early SKF-funded study which found that the drug reduced bed-wetting, probably through making sleep lighter rather than affecting the bladder directly.[9]

In any case, although there was ample scientific evidence (by the standards of the time) to support claims that amphetamine could boost school performance for at least some children, this use of the drug did not catch on for another three decades (as we shall see in chapter 8). SKF would not market their new drug for this purpose. Publicity problems presented an obstacle, as university students had begun to use Benzedrine to aid the time-honored practice of last-minute "cramming" for exams. This form of nonmedical use may well have started with students recruited for psychological testing of amphetamine. At the University of Minnesota, for instance, in early 1937, campus doctors were already warning of the popularity of Benzedrine Sulfate "Pepper-Uppers." In April 1937 the *New York Times*, covering a scientific meeting, trumpeted the power of Benzedrine as "high-octane" "brain fuel," and *Time* magazine luridly covered the student story the next month, condemning promiscuous use of the "powerful but poisonous brain stimulant." *JAMA* also commented on it in an editorial, predictably scolding the press coverage and condemning abuse —or "misuse" as more commonly said at the time—of Benzedrine without physician supervision. There were similar stories of misuse circulated about British university students. One psychologist noted that students "have come to cherish this drug as a gift of the Gods." Though SKF did what it could to contain the damage and manage professional opinion, complaining, for example, to *Time* magazine about calling their product "poisonous" and contacting student health service doctors who had published statements against Benzedrine, by the end of 1938 the student misuse issue, together with new worries about addiction (discussed below), had effectively blocked the marketing of amphetamine for mental performance enhancement.[10]

A Change in Mood

"If we haven't got a bearcat by the tail, then I'm a Dutchman," wrote SKF research manager Richard Webb after a Boston neurology meeting in March 1936. Webb had perceived exciting possibilities for Benzedrine Sulfate there. The meeting had featured the official debut of Prinzmetal's latest work, this time on the beneficial effects of amphetamine on a certain form of Parkinson's disease. More interesting to SKF, however, were three papers presented by Abraham Myerson, a professor of neurology at Tufts Medical School and of clinical psychiatry at Harvard, and also the research director at Boston State psychopathic hospital (Figure 9). Experimenting on "passive" inpatients at the mental hospital, Myerson had tried amphetamine along with other drugs that alter nerve activity, finding, for instance, that amphetamine counteracts sleep induced by barbiturates. He also measured amphetamine's action on the digestive organs. Most significant, Myerson also studied the drug's effects on mood. "Normal" medical students liked amphetamine, as did Myerson himself; he found that the drug improved his lecturing, or at least made it more pleasant. And, as we shall see, many neurotic, depressed patients in his clinic responded extraordinarily well.[11] In Myerson SKF had found what the drug industry now calls a "key thought leader": a top specialist whose ideas and influence could make Benzedrine Sulfate's future in his field. The firm was not slow in recognizing his potential value. Indeed, by the time of the 1936 Boston meeting, SKF was already funding Myerson, having offered him an unrestricted grant when he first approached the firm for drug samples in late 1935.[12]

Myerson was a very eminent man, even apart from his Harvard and Tufts professorships. At Boston State mental hospital, he headed one of the best-equipped labs in the country for studying the human nervous system, through generous funding from the Rockefeller Foundation, the most important supporter of medical research in the Depression era. Myerson was also a public intellectual famous for taking on big political issues, such as eugenics. Eugenics in 1920s America was a massively popular, pseudo-scientific movement that blamed a host of social ills on bad heredity—especially crime, insanity, and "imbecility" (a vague category that included Down Syndrome as well as mental retardation generally). Along with strict limits on immigration from "inferior" nations, sterilization was the movement's favorite proposal for cleaning up the gene pool. Half the states in the Union enacted laws to sterilize "imbeciles" and certain criminals, making America a model for racial purification that Hitler himself cited when he came to power in 1933. The eugenicists were powerful, and at a time when many scientists failed to take any public stand, Myerson assailed their scientific credibility. He did not dispute that genes and other biological factors largely determined mental traits, but he argued that the way that eugenicists drew the connection was rubbish. For instance, Myerson pointed out that studies allegedly showing that certain races are mentally inferior, including Jews like himself, actually measured cultural assimilation: test scores of immigrants, he found, rose the longer they lived in the U.S. In short, Myerson was an outspoken opponent of racism. He was also known for a popular 1920 book, *The Nervous Housewife,* where he argued that the passive housewife role imposed on middle-class women was unhealthy, as was their indoctrination with vanity, emotionality, and unrealistic expectations from marriage. For his time, this thinking qualifies Myerson as a feminist.[13]

More important for our story than his politics, Myerson was an expert on depression and the author of a 1925 book titled *When Life Loses Its Zest*. There Myerson described a depressive "symptom complex" he dubbed "anhedonia" (thus reviving and reinterpreting a nineteenth-century term), literally meaning "lack of pleasure," characterized by reduced interest in sleep, food, sex, and a low level of the "energy feeling" that motivates us to work and play. Although a number of conditions shared these anhedonic symptoms, such as menopause and early stages of schizophrenia, he identified a chronic illness that he called "idiopathic anhedonia" as a neurotic disorder in its own right. Indeed, Myerson argued, this particular neurosis was growing to epidemic proportions, especially among women but increasingly among male "brain-workers" of the higher classes. Like the hysterias of married women he discussed in *The Nervous Housewife*, idiopathic anhedonia was best understood as a disruption or diversion of natural drives caused by the blocking of their natural fulfillment. Further, Myerson thought, this frustration often manifested itself in the unfocused way that we call anxiety, as well as in apathy and in the feeling that we call sadness but which is actually low "energy feeling."[14] Neurasthenia (literally, "nervous weakness"), the reigning concept of depression as a depletion of nerve force, should be discarded and replaced with anhedonia, argued Myerson, because apathy is more fundamental than weakness or sadness. In Myerson's hands, depression thus became a disorder of frustrated drives and lack of fulfillment, rather than the exhausted nerves and fatigue it had been in the age of neurasthenia.[15] However, the medical world was not quite ready to embrace his radical theories about depression, judging from textbooks in the late 1920s and 1930s, which continued to foreground the "neurasthenia" concept and to treat anxiety as unrelated. But Myerson, together with SKF, would soon change that.

In the 1920s, Myerson had customarily treated anhedonic patients with a combination of occupational, physical, and talking therapies, all directed to restoring "pep, zeal, courage, concentration, interest," and pleasure. He would establish an unstressful routine of wholesome diet and moderate exercise, and then introduce an energy-restoring program of "graduated exertion" to bring the patient out of himself and into a realm of achievable goals (whether in crafts such as basket weaving or sports such as hunting or golf—options that say a lot about his clientele). He would talk extensively with the patient, not to encourage heavy introspection like Freudian psychoanalysts, but to "make the situation reasonably clear" to a patient and advocate a more adaptive "change of life" (rather like today's cognitive-behavioral therapists). And, to reestablish a regular pattern of activity and break the typical anhedonic's cycle of insomnia, he would also treat patients with mild sedatives at night and stimulants like caffeine in the morning. Because he saw mind and body as ultimately one, biological and talking approaches did not conflict for Myerson. As he wrote in 1922: "If the individual is depressed . . . you can change his attitude . . . by physical means just as surely as you can change his digestion by distressing thought . . . [D]rugs and physical therapeutics are just as much psychical agents as good advice and analysis and must be used together with these latter agents of cure."[16] No wonder he became fascinated with a new pill which enhanced the "energy-feeling" that is the opposite of depression.

At the April 1936 Boston meeting, Meyerson described how Benzedrine Sulfate brought striking improvements to some of his anhedonic, depresssed outpatients (that is, people with milder, neurotic conditions, not inmates in the mental ward). The drug helped whether the source of the depression was "endogenous"—internal, presumably biological—or "reactive"—external, from distressing events. For instance, a fifty-two-year-old engineer, unemployed since the Depression began, was cured of the despondency and the overwhelming thoughts of suicide that had plagued him every morning since his early thirties. If Myerson switched him to inert placebos instead of his 30–40 mg of Benzedrine daily, the despondency returned. With two suicides in his immediate family, his case of depression was largely hereditary and endogenous. On the other hand, the case of a forty-year-old female schoolteacher seemed typically "reactive," brought on by life events. She had grown depressed following a divorce, and then developed a serious anxiety neurosis after a car accident. She stopped teaching, drank ten cups of coffee a day just to get moving in the morning, and had to take barbiturates for sleep. By the time she presented herself for treatment, she had "a hysterical tremor of the right arm, a sense of low energy with general depression of the appetite, the power to sleep, and [the] capacity for physical and mental work." Given 30 mg of Benzedrine tablets daily, she almost immediately cheered up and cut down on coffee, and soon returned to teaching. In short, the new drug seemed to work wonders. When he glowingly described these and similar findings at an American Psychological Association meeting in September 1936, Myerson recommended prescribing Benzedrine to such "gloomy, anhedonic" depressives as well as normal people with morning hangovers and low moods. *Time* magazine picked up the story of his experiments and reported the "favorable results" to a national audience, albeit in a small curiosity piece.[17]

Drug Meets Disease

Myerson was not the only "neuropsychiatrist" excited about Benzedrine's possibilities: this specialty accounted for at least one-third of SKF's list of doctors using the drug experimentally in 1936. As the name "neuropsychiatry" for the area of medicine covering mental health implies, between the wars American psychiatrists and neurologists were considered part of the same medical field, much more so than they were in Europe. This blurred division of professional labor fit well with a theory, dominant in the United States since the beginning of the century, that neurotic conditions (milder mental disorders, such as commonplace depressions and anxieties) differed only in severity, but not in kind, from psychotic conditions requiring hospitalization (like schizophrenia and manic depression). All were treated as disorders of "adjustment" to society and one's place in it. There was also much discussion of "psycho-physical unity" among American neuropsychiatrists, which, in practice, meant that the style was eclectic. Like Myerson, many blended physical regimens with "psychodynamic" talking methods, derived either from Sigmund Freud or Adolf Meyer, the leading American neuropsychaitrist of the early twentieth century. The psychoanalysts and biological psychiatrists would come to blows in the 1960s but—as few psychiatrists today and not all historians have appreciated—the previous generation lived in a less doctrinaire and more pragmatic intellectual environment where diversity flourished.[18] The decade of the 1930s was a particularly innovative time for biological approaches, with the new "shock therapies" like insulin coma and electroconvulsion quickly replacing old methods like hot baths and cold blanket wraps. "Psychosurgery," or lobotomy, was in the experimental stage and would come into fashion at the end of the decade.[19] Thus, amphetamine came on the market at just the time when psychiatric medicine was especially open to new ideas and methods.

Particularly after the first batch of clinical studies on Benzedrine's mental effects reached publication around the end of 1936, neuropsychiatrists grew very interested in the new drug. With the bold mood prevailing in neuropsychiatry, they saw in amphetamine a potential tool for precision intervention in the mechanisms of mind. Alles's friend, Nathanson, had gone beyond his first narcolepsy and circulation work, reasoning that a stimulant might help patients with the sort of mild depression characterized by low energy and difficulty performing mental and physical tasks—that is, old-fashioned neurasthenia. On 20 mg of amphetamine per day, four-fifths of forty such patients at Nathanson's general hospital in Minneapolis experienced some improvement in their chronic fatigue and exhaustion, as well as an improved feeling of well-being. As controls in the study, he also gave eighty hospital staff members 20 mg of amphetamine per day or placebos, and those taking the drug also found that their spirits were lifted. Notably, Nathanson reported that many of his subjects (both hospital staff and patients) on Benzedrine lost weight, perhaps from decreased appetite and increased activity—a foreshadowing of things to come.[20]

A team at the elite Mayo Clinic in Minnesota reported similar preliminary results on a group of one hundred patients with mild to moderate mood disorders, mostly neurotic depressions and anxiety conditions, who were given amphetamine even for just a few days. More than two-thirds of those with chronic exhaustion and other depressive symptoms showed improvement. Some seemed instantly cured. For example, one forty-five-year-old man, recovering after several months in a state mental hospital, laughed for the first time in an entire year when he went to the movies with his wife on the first day he started taking Benzedrine. A twenty-seven-year-old man whose feelings of weariness had caused him to drop out of law school was given 20 mg of Benzedrine with breakfast and then again with lunch. On the afternoon of his first day on amphetamine he felt like "a cloud had been lifted from his brain," and he played twenty-seven holes of golf whereas nine holes was his previous limit. After a few months on 30 mg per day he was feeling much better and had returned to law school. So neuropsychiatrists with more conventional ideas about depression, those who preferred "neurasthenia" instead of Myerson's "anhedonia" to define the condition, also liked the drug. This boded well for amphetamine's commercial prospects.[21]

Experiments with long-term psychiatric inpatients were also encouraging at first, though not nearly so much as those with neurotic outpatients. Eugene Davidoff at Syracuse Psychopathic Hospital compared Benzedrine tablets to placebos and ephedrine with thirty seriously "self-absorbed" schizophrenics. Almost all the Syracuse patients grew more active and talkative on the amphetamine, but some became "surly" or "antagonistic"; for them, stimulation seemed a bad idea. But the drug brought improvement particularly for some of the "asthenic," depressed types, who became more outgoing and accessible to talking psychotherapy, easier to deal with, and more productive in the work they did around the institution. For instance, when amphetamine was given to one nearly catatonic patient who was generally "dazed, inaccessible, and . . . almost mute," he "began to initiate conversation, spoke rather freely, [and] became an efficient worker on the farm." Though he remained introverted, his mood improved and his hallucinations did not seem to bother him as much. But although one-third of the patients showed this sort of improvement, the difference seemed to be superficial, the drug bringing no real change in personality or in the subjects' basic mental illness. Alles's contacts at London's Maudsley Hospital, who had begun by investigating the effects of blood pressure on mental conditions, similarly found that depressive inpatients benefited somewhat from Benzedrine—a few of the severe melancholics but mostly the milder neurasthenic types. As with the others, this British group found that 10–20 mg per day was sufficient for the psychic effects without affecting blood pressure.[22]

For the rest of 1936 and 1937, SKF awaited further results from the doctors trying amphetamine at mental institutions across the United States, from Bellevue in New York to Elgin State in Illinois to Colorado State. The firm no doubt hoped that their new product would prove to be a promising treatment for schizophrenia, manic depression, or another of the major psychiatric conditions. Meanwhile, the results so far on neurotic patients, along with the general enthusiasm for the idea of a scientific drug for treating mental illness, were promising enough for SKF to move tentatively ahead. Around the start of 1937, SKF crafted a circular summarizing current research and stating that "the main field for Benzedrine Sulfate will be its use in improving mood," which the firm sent to a mailing list of ninety thousand doctors. Given that the American Medical Association had barely one hundred thousand members at the time, the mailing must have reached the great majority of physicians in the United States, which can only mean that the firm hoped that their new product would be prescribed in ordinary office practice.[23] Such science-based direct marketing was one of the methods the drug industry was learning to adopt for creating a buzz around new would-be miracle drugs.

In addition to the clinical trials, theories about the way that amphetamine affects the brain were also important to winning acceptance of Benzedrine Sulfate as a drug for neuropsychiatric use. The late 1930s marks the start of mainstream medical belief that the nervous system works largely through chemical, rather than strictly electrical, signaling. In 1936, Henry Dale shared the Nobel Prize with Austrian physiologist Otto Loewi for identifying acetylcholine as the chemical "neurotransmitter" (or neurohormone) carrying messages between the peripheral nerves. Their work specifically focused on the parasympathetic nerves, which help regulate automatic functions like the pupil, the digestive system, and blood pressure. The sympathetic nerves, which, as noted earlier, help regulate many of the same automatic functions, were believed to use adrenaline or one of its close chemical relatives. Thus, numerous involuntary functions were understood by many, including Myerson, as controlled by the balance of what Dale called "cholinergic" (acetylcholine) and "adrenergic" (adrenaline) nerve circuits of the peripheral nervous system. Similar views about chemical signals in the sensory nerves, and in the motor nerves controlling voluntary movement, were winning some acceptance. This left in question only the place of chemical signaling in the the brain and spinal cord, and even here the new chemical paradigm was gaining ground, although particular nerve circuits in the brain could not be dissected out in animals and studied in isolation to prove it. At Harvard, physiologist Walter B. Cannon had become world famous for relating the sympathetic nerves, and the involuntary actions they control, to strong emotions such as rage and fear. When frightened, a person's pupils widen, the blood pressure rises and sinuses clear, and the bladder and intestines relax. Cannon dubbed this the "fight-or-flight reaction," and he showed that this physical and emotional state is linked as a whole to a rush of adrenaline. The cholinergic functions that typically had opposite effects—narrowing pupils, lowering blood pressure, tightening bladder and gut—could be seen as governing a "rest-and-relax" reaction. Body and soul were becoming a unified, finely balanced, hormone-driven machine.[24]

Myerson's Boston circle played a key role in developing a rationale for Benzedrine's psychiatric use by putting the drug into this theoretical picture. Their concept was that the same balance of chemically driven nerve circuits existed in the brain, just as in the peripheral nerves, and that amphetamine worked in both center and periphery by strengthening the action of the adrenergic nerve circuits. Though neuropsychiatrists could not yet define the circuits of the brain, they could still identify the basic mental functions and determine which ones tended to be connected. For instance, there was a basic mechanism in the brain governing sleep and all the psychic functions linked to rest, akin to Cannon's rest-and-relax state of the peripheral nervous system. Whether this mechanism was stimulated by acetylcholine (and Myerson supposed it was), Benzedrine, with a waking effect powerful enough even to overcome narcolepsy and sleeping pills, obviously countered it. This, for Myerson, was the clue to its psychological effects: "The power to rest and recuperate and the power to get started in activity are fundamentally impaired . . . [in] most of the neuroses, no matter how produced." Thus, neuroses were states of brain imbalance, as well as frustrated drives. By strengthening the brain circuits that spurred activity and suppressing the sleeping mechanism, Benzedrine rebalanced and cured depressive neuroses, in which resting circuits were dominant and activity circuits weak.[25]

Wilfred Bloomberg, another Harvard neuropsychiatrist who conducted several studies on Benzedrine combined with psychotherapy to treat alcoholism, made the connection with Cannon's theories even more strongly than Myerson. He proposed that "Benzedrine is either closely akin to, if not actually identical with, a substance which is elaborated within the body," presumably "sympathin" (Cannon's word for the adrenergic neurohormone). Or if amphetamine did not function as an adrenergic brain hormone itself, it might work by blocking the action of enzymes that break down the natural hormone, thus boosting adrenergic signaling. Based on this kind of speculative reasoning, it made sense in the late 1930s to think of amphetamine, the artificial adrenaline, as shifting the balance of brain hormones in the active, wakeful direction, and thus as a medicine for stimulating the psychic drives oriented toward activities and projects.[26]

Although neuropsychiatrists had quickly found that amphetamine helped a great many milder, neurotic depressives, the exact way that doctors should prescribe the drug to "improve mood" still required some refinement in 1937. A second cycle of clinical studies reached publication that year, many funded by SKF, that helped define Benzedrine's proper uses for psychiatric medicine. The Mayo Clinic group came out with long-term results from their one hundred patients on Benzedrine. The amphetamine substantially benefited three-quarters of the Mayo's neurasthenics and other mild depressives, but it benefited few of their anxious patents, who generally became more anxious and irritable. The Maudsley group's ongoing studies essentially fit the Mayo findings: Benzedrine seemed to help people with mild depression, whether reactive or endogenous, but not those with severe depression, anxiety conditions, or schizophrenia. Frequently, the drug made these last two conditions worse. Other reports on the drug's effects upon severely ill, institutionalized patients were still less favorable. The Syracuse group's follow-up study found that the drug had a greater effect on normal controls and alcoholics than on severe neurotics, schizophrenics, and manic-depressives. Similarly, from Britain to California to Myerson's own wards at Boston State, psychiatrists reported that, essentially, the worse a patient's mental condition, the less likely he or she would benefit from Benzedrine Sulfate. By the end of 1937, expert opinion based on all this evidence held that amphetamine was not very useful for severe depression and other psychoses that typically required institutionalization. It was, however, a very promising therapy for less severe, neurotic depression. The new drug had finally found its disease: "mild" or minor depression.[27]

Amphetamine to Market

In mid-1937, SKF applied to the AMA Council on Pharmacy for permission to advertise Benzedrine Sulfate, waiting until evidence from Myerson's work was ready for submission. In December of that year, the AMA gave its approval to advertise the drug's use for narcolepsy and Parkinson's disease, and also for mood elevation in depression and other psychiatric conditions. Advertisements promoting prescriptions for these uses soon appeared in the major medical journals, and Benzedrine Sulfate sales responded, jumping from about $95,000 in 1937 to about $175,000 in 1938. In 1939, with heavier advertising specially targeting depression, sales nearly doubled again to about $330,000. Given that university students were already known to be misusing the drug to enhance their mental performance, it was no surprise that the AMA approval specifically excluded use of the drug by healthy people. More surprising, given the evidence that mildly depressed, neurotic outpatients benefited most, Benzedrine Sulfate advertisements carried a disclaimer that use should be restricted to institutionalized patients: depressive "psychopathic states" should only be treated in hospital, read a footnote in fine print. This odd outcome reflected a political compromise. SKF had sought general approval for fatigue and depression, and the AMA Council wanted the new drug to stay under medical control. Still, the warning footnote probably presented no great obstacle to amphetamine's market acceptance. Then, as now, physicians could write prescriptions however they wished for any drug on the market, and few would be likely to tell a customer he or she needed a stay in the mental ward just to try some new tablets.[28]

Like much pharmaceutical advertising then and now, the initial SKF campaign for amphetamine's use in depression aimed both to appeal to the medical profession's established attitudes and beliefs, and also gently to reshape them in a manner that could boost sales of the advertised product.[29] For instance, one common Benzedrine Sulfate advertisement from 1939–1940 features, in the largest type, "For the Patient with Mild Depression" (Figure 10). Below this headline is a list of four groups of signs and symptoms defining depressed patients. "Sensations of weakness" are listed among the key indicators of mild depression, linking the condition to traditional neurasthenia. Another key sign is anhedonia, "apathy or discouragement," along Myerson's lines. A third is subjective difficulty in thinking and acting. In extreme form this slowness was known as "retardation" and was traditionally suggestive of major depressive psychoses. And as the fourth main indicator of depression the advertisment lists hypochondria, even though standard psychiatric thinking of the time considered hypochondriacal complaints suggestive of neuroses in general and of anxiety conditions in particular. If taken seriously, this last criterion would hugely increase the number of diagnosed mild depressions to include large numbers of patients in general practice: a third or more of patient visits to the family doctor were (and still are) just like this, complaints lacking an apparent "organic basis." Taking all these definitions together—which, granted, no single physician was likely to do—the campaign thus promoted diagnostic criteria for neurotic depression that massively broadened the condition, and in several not completely consistent ways. Especially striking is that the advertisement gives Myerson's thinking top billing, listing "apathy" first.[30] As we shall see, anhedonia and apathy continued to play a prominent role in SKF's marketing for more than decade, and amphetamine sales grew hand-in-hand with the increasing significance of anhedonia in thinking about depression.

A tempting question we might ask at this stage is how much amphetamine's medical acceptance as treatment for depression owes to SKF. On the one hand, amphetamine and Myerson, with his long-standing interest in physical treatments to enhance "zest for living," were made for each other. He might have tried any promising new stimulant as soon as he heard of it, with no encouragment necessary. On the other hand, Myerson might never have heard about amphetamine without SKF's involvement. And even if he had, and tried it on his own, he might not have achieved any greater success in interesting the broader field of neuropsychiatry than he had in spreading the anhedonia theory beyond his immediate circle. SKF helped amplify Myerson's theories and amphetamine results to increase their impact. SKF also funded and encouraged dozens of other neuropsychiatrists (among other physicians) to experiment clinically with Benzedrine Sulfate, and thus helped put results in the medical literature. Pharmaceutical firms would not take such measures if drugs could always be expected to catch on without effort. But even if we suppose that eventually amphetamine would have been tested thoroughly in neuropsychiatry without any effort from its maker, SKF's advertising to doctors, strategic fostering of particular clinical studies, and distribution of amphetamine to pharmacies everywhere surely played some role in accelerating the drug's use.

Furthermore, to manage their products' images and make them successful in medicine, drug companies did more than just manufacture, distribute, advertise, and ensure that clinical research into the safety and effectiveness of their products was conducted. The situation in the 1930s bears comparison to that prevailing today, when pharmaceutical companies are widely criticized for such far-reaching effects on the medical literature that, some say, the scientific knowledge base on which health care depends has become nothing but an advertising medium dominated by the biggest spender.[31] The period between the First and Second World Wars, in contrast, tends to be viewed as a golden age of innocence, when upstanding medical scientists pursued the truth without commercial distractions, and fully reported results in medical journals free of the commercial "debauchery" that plagued the previous generation. Certainly, elite medical scientists like those who served on the AMA Council on Pharmacy saw themselves as champions of the medical literature's purity, victors over the drug industry's once dire influence.[32] However, the history of amphetamine offers a glimpse behind the scenes, suggesting that the medical elite may have been overconfident in this golden age, and that drug firms were already developing those more subtle influences on the biomedical literature that are only today arousing scandal.

By the 1930s, to be sure, the blatant paid testimonials that once cluttered medical journals were largely a thing of the past. Drug firms now funded reputable researchers to produce the kind of clinical studies on safety and efficacy they needed to impress the AMA. However, these studies were routinely designed by the firm's medical or marketing staff and then presented to potential collaborators for execution. In 1935, for instance, in planning studies to expand the range of proven uses for the Benzedrine Inhaler, SKF's assistant director of research, Ted Wallace, prepared "an outline of a possible article for Dr. [Louis] Sulman," a University of Pennsylvania otolaryngologist. An article by Sulman appeared at the end of that year, and it suggested, on weak evidence, that the Benzedrine Inhaler might prevent colds.[33] After commissioning a clinical trial, sponsoring firms retained considerable control. The sponsor might even micromanage the trial as did SKF with Dyer's Benzedrine Sulfate safety study discussed above, when the firm decided in September 1936 that there was "no need for Dr. Dyer to test blood pressure effects in normals further, but he should continue his experiments on hypertensives" with 20 mg doses, and then, a few months later, told Dyer to try 30 mg doses on the hypertensives, and to recruit normal and hypotensives for these high doses as well.[34] The sponsor's active involvement sometimes extended even beyond the design and execution of the study to its publication. For instance, SKF would prepare illustrations for Joseph Scarano, a Philadelphia office practitioner and regular collaborator with the firm, and submit publications to journals for him, presumably after helping with the writing or editing (since there seems no other plausible explanation why Scarano did not directly submit his articles to the journals). With only rare exceptions, proving that journals themselves were not responsible, the funded publications, such as these by Scarano and Sulman, acknowledged sponsoring drug firms either not at all or only for donating drugs. They did not disclose their financing and other involvement with the pharmaceutical firm.[35]

Published studies with favorable results could be cited in advertisements and, of course, provided valuable evidence for a product's safety and efficacy. But when results were not what the sponsoring firm hoped, they tended to go unpublished, whether through a gentleman's agreement or through the explicit terms of a contract (becoming more routine by the 1940s).[36] For example, following on Sulman's suggestion that the Benzedrine Inhaler might prevent or shorten colds, University of Minnesota occupational health researcher Howard Diehl conducted a study for SKF. When he found that the product had "no particular value" for "aborting" colds, the results never seem to have been published—although Diehl did publish on the inefficacy of other cold remedies and vaccines. [37] So at least one of the mechanisms that can explain the bias in today's medical research literature seems already to have been in place in the 1930s, despite the often high quality of company-sponsored trials: selective publication only of favorable results. The typical fee paid to the researcher, either directly or as reimbursements for expenses (as he chose), was, in the 1930s, $500 to $1,000 per study. This amount, a substantial fraction of a medical professor's annual salary, can be regarded as compensation for the chance that his work might not yield a status-enhancing publication. Accepting funding under these conditions essentially made a clinical researcher into a contractor or, as I prefer to say, an "Efficient" hired to produce science designed by the firm to meet a specific commercial need. As the examples of Dyer and Diehl remind us, some of the most reputable figures in academic medicine participated in this kind of role: Dyer was a rising star in internal medicine and a Penn professor at the time of his Benzedrine safety study, and Diehl was widely recognized for his meticulous clinical trial design and would soon become professor of occupational medicine in Minnesota.[38]

On the other hand, drug firms welcomed interest in their new products from freelancers, researchers with ideas of their own, motivated purely by curiosity and a wish to help their patients. The "hunches" of doctors like these might reveal important new uses of a drug not anticipated by its manufacturer, so drug firms were usually happy to cooperate by sending a supply of drugs. This is why SKF complied when approached in 1936 for injectable Benzedrine by the Buffalo endodontist. Sometimes this distribution of research samples was just a way of providing free samples to prime the pump of prescription sales, while some samples, in contrast, went to what the firms themselves distinguished as "actual research."[39] In exchange for drug supplies, firms asked researchers to keep them informed of what was happening, and to provide a draft of any report submitted for publication. An article in a scientific journal was in itself regarded as publicity; indeed, SKF judged that even Benzedrine research articles by dentists, although not worth funding, were valuable as "advertising."[40] And whatever the freelance researchers' articles might say, their publication served another indirect purpose for drug companies; because they usually carried a footnote thanking the firm for providing drugs, exactly the same as studies designed and commissioned by the firm, freelancers helped disguise those studies that were conducted on an Efficient basis. In other words, to a reader without inside information, studies conducted independently and those the firm partly controlled could not be distinguished (although some considered it obvious, at least by the early 1950s, that a small footnote acknowledging a "gift of materials often means an unstated grant for research expenses").[41]

The medical elite behind the AMA Council on Pharmacy approval system, which compelled drug firms to arrange for clinical research meeting high scientific standards, seem to have been completely blind to the possible effects of drug industry collaboration on both researchers and the research literature. Even Harvard medical school professor Soma Weiss, though he served as chair of that AMA Council, evidently saw no problem with funding from SKF in a large number of articles in the late 1930s—generous support not just for particular studies in his laboratory but also a large five-year grant for his clinic at Boston's Peter Bent Brigham Hospital. Weiss's publications, which consistently lacked acknowledgments, even included a prominent review on the progress of pharmacology in which he endorsed Benzedrine as one of the most promising drugs ever developed.[42] Behavior like Weiss's would surely excite scandal today but evidently did not breach ethical codes of the time. Apart from a naïve belief in their own incorruptibility, medical scientists like Weiss might have considered it a major accomplishment simply that drug firms were backing their advertising claims with real research by qualified medical scientists. It would take two more generations to appreciate that one unintended consequence was to turn the medical research literature itself into a marketing medium.

That major drug firms like SKF had considerable influence on the medical literature does not, of course, mean that they could create medical opinion from thin air. Drug firms could only amplify and encourage certain medical trends and views over others less favorable to their interests. However, this sort of subtle intervention may have been enough to help both the Benzedrine Inhaler and Benzedrine Sulfate through some public image problems that might otherwise have killed amphetamine's medical use at an early stage. For instance, the Inhaler encountered sluggish sales growth shortly after its AMA approval and general release on the market. In 1935 SKF discovered, through interviews similar to the "focus groups" used by marketeers today, that consumers and druggists perceived the Benzedrine Inhaler to be dangerous, despite the fact that physicians had high confidence in its safety. The perception of danger was traced to a "Do Not Overdose" warning label printed on the Inhaler (put there for AMA acceptance). To justify removing the warning label, SKF commissioned a pharmacology professor to measure the exact dose obtained by sniffing amphetamine vapors. When a freelance researcher did some animal experiments suggesting that amphetamine could harm the tissues lining the nose, the firm commissioned a counterstudy by physiologists to show that no detectable damage to the nose could come from amphetamine vapors in the Inhaler's dose range. The new studies on the product's safety were cited in advertising. Both may also have come in handy when, in mid-1938, a doctor published a high-profile article claiming that a seriously mind-altering dose of amphetamine could be absorbed by heavy sniffing on the Benzedrine Inhaler. Despite mounting bad publicity from the product's abuse, the Inhaler remained available over the counter, and advertised directly to the public, for another decade.[43]

An even graver publicity crisis erupted around Alles's newly approved Benzedrine Sulfate tablets around the same time that the Inhaler overcame this first set of difficulties. In April 1938, SKF management flew into a panic over stories in both the medical and lay press saying that some people who had been prescribed Benzedrine tablets were becoming "addicted" to the drug. The previous month, the Council on Pharmacy had run a warning in *JAMA* against the emerging prescription use of amphetamine in dieting, not only because this use was still unapproved but also because some patients seemed to have trouble getting off the drug. To make matters worse, SKF probably knew that, in May, the Syracuse psychopathic hospital psychiatrists were publishing an article describing how amphetamine, though effective in treating chronic alcoholism, often became the new drug habit of their addiction-prone patients.[44] Since the dieting and alcoholism patients were taking Benzedrine tablets medically, unlike the university student abusers, these reports of addiction could not be dismissed by claiming that the new drug was safe if used as prescribed.

Originally the firm had not been terribly worried about addiction. As one 1936 memo from a new products manager put it: "Data on tolerance to the drug will be obtained with the continued rat experiment. The question of addiction will be worked out eventually with continued use by patients."[45] Why, then, the sense of alarm in 1938? Apart from the bad news that some patients might, after all, be getting addicted to amphetamine, drug firms in general had fresh reasons for concern about their public image. In early 1938, the industry had fallen under withering attack in Washington for selling unsafe products, after a late 1937 pharmaceutical disaster in which more than a hundred people died from one of the new antibacterial "Sulfa" wonder drugs. The manufacturer, it emerged, had made the medicine into a syrup using toxic antifreeze and had rushed it to market without even rudimentary tests on rats. This sulfa syrup catastrophe finally gave consumer activists and populist politicians, long pressing for stricter regulation, their breakthrough. At length, the 1938 Federal Food, Drug, and Cosmetics act passed Congress, giving the Federal Drug Administration (FDA) authority to require proof of safety before a drug was sold, and setting the stage for the government to replace the AMA Council on Pharmacy as the main regulator of pharmaceuticals.[46] In the context of the harsh spotlight on the drug industry and the higher standards of product safety being written into law, the reports of addiction must have raised grave concerns for Benzedrine's future as a medicine. Amphetamine was not listed as a narcotic nor yet regarded as especially dangerous, but, given the new atmosphere of public distrust, the fledgling product might even find itself legally classified as addictive and brought under the harsh provisions of the Harrison Narcotic Act.[47]

SKF responded with an effort in crisis management that tested the limits of the company's public relations powers. To silence the media, SKF management planned to retain a "super libel lawyer" to "threaten and possibly sue" the next lay publication suggesting that Benzedrine is addictive, according to minutes of a meeting in early April 1938. Dealing with the medical world required more care. Here the approach would be two-pronged: first, the firm planned to "see all doctors who publish statements on Benzedrine Sulfate's harmful effects"; and, second, the minutes continued, "get article written and perhaps published comparing addictive and habit-forming properties of various drugs including Benzedrine." This would be commissioned from one of several experts friendly to SKF. (There are surprising resonances here with the tactics that today's pharmaceutical companies presently use in manipulating the medical research literature, at least according to some critics.) Thus, the firm's strategy was to mold professional opinion, through both personal contacts and specially designed scientific literature, so as to distinguish between addiction and habit formation. Given a sharp difference between addiction and "habituation," the aim was to show that Benzedrine was not an addictive drug, strictly redefined as one exhibiting tolerance (that is, increasing doses needed to obtain the same effect) and withdrawal symptoms—both characteristics of heroin addiction that are physiologically measurable. Apart from the fact that a distinction between habituation and addiction was already recognized by some, SKF was also fortunate in that pharmacological opinion at the time regarded stimulants in general as nonaddictive, with the possible exception of cocaine. Chauncey Leake did his part with a 1938 piece in the popular magazine *California Monthly,* making this point about stimulants and pronouncing that the addictive drugs are all "repressants . . . and dull sensibilities, induce relaxation and even sleep," thus meeting the weak, addiction-prone personality's need for escape from stress. Furthermore, according to Leake, truly addictive drugs are only those causing physiological withdrawal symptoms, while other drug habits could be treated by psychological methods.[48]

Leake, unfortunately for SKF, was not a nationally recognized addiction expert. Mid-1938 found SKF looking for ways of "putting heat on [M. H.] Seevers" to write a review article about addiction, although with "EXTREME FINESSE." Seevers was an up-and-coming pharmacologist and authority on narcotic drugs, and one of the first to propose a distinction between habituation and addiction. In an influential 1931 paper, for instance, he had argued that "without abstinence symptoms on [drug] withdrawal, a drug can scarcely be considered to produce true addiction." He had further concluded that because cocaine apparently did not lead to withdrawal symptoms in regularly dosed dogs and monkeys, even this notoriously destructive and habit-forming drug was technically nonaddictive. Thus, SKF was anxious for Seevers to reiterate and stress the distinctive and uniquely dangerous properties of heroin and morphine addiction, compared to the mere "habit" that stimulants can produce.

SKF must have been greatly concerned to learn that an even more influential authority, Assistant Surgeon General Lawrence Kolb, was writing a high-profile article about his experience as head of the new federal narcotics prison in Lexington, Kentucky. When it appeared in May 1939, Kolb's article in *Scientific Monthly* said roughly what SKF management had been hoping for, with its insistence that, apart from cocaine, stimulants were not addictive because their use is self-limiting. "Artificial stimulation eventually becomes unpleasant, but sedation is always pleasant" because it meets the universal human need for escape, wrote Kolb. Even cocaine addicts eventually end up addicted to opiates, he argued, because of their greater attractiveness and capacity to cause physical addiction. Although Kolb broadly used the loaded term "addiction" to include conditioning-based "mental addiction" or habituation, the fact that he made light of it by saying it was treatable by psychotherapy, together with his dismissive attitude toward stimulants generally, appears to have helped quiet the alarm at SKF.[49]

I have found no 1939–40 review article on addiction and habituation by Seevers, but Myerson did address the topic in a prominent 1940 review article on amphetamine in psychiatry. There he followed Kolb's line closely, pronouncing that Benzedrine presents "not much danger of drug addiction" because only opiate sedatives like heroin and morphine were seriously addictive. Also, even though a few patients who were prescribed the drug did develop an amphetamine habit, they showed no signs of harm. A consensus had emerged, enshrined in the definitive 1941 pharmacology textbook by Goodman and Gilman, *The Pharmacological Basis of Therapeutics*: "habituation to benzedrine may occur . . . similar to the habit formation produced by caffeine and nicotine, but addiction in the strict sense of the word is unknown." This party line was still being defended in the mid-1960s by advocates of amphetamine as a pharmaceutical, including Leake.[50]

Another lasting consequence of the Benzedrine addiction scare may also have been a narrowing of the remaining possibilities for amphetamine's prescription usage. In late 1938, SKF decided to discourage clinical research with the drug for the treatment of opiate addiction, even though some neuropsychiatrists were excited about this possibility. An inherently limited market, narcotic addiction was dangerous ground as well. Studies on the relief of withdrawal symptoms from opiates had sometimes revealed the addictive properties of other new drugs, and sporadic reports of amphetamine addiction continued to arise. Like the use of amphetamine for mental performance enhancement, which the student abuse scandals made disreputable, this avenue for marketing amphetamine would not be pursued by SKF. And not until the late 1940s would the drug be sold for weight loss by the firm. From 1938 through the next decade, SKF's marketing focus for Benzedrine Sulfate remained on depression.[51]

Preparing the Next Big Thing

Today's standard wisdom says that the pharmaceutical industry did not become interested in antidepressants until the 1960s. This view clearly needs revision in light of amphetamine's story. By 1939, Benzedrine Sulfate was well on its way to becoming the first mass-market "antidepressant," if by this we mean a medicine prescribed to elevate mood indefinitely in neurotic outpatients. SKF even began to use this term in their advertising by the later 1940s. The firm helped amphetamine weather the first storms, thanks to good luck, well-measured and energetic public relations efforts, the fostering of favorable clinical research, and the cultivation of experts, like Weiss and Myerson, friendly to the the fledgling drug. As the product matured and gained prominence as a "milestone" of medical progress (Figure 11), SKF continued to manage publicity problems such as the spectacular collapse and death of a Purdue University student during an examination in 1939, attributed partly to the Benzedrine "brain tablets" he had been taking regularly.[52] And, while building the product's image and its sales as an antidepressant, SKF also began quietly preparing for the next steps in amphetamine's development—new uses for the same drug, and also a new product to succeed Benzedrine Sulfate in the depression field. One avenue was opened by Myerson, a solution to the problem that many depressed people were also anxious, which made them unsuitable for Benzedrine therapy since amphetamine often worsened anxiety. When testing Benzedrine in 1936 on inpatients at Boston State, he found that, with the right doses, amphetamine in combination with certain barbiturate sedatives made patients relaxed, yet cheerful and talkative. This combination would one day become a blockbuster (as we shall see in chapter 5), but Myerson's idea stayed on the back burner while SKF quietly commissioned a few studies on it, and also on the soon-to-be explosive use of amphetamine for weight loss.[53]

SKF also pursued one of Alles's recent discoveries as a potential new product. Many molecules, including amphetamine, are asymmetric in their structure, coming in left-handed and right-handed versions known as "optical isomers." When chemicals are manufactured, the two isomers are normally mixed together in equal quantities. Alles had tried chemical methods to separate the left- and right-handed amphetamine molecules from each other in 1932 and again in 1934, not fully succeeding. The task is tricky, since the left- and right-handed versions of a given molecule behave almost exactly the same chemically; when Louis Pasteur discovered optical isomers in 1848, he did so by noticing that crystals of a certain chemical came in two shapes, which he separated using tweezers and a magnifying glass. But SKF chemists eventually found a fairly practical process to separate the two forms of amphetamine and sent both to Alles in 1938. When he took the first 10 mg dose of the right-handed isomer, dextro-amphetamine, on July 13, 1938, Alles thought it felt much stronger than Benzedrine (an equal or "racemic" mixture of left- and right-handed amphetamine molecules). It also made him feel better than Benzedrine had, not as jittery as he might have expected. In contrast, milligram for milligram, the left-handed isomer, levo-amphetamine, felt considerably more jittery and unpleasant and was not as strong a brain stimulant. Thus, he concluded, a 5 mg dose of dextro-amphetamine would work roughly as well as a 10 mg dose of the racemic mixture (that is, Benzedrine) and without so many unpleasant side effects. In 1939, Alles prepared a patent application on dextro-amphetamine for SKF, and the firm began to plan clinical experiments with the drug, soon branded "Dexedrine."[54]

Work on Dexedrine would slow drastically, though it was pushed forward as circumstances allowed. Competing drug companies had begun working on amphetamines, and SKF needed to defend its lead by thinking ahead to new products. The major challenge to the growth of the firm's amphetamine prescription sales, of course, lay not with competitors but with the ominous events building in Europe. In early 1940, Germany's offensives overwhelmed France and threw Britain into full retreat, virtually overnight. In the United States, preparation for the impending struggle began in earnest, unleashing an economic boom that ended the Depression almost as quickly as it had started. Through the early 1940s, SKF would continue to market Benzedrine for depression, and to design and fund studies on amphetamine products that might pave the way for new marketing campaigns once business returned to normal. Meanwhile, however, there was a war to be won.

3

Speed and Total War

WHEN THE GERMANS attacked Poland in September 1939, they unleashed an entirely new form of warfare on the world called *Blitzkrieg,* or lightning war. It was all about speed and shock, about delivering the strongest, quickest blow and then covering lots of ground before the enemy could regroup. The soldiers who delivered the shock were powered by the latest technologies: tanks twice as fast as their British and French counterparts, paratroops that materialized suddenly behind the lines, Stuka dive bombers that flew bombs precisely to their targets so that advancing forces need not wait for lumbering artillery. Blitzkrieg was also a form of psychological warfare; for instance, the Stukas carried sirens and their bombs sometimes sported toy whistles to enhance the terror of their shrieking dive attack.

Poland was finished by October 1939. In April 1940, Germany resumed by taking Denmark in a few days and Norway, weakly supported by British troops, a few weeks later. In May, Germany overran Holland and Belgium, and without a pause moved on to France where, expecting a replay of the First World War, French and English armies were entrenching themselves on a long front between the Belgian coast and the rough Ardennes Forest. The main body of German tanks drove right around them, through the supposedly impassible Ardennes and then West to the Channel, cutting off the British and sending the French into full retreat. Between May 10 and May 21, German tanks covered 240 miles of countryside, driving hard for eleven straight days, always ahead of where they were supposed to be, always maintaining shock and surprise. Paratroopers often got there before the tanks, landing behind enemy lines in a state that British newspapers described as "heavily drugged, fearless, and berserk."[1]

Fearless and Berserk

The German Blitzkrieg was powered by amphetamines as much as it was powered by machine. In 1938, the Temmler pharmaceutical firm introduced to the European market a product called Pervitin, which was methamphetamine—a very close relative of amphetamine (see Figure 5), differing only by one extra carbon atom and slightly stronger per milligram as a stimulant. (The drug had been made, studied, and described in print by Japanese pharmacologists years before, so it could not be patented.) Pervitin was marketed to physicians for psychiatric uses along the same lines as Benzedrine, and the German medical profession quickly welcomed the product. Methamphetamine's fortunes would for decades ebb and flow in unison with those of amphetamine, the two drugs being essentially interchangeable for both medical and recreational use.

The academy of military medicine in Berlin did some rather casual tests with methamphetamine around the beginning of 1939, finding unpleasant physical reactions and mental disturbance in a few subjects, along with marginal performance gains on mathematical and other mental tasks. Authorities were already aware that the drug was being used by some soldiers, who were obtaining it on their own. Nevertheless, they officially listed Pervitin (in 3 mg tablets) among the medicines that physicians in military units could requisition in 1939—just in time for the campaign that crushed Poland. In the Blitzkrieg's opening months, German troops were widely issued the drug. Pervitin proved popular among Hitler's fighting men: the German military consumed 35 million methamphetamine tablets in April, May, and June 1940, the peak season of the Blitz. There were no orders from Berlin to use it in any particular way, so this consumption reflects demand among the soldiers and medics at the front.[2]

Pervitin soon began to raise doubts in high circles. For instance, even in the 1939 military academy trials it was noted that a number of the student subjects were not only familiar with the drug already but were regular abusers. Military medical authorities worried that too much extra time was needed for troops to recuperate after taking methamphetamine. The Luftwaffe (Germany's air force) also found that performance was not as good objectively as it seemed to those under the influence, and that the drug might even cause accidents by making pilots overconfident and attentive to the wrong things. Because of controversy over whether Pervitin genuinely enhanced performance, as well as their personal observations of its effects on soldiers, doctors in the German military soon adopted a much more cautious approach. By December 1940, military consumption of methamphetamine had dropped to a little more than a million tablets per month, only a tenth what it had been early that year. In mid-1941, Germany placed methamphetamine, along with amphetamine, under strict narcotics regulation so that the drugs would only be available by special prescription, declaring that the amphetamines depleted users' energy stores and were dangerously habit forming. Military consumption again dropped late that year, and declined further in 1942, when German medicine officially recognized the amphetamines as addictive (remarkably, three decades before the American medical profession!)[3]

Another perspective on why the military started to discourage the use of amphetamines is suggested by the following undocumented tale. One day, during the drawn out siege of Leningrad, an entire German SS infantry company—a hundred men or more—surrendered to the Soviets without a fight. The Russians taking them prisoner noticed the Germans seemed unusually nervous and jumpy, and that they were entirely out of machine gun bullets. Apparently the men had used up their ammunition the night before, when they fired it all in a collective methamphetamine-induced delusion that they were under attack. Though there were also stories of units saved by judicious use of Pervitin, the German military leadership understandably did not want soldiers taking the drug too freely.[4]

Ironically, about the same time that the Germans were cutting back sharply on the Pervitin, the British military officially gave its sanction to amphetamine use, and was rapidly developing a strong appetite for speed. The American military soon followed, although well aware that the Germans had classed the drugs as addictive narcotics.[5] As we shall see, the reasons the Allies took to amphetamine have everything to do with that complex set of psychological factors that, in military thinking, mingle in the deceptively simple term "morale." Morale has always worried military leaders, but the terrifying new killing technology introduced in the First World War created an unprecedented morale crisis. Vast numbers of men were falling out of action with no sign of physical harm, casualties of mental trauma on the battlefield. Psychiatric casualties could outnumber surgical cases, in some battles. What could armies do with these broken men—some mute and others gibbering, some suffering hysterical limps and others totally paralytic? Were they really unable to fight? The traditional approach of shaming them as malingerers and threatening them with firing squads did not help. Sending them back to the trenches, where they were sure to panic under pressure, undermined the morale of the men still trying to fight. The military eventually turned to medicine for help. Some doctors thought "shell shock" was caused by nervous system damage and others by unbearable psychic experience, and there were various theories in between. Shell shock was treated with the occupational, rest, and talking cures that were standard for psychiatry and neurology of the day.[6]

When the Second World War came the Allied military recalled this problem and, in the United States especially, took psychiatry into account. Leading American psychiatrists like William Menninger and Harry Stack Sullivan helped establish mental health screening procedures for recruits, promising dramatically to reduce the numbers of servicemen—especially highly trained men like pilots—likely to suffer "psychoneurotic breakdown" in combat. Then once hostilities began, and the condition again reared its head despite all the rigorous screening, the military had to re-learn that every man, and not just weaklings, could only take so much punishment and horror before cracking. With some initial reluctance, psychiatrists were called to the front to treat the victims, in much the same way on both the British and American sides.[7]

For treating such cases of what today we would call Post-Traumatic Stress Disorder (PTSD), a key advance was treating men near the battlefield, and quickly. After some rest and talk with the psychiatrists, both sometimes assisted by sedatives, many were eager to return to their buddies, recovered from the "condition euphemistically and by intention vaguely called 'operational fatigue,'" in the words of pioneering combat psychiatrist Roy Grinker. There were other names for the condition too, like "battle fatigue," "combat exhaustion," and especially "combat fatigue." Psychiatry's success in returning men to combat depended crucially on some euphemism of this sort: it made the traumatic disorder sound like a cold, a temporary ailment that a little time out could fix. As John Spiegel put it, in 1942 he learned to diagnose combat-related acute anxiety and depression as "combat fatigue," "to avoid stigmatizing" his patients, and to avoid antagonizing military brass skeptical about the value of psychiatry. In the 1940s neuropsychiatrists like Spiegel actually called it "war neurosis" but only among themselves. In reality, the condition was "about 50 percent [physiological] fatigue and 50 percent emotional illness," according to combat psychiatrists David Hastings, Donald Wright, and Bernard Glueck. So the euphemism was half-true.[8] And the link between physical exhaustion and war neurosis was hormonal.

According to psychoanalyst Abraham Kardiner, the leading American authority on the condition between the wars, shell shock or war neurosis was ultimately caused by the "severe blow to the total ego organization" that a soldier suffered from his inability to escape or alter his threatening situation. Straying from Freud's own views on how this occurred, Kardiner believed the condition could be caused not only by acute trauma, such as being buried by a shell burst, but also by a combination of chronic anxiety and physical exhaustion. His theory was typical of American psychiatry's eclectic style between the wars. Man, like any organism, handled perceived threats with heightened psychic and physical preparedness, involving Cannon's fight-or-flight response. The adrenaline-fired state of arousal aided survival in the short term, but in the long run it depleted the nervous system and eroded the resilience of the psyche, eventually producing psychoneurotic breakdown. Major early symptoms of war neurosis included anxiety and irritability, and, as the condition worsened, psychomotor retardation (slowed action and responsiveness). These were also the signs and symptoms that indicated ordinary depression. To Kardiner and other psychiatrists, and likewise to medics like Dean Andersen at the front, combat fatigue was a depressive condition.[9]

This wartime medical common sense linking adrenaline, anxiety, arousal, and physical exhaustion to war neurosis made amphetamine an obvious possibility for preventing and possibly treating the condition. The artificial adrenaline—and the first and only antidepressant—might temporarily bolster the adrenaline circuits behind the fight-or-flight reaction, staving off incipient breakdown and alleviating its depressive symptoms. Thus we can understand why psychiatrists like Moses Kaufman, having read about Grinker's work in North Africa, shipped off to the front with luggage stuffed full of barbiturate sedatives and Benzedrine to treat combat fatigue cases using the latest methods.[10] How many others adopted this thinking as grounds for treating soldiers with amphetamine to prevent or treat combat fatigue, only extensive research into wartime diaries of medical officers can

show. Still, we can say with some assurance that the same useful ambiguity around "fatigue" that allowed psychiatrists access to the front,
together with the eclectic style of American psychiatry in the 1940s,
created a hazy zone that would have made the psychiatric use of amphetamine on fighting men during the Second World War easy to ra-
tionalize medically.

To state that amphetamine was used to fight fatigue among Allied
troops may, therefore, be to say much more than first appears: wherever combat fatigue was understood as a variety of fatigue, using amphetamine against fatigue was tantamount to using it as a psychiatric medication, for its mood-altering effects. Amphetamine alleviated sensations of tiredness, or physical exhaustion, as well as the
emotional signs and symptoms common to both depression and combat fatigue. Military common sense, confirmed by wartime psychiatric
research, also fit this with the fuzzy medical logic around combat fatigue sketched above, and related it to older morale concerns: physical
exhaustion tended to increase psychoneurotic breakdown, whereas
traditional morale-building factors like adequate rest, good rations,
bonding among men in a unit, and faith in commanding officers
tended to reduce it.[11] This cluster of ideas about combat fatigue, and its
vague boundaries with physical exhaustion and morale, can help explain Allied amphetamine use. For morale and soldierly conduct, not
just the problem of alertness, figured prominently in the decision of
the Allied armed services to supply Benzedrine. Furthermore, this decision did not depend greatly on careful studies into the effects of amphetamine conducted by scientific experts, the results of which were
late in coming, and never firmly established that the drug objectively
improved physical endurance, coordination, or mental efficiency.

Fatigue, Morale, and Britain's Finest Hour

Whether one defines the problem as one of morale, fatigue, or war
neurosis, it is easy to see why the British military would welcome
some chemical fortitude in the early part of the war. Britain barely survived the 1940 Blitzkrieg that crushed France. At the end of May 1940,
more than three hundred thousand British soldiers narrowly escaped
to England from the French town of Dunkirk, in a rag-tag fleet of fish-
ing boats and pleasure craft. While German tanks were closing in, the

milling crowds waiting on the beach underwent vicious bombing and strafing by the dreaded Stukas. Although the British army was saved, it had no equipment left to fight off a German landing in England. Nor could the British fleet be relied upon to defend the homeland, because German planes could destroy any ships the Royal Navy sent down the Channel. Only the Royal Air Force (RAF) prevented Nazi invasion. So, after a short lull while Hitler waited for Churchill's surrender, the Luftwaffe spent the late summer assaulting Britain's air bases and cities almost every day with hundreds of planes. In the two weeks between August 24 and September 6 alone, the British lost about 500 fighter aircraft, and 220 pilots were killed or wounded as the RAF struggled to keep its Spitfires and Hurricanes aloft. But the Germans took similar heavy losses. After three months of all-out struggle for control of the air, Hitler had to cancel the invasion, switching the Luftwaffe to less costly night raids on cities just to terrorize the civilian population. It was an intense collective trauma, but the British spirit, like London's Underground system, proved durable.[12]

In these dark days, rumors ran wild about the secret weapons that made Hitler's forces so invincible. The British War Office took seriously the ones about drugged paratroopers and the "Stuka Tablets" that made it possible for dive-bombing pilots to fly straight down into the ground and then pull out violently, right back up to 10,000 feet. This made physiological sense: G forces were tremendous during the pullout, and any drug that raised blood pressure might help the pilot stay conscious. In late June 1940, during the daily pitched battles over the airfields of southern England, pills had been recovered from downed German planes. The eminent physiologist Henry Dale was called in, and in September 1940 he correctly identified the drug as methamphetamine and cautiously recommended that it be studied for British use. This confirmed what the RAF had heard from intelligence sources earlier in 1940, that the German pilots were using Pervitin. At the request of the War Office, in late 1940, a contingent of elite British medical scientists, called the Flying Personnel Research Committee (FPRC), launched several studies evaluating "Benzedrine-series drugs."[13] From the outset, the military hoped not just for a new "wakey-wakey" pill but for true performance enhancement. Sports physiologists were aware that Benzedrine was already prized among long-distance bicycle racers and similar endurance athletes, who had long been using cocaine for a competitive edge.[14]

Two of the earliest British studies, completed in January 1941, reported ambiguous effects of Benzedrine in thirteen psychological and hand-eye coordination tests. In many experiments, such as message-decoding or rapidly placing pegs in particular holes on a board, amphetamine did not consistently improve performance. There were two exceptions, however. The lab test with the most direct military relevance was probably the "pursuit meter," a device with crosshairs to track a moving target, and here the study found not only that subjects scored higher on the drug, but that they showed greater improvement in repeated testing. In another test, in which subjects continually squeezed a spring-loaded grip that measures force, amphetamine significantly slowed the decline in exertion over time. The researchers concluded that the drug-induced improvement with the pursuit meter and the grip tester reflected the subject's mental attitude: amphetamine gives people greater interest in these simple challenges. Because they get less bored and feel more confident, they maintain effort and do better—just as psychologists had already concluded about amphetamine's effect on students taking exams and standardized tests. The military might use this attitude effect to advantage, researchers thought, even if the drug did not actually improve the body's mental or physical capacities. However, as the British scientists judged, caution was needed: along with the usual subjective effects such as "feeling of well-being" and "elation," fully 10 percent (6/64) of the subjects reported unpleasant experiences on doses of only 10 mg—SKF's standard commercial Benzedrine tablet.[15]

The Machine Outstrips the Man

By the time these early academic studies were done, the RAF had expanded its priorities from keeping the Spitfires flying to helping escort and defend shipping. Freighter convoys were Britain's lifeline, feeding and re-arming the island nation. After March 1941, when President Franklin D. Roosevelt finally managed to persuade an isolationist Congress to provide materiel on a "Lend-Lease" basis, many of these convoys came from the United States through the North Atlantic. To protect them, the RAF flew anti-submarine patrols with its longest-range planes, Catalina flying boats as well as obsolete bombers fitted with extra fuel capacity. These patrol flights were extraordinarily lengthy: Catalinas could fly for up to thirty-six hours, and the Whitley bomber eleven hours. They were also extraordinarily monotonous, consisting of nothing but staring at empty ocean for hours on end. Planes often disappeared without a trace, lost to accidents when attention lapsed. Aviators had started taking Benzedrine to stay awake, on their own initiative. According to R. H. Winfield, the medical officer from the RAF's physiological laboratory who was assigned the problem, since Benzedrine's "surreptitious use in the Service" was growing the RAF needed to study the drug and take an official position on it.[16]

Winfield, a former general practitioner and ship's surgeon with a keen taste for adventure, flew fourteen missions with RAF Coastal Command crews between April and October 1941 to test amphetamine in the field.[17] He was also asked to test methamphetamine, because it was available from the British firm of Burroughs-Wellcome under the brand name "Methedrine," whereas Benzedrine was well defended by SKF patents and had to be purchased from the U.S. On each of his flights in this study, Winfield would give crew members one of the two drugs or else placebo "dummies." He would interview the men after the flight and, of course, observe "objective signs of fatigue" during it, such as irritability and forgetfulness. Sometimes such signs were obvious. For instance, "on one occasion after flying through the night, poor visibility made it necessary to fly within fifty feet of the sea . . . the pilot flying the aircraft started to nod off and was roused only by a judicious nudge in the ribs." Summarizing his results, Winfield found that none of the men reported a bad reaction, and all who noticed the drugs approved of them. A dose of 8 mg of methamphetamine—a higher dose pharmacologically—was about as effective for keeping men awake as 10 mg of amphetamine. The Benzedrine, however, gave a more "marked feeling of well-being" than Methedrine, and this mood effect made it the better drug. (Although the study was not double-blind, and this view may reflect Winfield's expectations rather than a real difference between the drugs, his observations show the RAF was always studying the mood-altering "morale" effects of the drugs.) The RAF quickly put Winfield's recommendations into action, approving the use of two 5 mg Benzedrine tablets on long flights.[18]

The Atlantic convoys held the greatest strategic importance, along with the war raging in the Middle East over Britain's Suez link to the

East. However, in mid-1941, RAF Bomber Command was the only branch of the armed forces that could bring the fight to the German people, and avenging the Blitz had crucial psychological significance. To get to the heart of Germany with maximum safety, bombers had to fly at the highest possible altitudes and at night, despite the difficulties of finding targets in the dark. Radar helped with navigation, and the new four-engine heavy bombers that the RAF was introducing would take the airmen higher, faster, and further into enemy territory. But, in the words of Dr. Charles Stephenson, a U.S. naval officer stationed in London as an observer at the time: "the machine has far outstripped the man" in aviation.[19] Just as fighter planes were now capable of acceleration that pushed pilots beyond consciousness, so the cold and rarified atmosphere in which the newer bombers operated made for exotic medical problems. Bare flesh froze instantly to controls and other metal, and the air was too thin to think straight. Research on better controls, heating, oxygen supply, and (eventually) pressurized cabins would soon occupy many scientists.

In addition to adjusting the plane to the needs of the aviator, war research also worked on modifying the man to fit the machine. Special suits to prevent blackouts under high G forces were one major project. Another was biological enhancement of fliers: vitamin supplements were studied, as was testosterone for its reputed strength-building powers. However, the steroid hormones of the adrenal gland commanded the greatest attention. By releasing extra sugar supplies into the blood, improving circulation, and a host of other subtle actions related to the emergency function of the adrenal, these hormones were believed to improve the body's performance under strain. Such ideas were already in the air, but a faulty intelligence report in the spring of 1941 touched off a frenzied effort by the Allies to identify and manufacture the adrenal steroids. Sources said that the Germans were shipping 50 tons of frozen adrenal glands from South America in a giant submarine to manufacture hormones that allowed pilots to fly at 40,000 feet (12 km) without oxygen.[20]

Given this context in which everyone was prepared to believe that German research was producing Supermen and that adrenal steroids (particularly what we now call cortisol-type "glucocorticoid" hormones) were key to their success, amphetamine seemed another likely possibility for high-altitude performance enhancement. After all, the drug was understood as an artificial version of adrenaline, the adrenal gland's other main type of hormone. However, mid-1941 experiments with an experienced—and obviously brave—pilot performing extreme dives showed that nothing did much to prevent blacking out, neither a 25 mg Benzedrine injection nor ephedrine nor adrenal steroids. The idea that amphetamine boosted work output crumbled around the same time as did the notion that it enhanced resistance to acceleration: as Cambridge psychologist F. C. Bartlett told the FPRC, his studies proved that, on Benzedrine, "individuals were disposed to try to make greater efforts; they thought they were working harder, whereas they were doing exactly the same amount of work."[21]

But as one set of claims about amphetamine's performance-enhancing effects collapsed under scrutiny, another slightly different set arose in its place. Though amphetamine does not do much for rested people under normal conditions, the new view held, it prevents the decay of performance over time at high altitude and under other strains. In one British study with a flight simulator, for example, maneuvering accuracy declined quickly when pilots had to breathe low-oxygen air like that found at 16,000–17,000 feet (5 km). Caffeine did not help simulated flying performance under either low- or normal-oxygen conditions, and Benzedrine did not improve performance in normal oxygen, but it did seem to help significantly at simulated high altitude. It remained unclear whether Benzedrine's effect was physiological, in that oxygen was somehow used more efficiently (unlikely given earlier FPRC experiments showing that the drug did not improve rat survival in low oxygen), or simply psychological as in the earlier human tests.[22]

Would the drug also help fliers in actual high-altitude combat, particularly in bombing raids? The RAF turned again to the intrepid Wing Commander Winfield to find out. For Bomber Command boredom was not the main problem. In addition to low oxygen and cold, the extra strains of bombing missions included "the tension which is experienced before the flight" when air crews waited to hear when and where they were flying, and the anxious anticipation of the enemy fighters and anti-aircraft guns that gave them an average 5 percent chance of not returning from each mission in one piece. Strains also included the psychological toll taken by "the excitement which is evident while actually in the target area," where terrific concentration is needed to identify and bomb the target despite searchlights, flak, and night fighters. Then there was the premature sense of relief on the return flight, where hazards like anti-aircraft fire and enemy fighters were as great as ever. Accidents frequently occurred during landings, with pilots too eager and relieved to be home. Winfield accompanied crews in Whitley and Stirling bombers on twenty missions between August 1941 and July 1942, including night raids on Kiel, Hamburg, Cologne, Essen, Rostock and the Ruhr valley, and a daylight attack on Lubeck.[23] Air crews were given either Benzedrine or placebo tablets at the beginning of a mission, and told that they had even chances of getting the dummy or a new caffeine-like drug. As in the submarine patrol study, Winfield observed the men during the mission and interviewed them afterward to see whether amphetamine had desirable subjective effects.[24]

Results exceeded expectations. In many fliers, the drug seemed, according to Winfield, to boost vigilance on the way home, and perhaps effort as well. For example, when one pilot suggested turning on the automatic pilot after reaching the coast on the way home from the Ruhr, his co-pilot insisted on piloting the plane himself and practicing his instrument flying (in contrast to his five previous, drug-free missions, when he was happy to do the minimum). Gunners, isolated in their frigid turrets and prone to dozing, especially appreciated the drug. On Benzedrine, one "gave an extremely detailed and accurate account of the defenses through which the aircraft had passed, although as a rule he was silent" in post-mission debriefing.

The effects on mood and attitude, which Winfield had already identified as an advantage of amphetamine over methamphetamine in his Coastal Command work, impressed him still more than the drug's effects on alertness. As Winfield put it: "In some people the drug may increase determination in circumstances of acute anxiety," although not generally to the point of "recklessness" that would be undesirable (at least in combat). For example, on the mission over Cologne a pilot decided that instead of "bombing from 15,000 feet through eight-tenths cloud" like most of the planes, he should "press home the attack and bomb below the cloud layer" at 8,000 feet where flak was heavy. And "although the aircraft was hit just before the bombs were released, a direct hit on the target was made" by this Benzedrine-assisted crew. During an air raid against the Renault factory outside Paris in March 1942, an air crew on Benzedrine swooped in at a tree-trimming 200 feet to strafe and kill an enemy anti-aircraft team with their ungainly bomber, impressing Winfield deeply. Air crews on Benzedrine would even fly their heavy bombers right down a searchlight beam to dive-bomb an anti-aircraft emplacement that had the plane in its sights.

Winfield concluded that since about half the men taking Benzedrine functioned better (that is, behaved more like fighting men were meant to), and since habit formation seemed unlikely during a regular Bomber Command tour of duty, the drug should be made available to all air crews. There was no effort to distinguish the effects that the drug produced through mood and morale and those it produced by acting directly on the nervous system. He recommended two 5 mg doses, one taken as the plane entered enemy airspace and another soon after the bombing run, for the return flight. He also suggested men should take a trial dose on the ground their first time to check for adverse reactions. In 1942, RAF Bomber Command adopted Winfield's recommendations (Figure 12).[25] As we shall see, continuing research during the war never found good evidence that amphetamine measurably enhances or preserves physiological function in low oxygen, nor evidence that the drug provides any objective performance advantage in exhaustion other than prevention of sleep, which caffeine also could accomplish.

Nevertheless, Bomber Command kept issuing Benzedrine. What seems to have mattered most were amphetamine's behavioral and emotional—that is, strictly subjective—effects. In Winfield's words, to reach "peak efficiency, a squadron must be possessed of the highest morale, and morale depends upon the sum total of all those things that affect the minds and bodies" of the aviators.[26] Although these were Winfield's postwar reflections on morale and efficiency generally, it is easy to see how Benzedrine would appear a reasonable psychosomatic morale enhancer from this medical perspective, especially in the darker days of the Second World War. So impressive are Winfield's studies in the military imagination that they are still, six decades later, cited by the U.S. Air Force to support the continued use of amphetamine by combat pilots as part of its official "warfighter endurance management" procedures.[27] One might have hoped that the American military could cite recent and superior authorities, but perhaps nothing carries as much weight as Winfield's participant observations that amphetamine gives airmen the right combination of optimism and aggressiveness to achieve "peak efficiency" in combat. Whatever impairment of judgment or distractibility the drug might also cause—reasons the Luftwaffe abandoned regular use of methamphetamine early in the war—evidently were and are still outweighed by such effects on "morale."

Snap and Zest: Amphetamine in the British Army

Though Air Council approval came almost a year later, by early 1942 the British military, according to U.S. officials in a position to know, had already bought several million Benzedrine Sulfate tablets from SKF.[28] Of course, the British military's Benzedrine shipments went not just to the RAF. Paratroops and special forces used the drug too, just as on the German side; Churchill personally suggested that Benzedrine should be used by his commandos in a March 1941 operation in Greece. Although it never established a formal drug testing program, the Royal Navy seems to have done its own informal trials with both methamphetamine and amphetamine by mid-1942. The navy found that both amphetamines were useful for situations such as long, high-alert watches on convoy escort missions and that objectionable side effects were rare. One of the exceptions was an officer on watch who, having gulped down seven Benzedrine tablets at once—5 mg rather than 10 mg each, one hopes—"was thought to have reported seeing rather more enemy submarines and aircraft than actually existed."[29] (This was not the first and certainly not the last piece of ignored evidence that showed amphetamine capable of causing paranoid hallucinations, even with a single dose.)

The British Army too was no stranger to the drug. In this case also, as with the RAF and the navy, the British military adopted amphetamine without scientific evidence that the drug objectively improved performance, although plenty of good science was done. By August 1941, the "Subcommittee on Analeptic Substances" of the Military Personnel Research Committee (MPRC) had begun to organize amphetamine studies for the army. Like their counterparts on the RAF's fatigue research committee, who were only slightly ahead in their experiments, this MPRC subcommittee was made up mainly of university professors. In October 1941, these scientists organized their first large experiment with Benzedrine made up in chocolate "emergency rations" with a British unit on maneuvers. (Like the RAF, they had intended to test methamphetamine since it was not controlled by an American company, but Methedrine was not available from Burroughs-Wellcome when they ordered the supplies, whereas Benzedrine was). The October test produced no meaningful results because, MPRC researchers complained, army officers had not cooperated.[30]

Not so easily discouraged, the scientists organized an extensive series of tests, many employing placebos, statistics, and the latest in clinical research methods. Much like the FPRC experiments, one after another of these careful MPRC studies failed to show that amphetamine improved performance or helped with fatigue, defined as measurable performance loss due to lack of rest. For example, one January 1942 experiment found no distinction between Benzedrine-drugged and undrugged Canadian infantry doing sets of marches, drills, obstacle courses, and so forth, over about thirty-six hours. Another 1942 study used 15 mg of Methedrine on soldiers made to go on night exercises and marching maneuvers. Despite this rather high methamphetamine dose, these men also showed no great difference in marching performance. Moreover, one officer "showed considerable error of judgement" on the drug. In these studies, negative results were explained away as due to insufficient exhaustion of the men. Another trial with a Canadian unit on maneuvers near the end of 1942 finally found a gain, of marginal statistical significance, in the physical performance of exhausted men on Benzedrine.[31] Then, at the beginning of 1943, a careful study of Benzedrine's effects on officers doing calculations and complex paperwork tasks almost continuously for seventy-two grueling hours found no significant gain in efficiency. Remarkably, the experimenters concluded that if officers wanted to use the drug on duty, they should be allowed to take it (rather than asserting that amphetamine should not be used, since it did not help). The burden of proof implicit in this conclusion suggests that, as in RAF Coastal Command, Benzedrine was already being used by officers in the British Army.[32]

In sum, studying drugs carefully for a year and half under controlled conditions back in Britain, top scientists could find very little objective evidence to recommend amphetamine use over caffeine. But by mid-1942 the British Eighth Army was mired in North Africa and desperate for a boost, and like Bomber Command it did not wait for scientific approval. Since early 1941, when the brilliant German general Erwin Rommel arrived to help the floundering Italians, the North African campaign had gone badly. With his comparatively small but well trained and equipped German force, Rommel quickly turned the tables on the previously victorious British and by midyear drove the Eighth Army three hundred miles eastward across Libya to the Egyptian frontier. Then fortunes reversed, and in January 1942 the Eighth Army had retaken this terrain and were driving the Germans west across Libya. But just when he seemed defeated, wily Rommel suddenly counterattacked and in just two weeks drove the British four hundred miles eastward, almost back to the Egyptian border. This was the Blitzkrieg all over again, and it would be surprising if Rommel's troops had not been taking any Pervitin. At last, in early July 1942, the Eighth Army stopped the outnumbered Germans at an Alexandria suburb called El Alamein, virtually the doorstep of the Suez Canal and a thousand miles from Rommel's main supply port. But the Germans dug in and held their position, once almost breaking through to Cairo.

Because nothing they did seemed capable of beating Rommel and ending the tug-of-war, the British forces in North Africa underwent repeated changes of leadership. Bernard Montgomery, who took charge of the Eighth Army in August 1942, immediately conducted his own informal Benzedrine studies in the field. The problem he hoped to address was, to him, largely one of morale: made cagey by their experience with Rommel and his formidable Afrika Corps, the Eighth Army seemed lacking in fighting spirit (that is, they showed an absence of aggression or a great deal of good sense—depending on one's perspective). Montgomery wanted full-throttle tank charges spearheading infantry offensives, but he was frustrated by his generals, who considered this a wasteful and ineffective tactic. In short, Montgomery wanted to adjust his army's attitude so that both officers and men would snap to his command and attack energetically, and Benzedrine interested him greatly.[33]

Montgomery's tests were not carefully controlled trials. One practical study with the Eighth Light Field Ambulance, conducted in Egypt for forty-eight hours starting on September 7, 1942, found that both amphetamine and methamphetamine seemed to improve marching speed slightly compared to placebo, and scores in arithmetic tests somewhat more. Another, done at the end of September 1942, involved two infantry squads put through fifty-six straight hours of exercises, including rifle shooting, trench digging, and arithmetic, as well as specialty testing (such as code signaling and machine gun reassembly), with short rest periods but no sleep. At the end of the test, both drug and placebo groups did a competitive seven-mile march. Not only did the "Benzedrine squad" win by eleven minutes, and report feeling more energy and clearer thinking, but they also marched with a "snap and zest" "conspicuously absent" in the other squad. This sort of result was good enough for Montgomery. For the massive offensive he was planning, where he would throw everything he had at Rommel to break through at Alamein, he ordered amphetamine supplied to all the combat units—one hundred thousand tablets for the initial Allied attack of October 23, according to an official source.[34]

Although Benzedrine was in general use at Alamein, some British soldiers there were participating in a medically monitored field experiment, rather like Winfield's bomber trials in the RAF. The 41st, 45th, and 47th Battalions of the 24th Armoured Brigade were dosed with measured quantities of Benzedrine in combat, between October 24 and 28. According to a brief communiqué back to the MPRC, "the reports of the tank crews were in favour of the tablets, and the Brigadier and two Brigade staff too, who took them, were greatly benefitted."[35] These few dry lines do nothing to convey the tank unit's experience. After creeping through minefields through the entire opening night of the battle, the Brigade spent October 24 driving among milling crowds and under confusing orders, and then in the evening was hammered by an air strike. Regrouping during the night, on the morning of October 25, the Brigade charged over a key hill called Miteirya Ridge into the teeth of a panzer division, and spent the whole day in battle without cover, one after another of their new Sherman tanks erupting into flame like the Ronson cigarette lighters they were nicknamed for. The survivors spent that night and then the entire next day picking their way through more minefields, finally stopping on the night of October 26 behind a small rise in the desert called Kidney Ridge—their first chance to sleep in four days. The plan was for them to advance at dawn to support British infantry, who were moving overnight into a forward position named "Snipe."[36]

They were slow to start in the morning of October 27, and given that the medical reports indicated that they took Benzedrine through October 28, these exhausted men may well have taken the drug with breakfast. When the 24th Armoured Brigade charged over the ridge, they encountered a battle already raging, and the tanks in the lead returned blistering fire. More than half an hour later, once a British runner somehow struggled through the no-mans-land, the 24th

Armoured received sharp new orders to stop: the men they were shooting at were actually British infantry dug in at Snipe. The tanks then fought their way through to the infantry position in an effort to help, attracting a heavy artillery barrage that quickly incinerated more of their number and made them unpopular with Snipe's defenders. As they withdrew back up toward the ridge, still firing on the enemy tanks swarming the Snipe position, many more tanks of the Brigade were smashed by heavy German guns. Of the 153 working tanks with which the Brigade had entered Alamein on October 23, just over two dozen remained by October 28, at which point the few survivors were sent to reinforce other units.

The 24th Armoured Brigade could not have fought longer or more fiercely—until the unit ceased to exist, almost to the last man. One cannot help but wonder whether Benzedrine had something to do with that. One also must question whether their chemical assistance explains why they nearly cost Montgomery victory at Alamein. Fewer than a hundred in number but well armed with antitank guns, the soldiers dug in at Snipe unsuspectingly stood in the way of Rommel's main tank counterattack.[37] If the 24th Armoured had done them any more harm, so that the infantry had not remained in place later on October 27 to blunt the panzer advance, Rommel might have turned the tables yet again on the Eighth Army.

There is certainly some evidence of mixed feelings about Benzedrine's impact at Alamein. In 1944, one captain reported to the MPRC that the Benzedrine tablets were helpful in his unit during the battle, although "it was abused by certain units with deleterious results." The enhancement of aggression, the paranoia, and the hallucinations that amphetamine can cause in exhausted men can only have increased the risks of "friendly fire." Indeed, in a follow-up study conducted in the Eighth Army around the end of 1942, where tank crews took Benzedrine during two days of hard driving and maneuvers in the desert, some did report hallucinations such as seeing tanks driving sideways. However, the majority of the men liked the pills, reporting greater confidence and energy to medical officers.[38]

In any case, Montgomery's overall impression of the drug's effects must have been favorable since, in November 1942, British Middle East Forces were given standing orders authorizing Benzedrine use, roughly coinciding with the Air Ministry's approval of amphetamine for regular use on bombing missions. Montgomery approved much higher levels of drug consumption, however. To relieve fatigue, not more than 20 mg of Benzedrine per day were to be used, in 5 mg doses, and for periods not exceeding five days straight (or half that dosage for officers who were fatigued only mentally).[39] According to medical opinion then and even now, 100 mg of amphetamine over several days does not qualify as an enormous amount, but five solid days awake on Benzedrine is likely to produce unusual behavior nevertheless.

British military demand for amphetamine—Benzedrine from SKF —was substantial, amounting to a wartime total of 72 million tablets. Since military personnel were forbidden to use the drug on British soil without special permission around the time the Air Ministry and Middle East Forces officially adopted amphetamine, this consumption represents use in combat theaters almost entirely.[40] As British experience accumulated, an increasingly cautious attitude toward the drug emerged. One mid-1943 Air Ministry booklet on fatigue issued to RAF medical officers and squadron commanders recommends amphetamine use only in occasional emergencies, and warns of impaired judgment: "Benzedrine has the effect of causing the individual to feel on top of things and able to carry on with his duties without rest: he feels that he is doing well, when in fact he is making all sorts of mistakes."[41] Early hopes that amphetamine enhanced performance biologically— boosting resistance to G-forces, oxygen efficiency, and muscle work capacity—had all been dispelled by scientific studies even before the Air Ministry and British Middle East Command approved the routine use of the pills around November 1942. Later testing found little or no significant superiority to caffeine by other objective measures. But as Winfield's studies and Montgomery's field tests indicated, since the drug raised morale and mood (making men more cheerful and optimistic, more aggressive or "determined" to fight) it was nonetheless useful in combat. In other words, the British military used amphetamine largely because its consciousness-altering properties made men fight harder, and the men liked it. The drug was simply too useful for the military to do without, regardless of what science had to say.

American Research: Outdoing the Nazi War Machine

The U.S. military reached a piecemeal decision to supply its men in combat with Benzedrine in much the same way as the British had, and for similar reasons having little to do with scientific evidence. Aware of the British research, the Americans also conducted many of their own studies: careful laboratory experiments at universities by top medical researchers, as well as much less scientific field studies by the services themselves. From the beginning, performance enhancement, and not just prevention of sleep, was the result that both kinds of study sought. In the words of University of Minnesota physiologist Ancel Keys in mid-1940, to achieve maximum performance with nutritional supplements, cocaine, or other drugs, "it will probably be necessary to rediscover facts already being utilized by the Nazi war machine but there is no reason to believe that we cannot go further." (Ironically, Keys's major wartime contribution was the K-Ration, containing crackers, tinned meat, chocolate, and cigarettes—more an economic rather than nutritional breakthrough, since these last items were universally tradable.)[42]

Keys's call for research came in a discussion among an elite committee of the National Research Council (NRC) of the U.S. National Academy of Sciences, set up to oversee research in preparation for war. Like no American conflict before, the Second World War would be a scientists' war, forging a tight link between the nation's universities and the military that would play a key role in the long era of U.S. world dominance that followed. When the NRC established medical advisory panels for the military in mid-1940, it made fatigue treatments and performance boosters top research priorities. In September Chicago physiologist A. C. Ivy surveyed the state of the art for the NRC, reporting that "the Germans give Benzedrine to dive bombers before the takeoff, to their panzer units and shock troops, and that captured parachute troops are equipped with Benzedrine and that the drug was tested on a divisional scale with favorable results in the Polish Campaign." In preparing his survey, Ivy had consulted SKF, Leake, and Alles, which may account for his belief that the Germans owed their success to amphetamine rather than methamphetamine as was actually the case (and as the British already knew).[43]

The NRC appointed Ivy their "impressario" of fatigue science, and he served as the central manager of U.S. amphetamine research much more than any single scientist among his British counterparts. He monitored the ongoing British research on amphetamine and aviation medicine, and the German work as well, insofar as it could be traced in medical journals. He also did a number of experiments in his own laboratory at Northwestern University's medical school, and oversaw research by other American scientists. His main explicit goal was to remedy a gap in scientific knowledge that he identified in January 1941 review of the literature on amphetamine's effects: while the drug unquestionably was effective in keeping people awake, and its mood-elevating power well established by psychiatrists, Ivy saw the psychological literature on amphetamine's intellectual and psychomotor (hand-eye) performance effects as inconclusive and in any case inadequate for evaluating the drug as a substitute for caffeine in military operations, since the experiments typically did not study strained or exhausted subjects. Was the drug measurably better than caffeine for boosting or maintaining physical performance in men deprived of rest? If not caffeine seemed a wiser choice to Ivy, given amphetamine's novelty, its unknown effects on men experiencing anxiety as in combat, and its known habit-forming potential.[44]

Ivy brought a particular, sophisticated perspective to the question of drugs and fatigue. Along with Keys and David Bruce Dill, his collaborator for some of the amphetamine work that he did during the war, Ivy belonged to a circle associated with the Harvard Fatigue Lab. This institution in Harvard's Business School featured a distinctive approach connecting the psychology and biology of work. The lab's cofounder, Elton Mayo, is still famous for showing that factory workers improved productivity more in response to management attention—a morale intervention—than better physical work conditions. A basic principle of the Harvard Fatigue Lab was, in fact, that there is no such thing as fatigue, if this refers to a single physical reaction to the strains that can impair efficiency.[45] Just as Mayo might have done, Ivy sought to understand the problem of military fatigue broadly, taking into account but not confusing issues of training, individual and group psychology, physiology, and engineering factors.

Already in late 1941 a number of amphetamine studies were under way, both by Ivy's own lab group and by others. Ivy's early studies looked strictly at the influence of the drug on physical exhaustion, using medical students as guinea pigs in the time-honored tradition. For instance in one experiment Ivy compared the effect of caffeine, 10–15 mg amphetamine, and 5 mg methamphetamine. The study included a small group of medical students, but they were standardized by living at the hospital on a fixed diet, and they were made to do an exhausting routine on an exercise bicycle three times a week, for more than three months, before the experiment began. Then, in the experimental sessions, the young men were given an injection of drugs (or a placebo injection) and put on their usual exercise bicycle. Ivy again found that amphetamine neither increased total work output nor speeded recovery after exhaustion. Caffeine, however, increased total work output, and there was some indication that methamphetamine did also (at least in one of the students who especially liked the drug). These studies were funded by the Illinois drug firm Abbott Labs, which was eyeing the possibility of selling methamphetamine, unprotected by patents, to the U.S. military. Ivy did not immediately recommend methamphetamine or amphetamine. Evidence supporting the use of either drug for physical exhaustion still seemed weak to him, and he thought it better to wait for studies that more accurately represented exhaustion in real military situations.[46]

For studies under the auspices of the NRC's panel on aviation medicine, researchers set up airtight chambers to experiment on men in rarified atmospheres that simulated high altitude, both at City College of New York and at Northwestern where Ivy himself worked. Here the focus was not mainly on muscular work but on psychomotor performance, especially hand-eye coordination tasks representative of flying. Between January 1942 and the end of that year, the scientists gathered extensive data on the effects of six drugs at normal atmospheric pressure and at low pressures simulating altitudes up to 18,000 feet: caffeine, amphetamine, methamphetamine, a caffeine-amphetamine combination, an amphetamine-methamphetamine blend, and dextroamphetamine—SKF's newly introduced Dexedrine product. Where statistics were used to gauge differences, performance on the various drugs did not in general differ significantly, except that caffeine definitely was worse for hand tremor at altitude, while on the other hand it significantly boosted overall work output. Nevertheless, Ivy felt that the data showed trends suggesting genuine differences in psychomotor performance. In some tests of hand-eye coordination and perception, methamphetamine seemed to help performance at high altitude more, but in most of them the two forms of amphetamine seemed best. (Recall that Benzedrine and Dexedrine are the same basic chemical, amphetamine: Benzedrine is an equal mixture of left- and right-handed amphetamine molecules, Dexedrine only the right).[47]

Ivy now reasoned that it did not matter whether differences between the drugs were statistically significant, and whether amphetamine genuinely boosted performance compared to caffeine: so long as it did not produce *worse* performance at high altitude than caffeine, there was no reason *not to use* Benzedrine for its waking effects (despite the lack of demonstrable difference between the two drugs' waking power, apart from how often one needed to take pills). And Ivy was now unworried that in "in ordinary doses" amphetamine might impair skill, coordination, or judgment—although he did not evaluate judgment specifically in any test—or lead to habit formation. Why and how Ivy came to lose his scruples over amphetamine's safety between early 1941 and early 1942, accepting a shift in the burden of proof from not using amphetamine unless it was better than caffeine to using it unless it proved worse, remains a mystery. Perhaps he was under pressure to provide scientific support for a decision that had already been made on other grounds. At the end of 1942 Ivy concluded his flight simulator and pressure chamber studies with an endorsement of Benzedrine as "the drug of choice for aviators," finally winning the concurrence of the aviation medicine panel (which had rejected the same endorsement earlier in the year, demanding more evidence). But by the time the NRC experts reached this determination, the military was already buying the drug from SKF in significant quantities for Air Force use, implying that science was not driving that decision.[48]

Drug research with pressure chambers continued into 1943, because huge new bombers like the B-29 "Superfortress" were being introduced, accelerating the rate at which "the machine outstripped the man." At the maximum altitude of the Superfortress, almost twice 18,000 feet, men could not function without an oxygen supply. The cabin was pressurized to raise oxygen levels, but if the plane was damaged, all that extra air might escape. So Ivy's team and at least one other group of physiologists (at the University of Cincinnati) tested drug effects on the "bends," or decompression sickness, long a problem among divers and now threatening aviators. They found that dextroamphetamine helped reduce incapacitating "bends" and "chokes" when people—mostly medical students yet again—were subjected to rapidly thinning atmospheres as extreme as 40,000 feet in the pressure chambers. This time, the researchers explicitly attributed the improvement to the drug's subjective, mood-altering effect ("willingness to endure" and "feeling of well-being"), rather than anything to do with nerves or circulation.[49] The profile of amphetamine emerging in the scientists' hands was that the drug might measurably improve test performance in thin atmospheres, but that it did this mainly by altering mood so as to increase effort.

The American military's commitment to amphetamine probably had much more to do with their own internal research, and perhaps also the British testing and use of the drug. Starting around December 1941, the Army Air Force did a number of its own more practical tests focusing on physical exhaustion, many by David Bruce Dill, who had just left Harvard's Fatigue Lab for the military's Aeromedical Laboratory. The Air Force scientists compared bombing scores of crews tired by ten hours of flying maneuvers and then given drugs. They also tested pilots for hours with the hand-eye pursuit meter and with flight simulators, on amphetamine, methamphetamine, dextroamphetamine, and caffeine (tellingly, just as in some RAF studies caffeine was sometimes omitted from testing, suggesting a mindset that had already decided to choose one or another amphetamine). Little effort was made to distinguish true drug effects on capabilities from effects on motivation, and in any case few clear-cut differences were found, an outcome usually attributed to the small number of test subjects and the lack of fatigue extreme enough for drugs to help. In the "flicker fusion" test of visual discrimination (which measures the ability of the eye to distinguish a rapidly flashing from a continuous light), however, amphetamines gave a fairly reproducible improvement over caffeine. Despite the weak evidence overall, by mid-1942 the Air Force scientists concluded that 5 mg of amphetamine, taken every few hours, was the best way to alleviate a range of fatigue effects in aviation.[50] As noted the military started purchasing Benzedrine in the last quarter of 1942, in advance of Ivy's conclusions (although Dill and Ivy no doubt talked), so the Aeromedical studies may have contributed to that decision. By 1943 amphetamine was widely issued to crews flying long missions, and packages of 5 mg Benzedrine pills were in the emergency kits in every American bomber.[51]

The Air Surgeon, the top medical officer in the Air Force, cautioned crews that Benzedrine should not be taken regularly, only with medical authorization and only in special circumstances as determined by commanding officers. But "special circumstances" must have been commonplace, since by all indications amphetamine use was routine, particularly among bomber crews. A March 1945 *New York Times* feature on the long-range bombing campaign against Japan,

"With a B-29 over Japan—A Pilot's Story," captures how normal it had become to take the drug on these long flights. The navigator "just rubs his tired eyes, takes some more Benzedrine and goes to work again" over the whole fifteen-hour flight, whereas the pilot and co-pilot could take turns sleeping and use the autopilot for long stretches. General Curtis LeMay, leader of the U.S. bomber force in the Pacific, flew a Superfortress from Japan to Chicago in late 1945 to set a long-distance aviation record (and, incidentally, flex American muscle in the developing Cold War), fuelled by his standard flight diet of "cigars, K-rations, and Benzedrine." Moreover, it was not just bomber crews that took the drug. In a May 1945 survey of fighter pilots in the European theater, who regularly flew bomber escort missions five or more hours long, thirteen of eighty-five (around 15 percent) acknowledged frequent Benzedrine use. Of this group that regularly used the drug on missions, some took it half an hour before and again after leaving a target area as officially recommended, but more pilots said that they "made their own policy" and took it "when they felt like it," rules notwithstanding.[52]

The Tough Get Going

While his aviation experiments were underway in 1942, Ivy and his Northwestern collaborators also carried out a series of practical drug experiments for the U.S. Army on infantrymen, tank drivers, and truck drivers at domestic military installations. In all the experiments, men were given identical "vitamin" capsules that contained either caffeine, or amphetamine (10 mg), or methamphetamine (5 mg), or else milk sugar as a placebo, and then made to do the work they were trained for under exhausting conditions. They were observed and also given a questionnaire at the end of the experiment. For example, men of the 502nd Coast Artillery Regiment at Fort Sheriden, Illinois, took pills before a single ten- to twelve-mile march with full packs, and in another test did two marches on consecutive days. Drivers of heavy trucks at the Fort Knox, Kentucky, Army base were given pills, made to drive over difficult roads for twenty miles without lights, and then tested for perception and coordination with devices like the pursuit meter. In both experiments Ivy found that caffeine produced "subjective" effects in that men felt less tired, whereas methamphetamine brought "objective," measurable improvements to hand-eye coordination under fatigue; amphetamine, however, seemed the superior drug because it had the best "subjective" effects on mood and alertness and also showed some evidence of "objective" improvement. Ivy and his team also looked at drug effects on tank crews, first at Fort Knox and then at Camp Young, California, under conditions something like North Africa. At Fort Knox Ivy found that the drugs made no difference on a five-hour cross-country drive, but in six to seven hours of maneuvers in the desert, Ivy found that men on amphetamine did somewhat better in a few of his tests than undrugged men. With infantry in the desert, the drugs made no difference in the speed of overnight, twenty-mile marches. Whenever he failed to detect any performance improvement from amphetamine, as in this and many other experiments, Ivy blamed insufficient fatigue, rather than abandoning faith in the drug.[53]

Evidence supporting the idea that amphetamine provided any measurable, objective performance enhancement in physical exhaustion was feeble at the beginning of 1943, and not getting any stronger. Nor were amphetamine's mood effects ever ruled out as the cause of such differences in test outcomes as sometimes occurred. Not that Ivy forgot the psychiatric component: in a late 1942 document summarizing his research and issuing recommendations on how to use the drug he affirmed that amphetamine "increases confidence" and "raises morale which has suffered from fatigue and sleepiness" because issues like " 'sore feet' tend to be disregarded due to general elevation of mood." And when men in his Army experiments asked about "obtaining capsules for use on other occasions, such as weekend leaves, when they might wish to obtain the same desirable effects," this only proved to Ivy how good a choice amphetamine was. Ivy's conclusions that Benzedrine was the drug of choice for regular Army operations, just like his endorsement of the drug for the Air Force, ultimately rested in large measure on the drug's subjective effects: amphetamine made men try harder and feel better.[54]

Beginning in 1943, amphetamine was issued widely throughout the Army in combat first-aid kits, with instructions that one 5 mg Benzedrine tablet should be taken every six hours for "extreme" mental fatigue, or two tablets for "extreme" physical fatigue, up to three times (eighteen hours) running. As *Business Week* magazine wryly observed in early 1944, based on the "huge laugh" a comedian touring the European front evoked from a joke based on Benzedrine, plenty of soldiers must have encountered fatigue "extreme" enough to take the drug.[55]

Aware of developments elsewhere, the U.S. Navy initiated its own tests of amphetamine with the Marines in mind. After all, the Marines had to storm hostile islands, and rather like paratroops might have to fight continuously against a surrounding enemy for days on end. A particularly thorough study was conducted in April 1943 at Camp Lejeune, North Carolina, to measure the effect of fatigue on small arms fire, and how Benzedrine might affect it. One hundred Marine volunteers were broken into squads of ten, and an officer heading each squad kept a log of impressions during the experiment. On a Monday morning, all the men did target practice with the standard M1 rifle and were ranked according to their scores. They were then divided into two groups of similar marksmanship, by placing those of odd firing rank in "A Group" and those of even rank in "B Group." After a full day of various exercises and work, the squads of mixed A and B men made a forced march of twenty-five miles with full combat equipment, until 5:00 the next morning. During the evening march, they began taking capsules every six hours, 10 mg Benzedrine for the B men and identical placebos for the A men. The men were then kept awake throughout Tuesday and Tuesday night with more marksmanship exercises, drills, calisthenics, and war games. On Wednesday there was more of the same, then marksmanship was again tested carefully, and the exhausted men were finally given a hot evening meal and allowed to sleep on Wednesday night.

The B men had taken 10 mg Benzedrine capsules seven times by this point, on roughly the same schedule recommended in Montgomery's Eighth Army, but double the dosage. In marksmanship testing at the end, fatigue actually seemed to increase everybody's firing accuracy, an effect attributed to relaxation, but men on Benzedrine scored somewhat higher on "fire power" defined as total hits per minute near the target center. This study met the highest standards of medical research for its day, with its (pseudo-) randomized, placebo-controlled design and careful statistics. Based on the numbers, the drug made no significant measurable difference other than in "fire power" in target practice (and naturally, the rate of firing in these test conditions would have to depend on enthusiasm for the experiment). But numbers did not tell the whole story.

Like the Army studies overseen by Ivy, the Marine study's most remarkable findings concerned amphetamine's subjective effects on attitude and behavior. Squad leaders observed that, by Tuesday, "A's were rather lethargic and the B's were full of energy," in "better spirits," "peppier," with less bloodshot eyes, presenting "a much more military appearance," and showing a "devil-take-the-hindmost attitude." As one officer on Benzedrine wrote, "on the march the pills were very exhilarating with the B's leading the parade, the A's eating dust and not liking it." Nor did any major misbehavior emerge, although a few cases of "overenthusiasm" were noted. On the face of it, the drug made men behave more like U.S. Marines are supposed to, enthusiastic but disciplined.[56]

Several cases of hallucination occurred among the drugged men on Tuesday night, when the B group were alert on their fifth and sixth 10 mg doses of Benzedrine, and the A men needed constant prodding to stay awake around their campfires. Said a captain on Benzedrine: "One fire became a burning bungalow, another a ruby bracelet. The trees are the corner-posts of a building inside of which I am. No conception seems too fantastic for acceptance." A medical observer reported: "One officer sent a marine to investigate the presence of 'girls' around one of the fires, while another cried out that the fire had become a waterfall. Several men stated that the fires had become "fireplaces," complete with mantels [sic], etc." In hindsight, we may recognize an important foreshadowing of what would become understood in the 1950s as amphetamine psychosis, but the Navy researchers attributed these visions simply to exhaustion rather than the drug (hallucinations were noted also in the un-drugged, exhausted group, though not described).[57] The "improved spirits," "pep," "military appearance," and soldierly "attitude" brought on by the Benzedrine carried the day.

In November 1943, Benzedrine played its part with the Marines at Tarawa, in one of the bloodiest battles of the war. The Allied counteroffensive to push back the Japanese had to pass through Tarawa atoll because of the Japanese air base there on the tiny coral island of Betio, which menaced ship movements through the Gilbert Islands area. Starting around 3:00 AM on November 20, troops of the 2nd Marine Division unloaded from ships into smaller craft for a scheduled landing at 8:30. Shallow reefs around Betio obstructed the landing craft, while elaborate defenses slowed the men coming ashore and took a gruesome toll. "Have landed. Unusually heavy opposition. Casualties

70 percent. Can't hold"; so a famous radio communication put it, from the few who established a toehold on the corpse-washed beach by 10:00 AM. Indeed, they barely held under blistering fire from thousands of elite Japanese soldiers, dug into emplacements and pillboxes covering the entire island. Wave after wave of Marines struggled ashore and fought through the entire first day and night just to maintain the beachhead, in many places nothing more than the strip of sand below a log seawall. All told, it took ten thousand marines and seventy-six hours of ferocious combat to end the fighting over this "one square mile of hell" (Figure 13).[58]

Almost all forty-eight hundred Japanese defenders were killed, and the Marines suffered thirty-four hundred casualties, more than a thousand of them killed. This level of carnage shocked the American public and stirred demands for Congressional investigation. The military scrutinized this battle so that its lessons could be applied in the rest of the war against the Japanese, interviewing many men and officers involved shortly afterward. Lt. Col. Kenneth McLeod, who spent the second night of the assault circling in a landing boat offshore with his battalion, and then the third day and night pressing home the attack against some of the strongest Japanese positions, reported that "Benzedrine tablets came in quite handy." Medical officers in his unit and some others dispensed the pills during the battle, but they were not carried by each marine, and this now was seen as a mistake. Donald Nelson, chief medical officer of the 2nd Marine Division, summarized his views after interviewing the medical corpsmen and doctors in the battle: "Benzedrine tablets should be furnished each man" in advance, for future amphibious assaults.[59]

Speed and the War's Lessons

The American military, like the British, widely issued Benzedrine for use in combat, supplying it via medical officers and also making it available in emergency and first-aid kits through most of the Second World War. Like their British counterparts, the American scientists evaluating amphetamine for the military consistently found that, by all but a few measures, amphetamine did not objectively improve or restore performance lost to physical exhaustion, lack of sleep, or low oxygen any better than caffeine. Users certainly felt that the drug boosted their performance, but subjective impressions seldom re-flected objective performance. Even where measurable gains were oc-casionally produced these were largely or entirely due to increased optimism and persistence in the contrived test conditions. This lack of scientific foundation did not deter the U.S. military. Even the halluci-nations many studies reported, and the loss of judgment these imply, seem not to have mattered much. Methamphetamine proved as good as amphetamine in most careful tests, even the small minority where caffeine was not as good objectively. Nevertheless according both to Ivy's own work and the studies done by the services themselves am-phetamine—Benzedrine—was the best choice because of the *subjective* lift in mood it provided. And this is precisely the point.

To Ivy, "fatigue," in the sense of physical and mental exhaustion, may have differed sharply from "battle fatigue" in the sense of psy-chiatric breakdown. However, encouraged by the psychiatrists' own deliberate vagueness, the military could view these as one problem begging a single solution. Thus, the U.S. Army, Air Force, and Ma-rines, just like the Royal Army in North Africa and RAF Bomber Command, adopted Benzedrine for its effects on optimism, aggres-siveness, military comportment, and the other aspects of emotional condition that figure in morale. To put it more baldly, the Allied mili-tary dispensed amphetamine for its mood-altering effects. The Japa-nese military did the same but were only more forthright than their American and British counterparts, calling the methamphetamine they issued their soldiers "Senryoku Zoko Zai" or "drug to inspire the fighting spirits."[60]

However, for the British military, in contrast to the U.S. military, the increasingly obvious gap between amphetamine's subjective and objective effects discredited the drug by war's end. As RAF scientist D. R. Davis wrote in a postwar summary of British aviation research, amphetamine can boost performance in tests of simple, repetitive tasks, but it reduces performance in complex tasks through poor judg-ment, inappropriate perseverance, and overly optimistic self-evalua-tion. Furthermore, since pilot errors in combat result mainly from anx-iety rather than physical exhaustion, observed Davis, only confusion around the term "fatigue" could make amphetamine use seem an ap-propriate solution. As for subjective effects, he concluded, "training and other measures which lead to good morale" can achieve at least as many of amphetamine's benefits without the drawbacks. The German

Luftwaffe had reached essentially the same decision early in the war, while, not long after, the German military as a whole turned away from amphetamines because of their abuse potential and addictiveness. But for the U.S. military, neither persistent difficulties in demonstrating a significant objective performance gain, nor the impact of the mood effects of amphetamine on perceived performance, nor confusion about the drug's relation to "fatigue" were ever acknowledged as problematic. Indeed, for the U.S. Air Force, amphetamine's mood effects remained the official explanation of the drug's military usefulness until the mid-1950s, when government researchers found some new, although still questionable, evidence that the drug did more than simply adjust attitude.[61]

Ivy's role in the American military's adoption and ongoing rationalization of amphetamine use for fatigue in combat personnel is ambiguous. On the one hand, Ivy always recognized that the mood-altering effects of a drug like amphetamine were distinct from its effects on wakefulness and physical exhaustion. On the other hand, despite flimsy evidence that the drug was measurably better than caffeine for performance loss due to lack of rest, he quickly forgot his early concerns about amphetamine's potential for habit-formation, and its unknown effects on soldiers experiencing anxiety in combat, endorsing Benzedrine as the "drug of choice" "for its waking effects" (albeit for "emergency use" only). He also endorsed the military use of amphetamine as a command rather than medical decision, just as Smith, Kline & French early in the war had urged. The drug firm had proposed in 1942 that the military design battle plans around "reinforcement of troops by re-energization," that is, ordering troops to take Benzedrine in unison as a combat tactic. Very close to the way Montgomery employed the drug at Alamein, this proposal of chemical reinforcement with the drug smoothly blended the psychiatric and physical senses of "fatigue" in a way that fit nicely with medical common sense about psychoneurotic breakdown and war neurosis: Benzedrine could "bring into play reserves of mental alertness and physical energy" and thus "postpone exhaustion and collapse." A Benzedrine advertisement from autumn 1944 seems to indicate that the company's proposal actually became official policy (Figure 14), aiming to reassure doctors in a situation where, in effect, nonmedical commanding officers were prescribing drugs.[62] However, official military policy (like medical theory) does not always translate into practice on the ground. Further study of wartime documents written by the men and medics using Benzedrine will be needed to clarify the typical circumstances of the drug's use in combat, and the experience of its effects.

Some explanation for the American military's commitment to amphetamine is certainly required since it was so poorly justified, in the face of acknowledged risks, by scientific and medical evidence. A series of personal visits and phone calls to Assistant Secretary of War John McCloy by SKF's chief executive Frank Boyer in July 1942, which lead to pressure from McCloy's office on Ivy's oversight committee to speed up the Benzedrine studies—coinciding nicely with the shift in the burden of proof in research on the drug's value—may well have had something to do with it. Further research is needed. And the quantities supplied by the military to US personnel, unlike the British figures never disclosed (to my knowledge), also call for further investigation.[63]

There was certainly enough to expose virtually all 12 million Americans who served overseas in combat theaters during the war, about a quarter of the adult male population, to abundant Benzedrine, since it was found in easily raided emergency kits found on planes, lifeboats, etc, as well as widely issued. And if the 1945 Air Force survey of fighter pilots is any indication, about 15% of servicemen offered the drug in military service would have become regular users.[64] But however many millions of Benzedrine tablets were taken by however many hundreds of thousands of American soldiers, it cannot be denied that the Allied military's endorsement and adoption of Benzedrine during the war years normalized and fostered amphetamine use on an enormous scale.

In 1945, amphetamine use in the military was not yet an issue of medical or public concern. Benzedrine Sulfate tablets still enjoyed a high scientific reputation—a "Milestone in Medical History" as one 1943 advertisement put it—as the first psychiatric drug specifically to treat mood disorders (see Figure 11). Amphetamine's use for depression was very far from peaking, and for weight loss the drug was not yet officially approved but already surging in popularity. The future of Alles's brain-child must have looked bright, as the miracle drug prepared to come into its prime in peacetime medicine. In 1945 a million amphetamine tablets poured daily into civilian distribution channels, marketed mainly for depression.[65] However, a problem that had been brewing silently for a decade was now emerging into public consciousness, menacing amphetamine's postwar prospects as a respectable drug.

β-Phenyl-isopropyl amine

Action on circulation - Man
— Subcutaneous administration.

Alles   6/3/29.   90 kg.

2:00   130-78/
2:05   126-76/
2:10   128-78/
2:15   126-72/
2:20   120-70/
2:35   118-70/
2:45   128-72/

2:46   50 mgm   β-phenyl-isopropyl amine HCl (1.0 cc 5% soln) injected sq.

2:51   128-80/
2:53   132-88/   Nose cleared, dry
2:56   132-94/
3:03   132-90/   Feeling of well being - palpitation
3:10   138-86/80 Dryness in nose more marked.
3:14   142-88/   Local edema at site of injection
3:20   140-84/
3:26   150-90/68
3:34   150-90/68
3:45   152-96/72
4:00   154-90/
4:17   158-90/
4:30   158-92/
4:45   154-94/
5:00   164-96/
5:15 . 154-94/76
5:30   156-92/
6:00   156-90/
6:15   158-90/
6:30   152-88/
7:00   152-90/
7:25   154-94/
7:55   136-80/
8:25   144-84/
9:15   144-84/
10:00   146-88/
11:00   140-84/

        Rather sleepless night. Mind seemed to run from one subject to another.

9:00 A.M. 6/4/29   128-82

FIG. 1. Record of the first amphetamine experience, Gordon Alles, 1929.
Courtesy California Institute of Technology Archives.

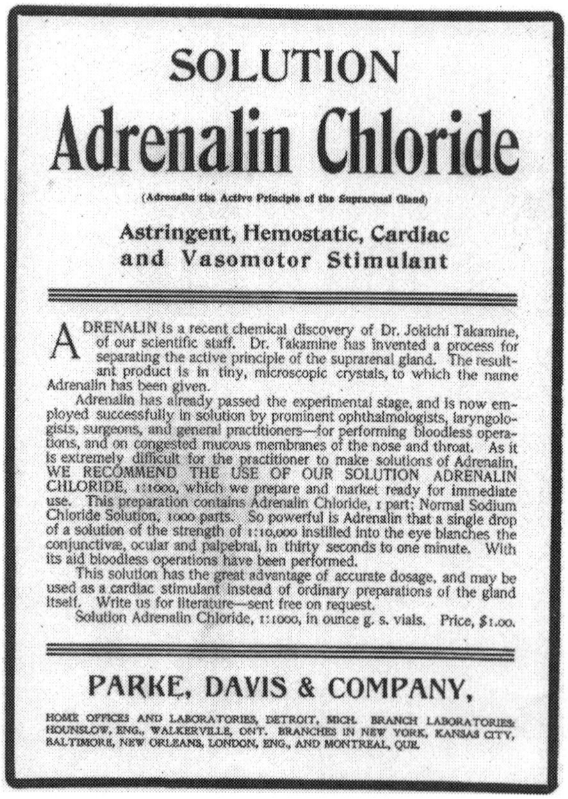

SOLUTION

Adrenalin Chloride

(Adrenalin the Active Principle of the Suprarenal Gland)

Astringent, Hemostatic, Cardiac and Vasomotor Stimulant

ADRENALIN is a recent chemical discovery of Dr. Jokichi Takamine, of our scientific staff. Dr. Takamine has invented a process for separating the active principle of the suprarenal gland. The resultant product is in tiny, microscopic crystals, to which the name Adrenalin has been given.

Adrenalin has already passed the experimental stage, and is now employed successfully in solution by prominent ophthalmologists, laryngologists, surgeons, and general practitioners—for performing bloodless operations, and on congested mucous membranes of the nose and throat. As it is extremely difficult for the practitioner to make solutions of Adrenalin, WE RECOMMEND THE USE OF OUR SOLUTION ADRENALIN CHLORIDE, 1:1000, which we prepare and market ready for immediate use. This preparation contains Adrenalin Chloride, 1 part; Normal Sodium Chloride Solution, 1000 parts. So powerful is Adrenalin that a single drop of a solution of the strength of 1:10,000 instilled into the eye blanches the conjunctivæ, ocular and palpebral, in thirty seconds to one minute. With its aid bloodless operations have been performed.

This solution has the great advantage of accurate dosage, and may be used as a cardiac stimulant instead of ordinary preparations of the gland itself. Write us for literature—sent free on request.

Solution Adrenalin Chloride, 1:1000, in ounce g. s. vials. Price, $1.00.

PARKE, DAVIS & COMPANY,

HOME OFFICES AND LABORATORIES, DETROIT, MICH. BRANCH LABORATORIES: HOUNSLOW, ENG., WALKERVILLE, ONT. BRANCHES IN NEW YORK, KANSAS CITY, BALTIMORE, NEW ORLEANS, LONDON, ENG., AND MONTREAL, QUE.

FIG. 2. In 1901 Adrenalin was introduced, the first pure hormone pharmaceutical and arguably the first drug based on advanced life science research (as opposed to chemical refinement of traditional botanical remedies). Adrenalin and similar preparations were popular for relieving acute asthma and allergy attacks, raising blood pressure, reducing surgical bleeding, and, as a nasal spray, for relieving congestion. Source: *JAMA*, June 22, 1901.

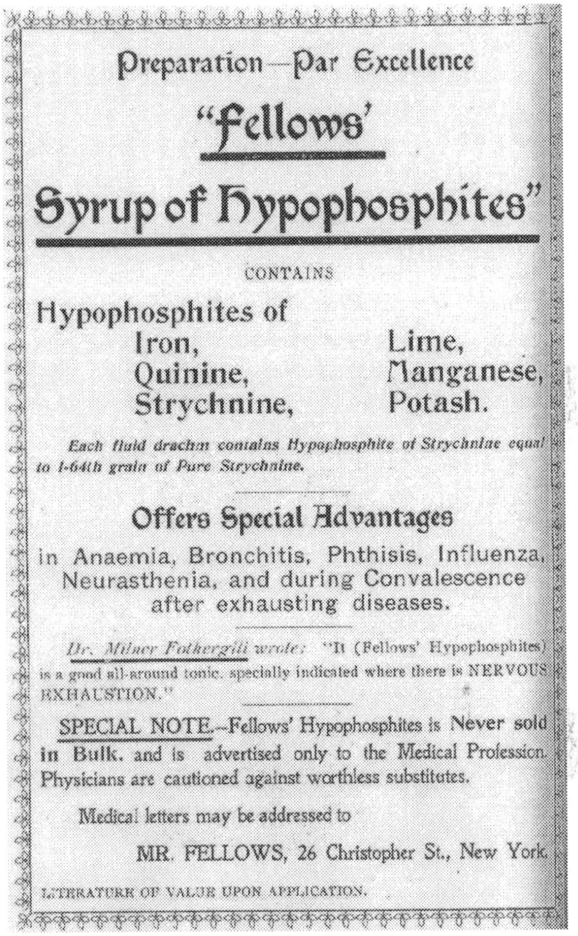

FIG. 3. In the early twentieth century, nerve tonics were top-selling prescription drugs. Source: *American Medical Journal*, February 1903.

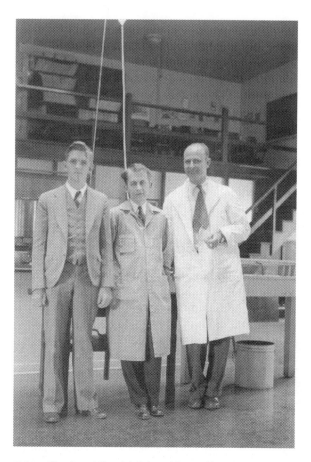

FIG. 4. Gordon Alles (*right*) and his colleagues in the University of California medical school's pharmacology lab in San Francisco: S. Anderson Peoples (*left*) and Peter Knoefel (*center*), 1932. Courtesy of Archives and Special Collections, Library and Center for Knowledge Management, University of California, San Francisco.

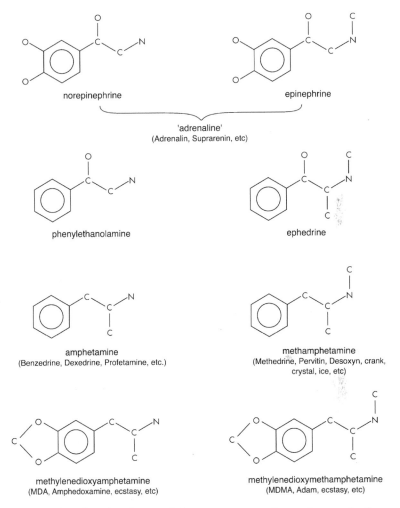

FIG. 5. Adrenaline (a mixture of the two compounds now known in the United States as epinephrine and norepinephrine) and its relationship to the amphetamines and certain other "sympathomimetic" amines.

β - 3,4-methylene-dioxyphenyl-isopropylamine hydrochloride

7/16/30
Alles
90 kg.

Light breakfast at 7:00
8:00   126-70 pulse 72
  36 mgm. taken by mouth
8:20   132-74 pulse 72
8:30   130-80   76
8:40   132-80   76
8:50   128-78   74
9:00   122-74   70
9:20   122-72   70
9:40   120-70   70
9:50   120-70   70
10:00   120-74   68
  90 mgm. taken by mouth
10:10   120-74 pulse 70
10:30   148-100   68   Nose and throat dry, very shaky
10:45   138-96   68   Very shaky, when relaxed room appeared to be filled
11:00   140-94   70   with curling smoke. Pupils markedly dilated. Arteries
11:15   136-86   70   in eye grounds contracted, also in gums.
11:30   136-84   70   Throat still dry, still very shaky, tendency to close
11:45   136-86   72   jaw tightly and grind rear teeth. Occasionally long
12:00   134-84   68   deep sighs. Can not think in long chains, thought
12:15   132-84   72   skips rapidly but seems quite clear. Visual accomodation
12:30   130-84   70   slowed. Can not focus at distances of over 3 blocks and
12:45   134-84   72   see double at short distances-6 inches. Feeling of
1:15   128-84   74   pressure in ears. Seem exceptionally aware of sound
1:45   130-84   74   perceptions can readily pick out minor sounds accompaning
2:15   128-94   80   louder sounds such as street cars. Generalized feeling
2:45   126-82   72   of well being when sitting relaxed, deep slow breaths
3:45   126-80   74   with rate decreased to 10 per minute. Considerable
4:45   128-84   72   perspiration throughout. Forehead rather pale.

  Went home

6:00   144-106   76
7 Light dinner eaten
7:45   134-86   76
9:15   130-80   68
10:45   126-76   66   Pupils still widely dilated.

  Slept readily, was tired. Woke early in morning but no undue mental excitement.
8:00 A.M. 124-82 pulse 66   Pupils normal, feel fine.

FIG. 6. Record of the first ecstasy (MDA) experience, Gordon Alles, 1930. Courtesy California Institute of Technology Archives.

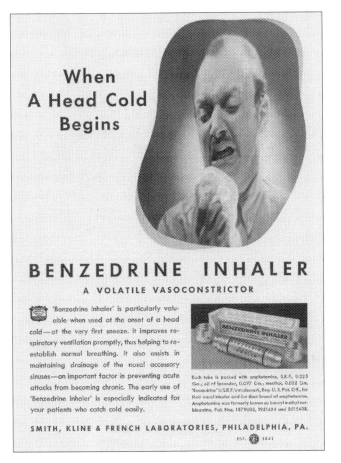

FIG. 7. Around 1933 Smith, Kline & French introduced volatile amphetamine base as a decongestant product. The firm's Benzedrine Inhaler, which contained 325 mg of amphetamine base in a perforated metal tube, was not intended to be taken internally. Source: *Journal of the National Medical Association*, November 1938.

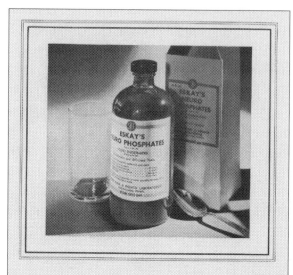

FIG. 8. Eskay Neurophosphates, a nerve tonic introduced in 1901, was the top-selling prescription product of Smith, Kline & French when the firm began marketing amphetamine tablets for depression in the late 1930s. Source: *Journal of the National Medical Association*, May 1939.

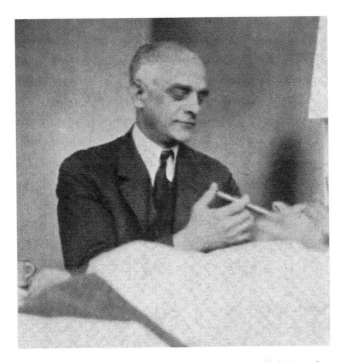

FIG. 9. Abraham Myerson (circa 1930), Professor of Neurology at Tufts Medical School and of Clinical Psychiatry at Harvard, and also Research Director at Boston State psychopathic hospital, was an expert on depression and an early champion of amphetamine use in psychiatry. Courtesy Tufts University Digital Collections and Archives.

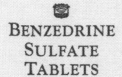
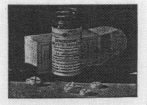
FIG. 10. Early advertising for Benzedrine (amphetamine) as an antidepressant, featuring Myerson's anhedonia concept of depression. Source: *New England Journal of Medicine*, July 18, 1940.

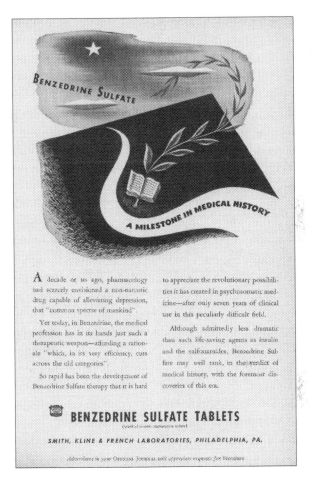

FIG. 11. By the time of the Second World War, amphetamine was widely accepted as the first specific "antidepressant." Source: *California Medicine*, August 1943.

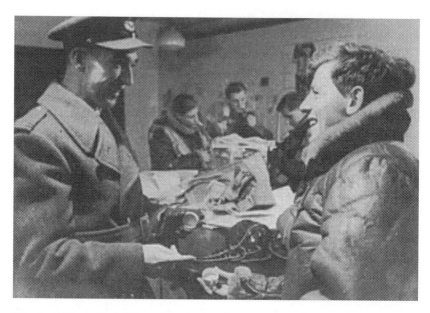

FIG. 12. RAF medical officer distributing "wakey-wakey" tablets to bomber flight crew. Amphetamine was widely adopted in place of caffeine by both British and American air forces. Source: *Short Bursts: Ex Air Gunners* newsletter, June 2001, reprinted by permission.

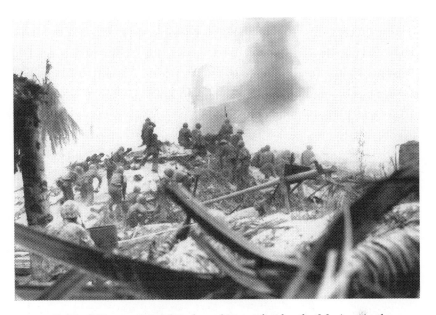

FIG. 13. Benzedrine was issued and used in combat by the Marines in the extended and bloody amphibious assault on Tarawa atoll in November 1943. Source: National Archives, USA (ARC image number 532517).

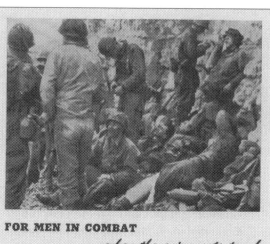

FOR MEN IN COMBAT

when the going gets tough

To save the lives of men in combat through sustaining their mental efficiency by overcoming the symptoms of fatigue, BENZEDRINE SULFATE TABLETS are available for issue in the Armed Forces.

The tablets are issued for combat use under strict medical supervision, and only on those occasions when intense or prolonged operations, without opportunity for normal rest, are anticipated.

Although this is, of course, a tactical rather than a therapeutic use of Benzedrine Sulfate, the physician will, we believe, be interested to know that this familiar, clinically established drug has such a unique military application.

BENZEDRINE
SULFATE TABLETS
Racemic amphetamine sulfate

SMITH, KLINE & FRENCH LABORATORIES—PHILADELPHIA, PA.

FIG. 14. Benzedrine was, in fact, widely distributed in the U.S. Army during the Second World War. Source: *Minnesota Medicine*, October 1944.

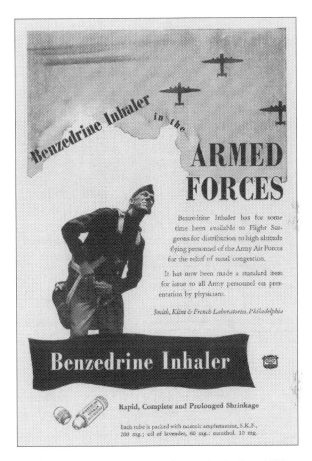

FIG. 15. Although the practice began in the late 1930s, recreational consumption of large amphetamine doses from Benzedrine Inhalers became more widespread among military personnel during the Second World War. Source: *Minnesota Medicine*, October 1944.

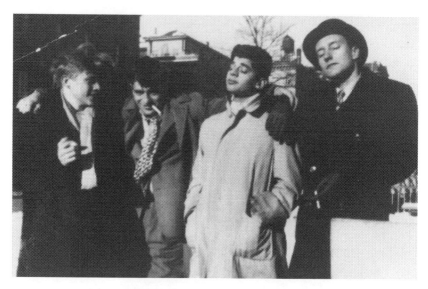

FIG. 16. The original "Beatnik" writers Jack Kerouac (*center left*), Allen Ginsberg (*center right*), and William S. Burroughs (*right*) enjoyed frequent use of Benzedrine pills and inhalers to spark creativity and alter perception in the 1940s. With Hal Chase (*left*), early 1940s. Image supplied by Bettmann/Corbis.

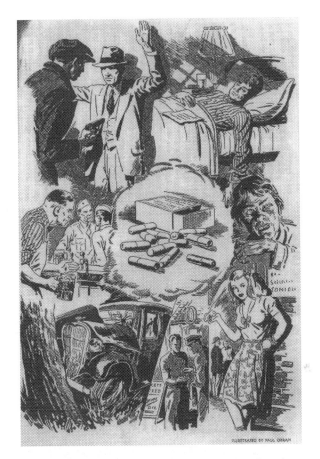

FIG. 17. Abuse of pharmaceutical barbiturate "goof-balls" became associated with crime, juvenile delinquency, and non-white countercultures during the 1940s. Source: *American Druggist*, September 1945.

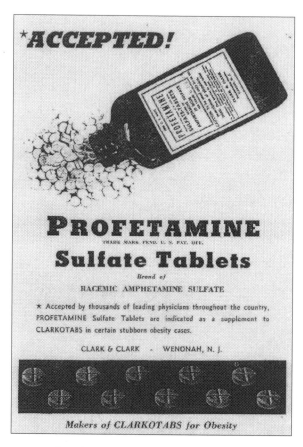

FIG. 18. The Clark & Clark firm was one of many small manufacturers that ignored the Smith, Kline & French patents on amphetamine and sold large quantities, such as these imitation Benzedrine tablets, to druggists during the 1940s. Source: *SKF vs. Clark & Clark* records, plaintiff's exhibits.

4

Bootleggers, Beatniks, and Benzedrine Benders

MOST DRUGS HAVE multiple effects on the body; of these, only one or two may be medically useful. The others might still be valuable for scientific research—as well as for other quite unscientific purposes. The early nonmedical users of amphetamine experienced an especially wide range of effects from which they selected a few as interesting or valuable, just like the first medical experimenters with the drug. In their 1930 self-experiments with amphetamine, Alles and his friends recorded feeling "peppy," "exhilarated"—the same type of effects later recognized as part of the drug's antidepressant action—along with related but less positive sensations like feeling "restless" and "jumpy." Feeling "jittery" was another negative sensation that subjects often reported in the first American clinical trials of amphetamine, whereas "more pep" was a typical positive patient reaction. The medical students and hospital staff who served as "normal" controls in these studies similarly experienced "increased energy," a "feeling of being very efficient," and, again, of being "pepped up."

One hospital staff member on Benzedrine demonstrated this pep when, an hour after ordering a flower delivery for a sick friend by phone, he grew impatient and walked several miles to the shop so he could deliver the flowers in person. ("I wanted action, and I got it!" he said). Another demanded that he be allowed to take an examination for which he was not eligible, and a third abruptly hung up on a superior while being reprimanded. Even these reactions, it is worth noting, were not perceived as negative; such assertiveness counted as valuable "pep" in an American cultural context putting a premium on hustle, drive, and ambition. Already by early 1937, when abuse of the drug first began to appear among midwestern university students, Benzedrine Sulfate had taken on an identity in the American popular imagination as "Pep Pills" or "Pepper-Uppers."[1]

The British have never taken much to American "pep," and they initially did not report any of it under the influence of Benzedrine. Instead, British subjects reported feeling "right as rain," "lively," and "more composed." Perhaps the most typical, distinctively British experience of amphetamine was one of unusual "self-confidence," as a "normal" subject put it. One mildly depressed subject even felt like "an exulted being" on Benzedrine, and another said "I felt like after a double whiskey, so full of energy and self-confidence." By early 1937, Benzedrine Sulfate was already known to the British public as "the confidence drug"—which may help explain why Montgomery and other military leaders were so interested in it early in the war. Not that there was any difference in the way British and American medical researchers objectively described Benzedrine's effects; increased talkativeness and activity, elevation of mood, and euphoria were the same on both sides of the Atlantic.

We can understand this cross-Atlantic difference in subjective effects through cultural differences, which sociologists have long considered to play a key role in drug experience. Of all the many sensations offered by amphetamine, Americans picked out the increase in "energy" to get things done—drive and motor activity, as the scientists put it—as most significant, because in the United States you never can have enough "pep." In Britain, they presumably felt more "energy," too, but people there worry less about advancing their careers and more about finding clever things to say, and saying them confidently. So Britons focused on the talkativeness the drug provided; on Benzedrine, one was never at a loss for something to say, whether it was witty or just "brittle, flashy gibberish" (as a later British article criticizing amphetamine overuse would put it). In Hitler's Germany, subjective experience differed in its own way, the first advertisements for amphetamines in 1936–37 claiming that users would experience such "joy in work" that they would feel like they had just returned from several weeks' holiday when using the drugs. People noticed what mattered most to them, given their cultural contexts, when they took amphetamine: in Britain, confident wit; in the United States, assertiveness and drive; and in Germany, devotion to work.[2] And these are just the varying intrepretations of low doses of amphetamines. Like many drugs, amphetamine has additional, quite distinct effects in higher doses.

The Benzedrine Inhaler: Escape in a Tube

Working in the military prison at Fort Benjamin Harrison, Indiana, at the end of the Second World War, psychiatrists Russell Monroe and Hyman Drell unexpectedly found themselves in the middle of an epidemic. Men would be sent to the clinic agitated, overly talkative, trembling, perspiring profusely, and with dilated pupils. Most said little about what was wrong and left as soon as possible. A few, however, sought help for the hallucinations and the deep depression and intestinal distress that usually followed. The mysterious problem turned out to be amphetamine. Although it was difficult to buy Benzedrine tablets in the prison, Benzedrine Inhalers were widely available without prescription both in nearby stores and supplied by the military. Guards smuggled them in and sold them for $.75 to $1.50, three or four times the drugstore price. One guard was caught with more than three hundred inhalers in his room. At this time each Benzedrine Inhaler contained about 250 mg of the volatile amphetamine base, down from 325 mg in the 1930s (Figure 15). The oily chemicals inside, representing a dose stronger than fifty of the 5 mg Benzedrine pills used in the military, were contained in a paper insert folded into eight sections. The men would break the tubes open—now plastic instead of the original metal—and eat the paper sections, each 30 mg strong, mainly by soaking in coffee and then drinking it down, paper and all. Taking most of a Benzedrine Inhaler all at once, instead of occasionally sniffing tiny doses of the vapors into the nose for congestion, made for a totally new kind of amphetamine experience.

The jailed soldiers who came to Monroe and Drell for psychiatric help said that huge numbers of their fellow prisoners also had an amphetamine habit. Many guards took Benzedrine in pill or inhaler form, too, and freely admitted this before the drug was banned at the prison. Clearly amphetamine had found popularity as a cheap high, and the doctors wanted to find out just how popular. They distributed an anonymous questionnaire, and more than a thousand completed forms were returned. A quarter of the prisoners admitted that they were currently using amphetamine inhalers recreationally, and although most had started abusing inhalers in prison, almost a third of the abusers had begun cracking inhalers in the military before being imprisoned. Although some had started abusing Benzedrine tablets or inhalers before the war, abusers were five times more likely than non-abusers to have been issued the drug in the service, in tablet form. Fully 89 percent had begun using some form of amphetamine in the past four years. Thus, Benzedrine abuse was an existing practice that wartime, and particularly military exposure, had amplified by an order of magnitude. Indeed, if this prison population were typical of the military, around one-twelfth of American servicemen must have been amphetamine abusers during the war. Of course, this population was not a typical sample of U.S. soldiers, since, as lawbreakers, this was an undisciplined group, "poorly adjusted" to military service. But neither were they highly abnormal young men in the opinion of the psychiatrists.[3]

Monroe and Drell considered Benzedrine Inhaler abuse a serious problem for society as a whole, more so than "indiscriminate" use of Benzedrine tablets. Not only were inhalers available everywhere cheaply without prescription, but they held the equivalent of a whole jar of pills and some people were taking the entire contents all at once. The toxic effects on the mind were obvious. One of their patients described what a Benzedrine Inhaler high felt like:

> After taking the contents I felt no effect for approximately an hour; then I began to feel as if I was mildly intoxicated, which lasted for another hour. Then I suddenly felt an intense pain at the base of my skull, which almost caused me to lose consciousness. I was rushed immediately to the station hospital. Shortly after my arrival at the hospital my pain subsided, but I became numb on my left side. [. . .] I became frightened and ran out into the ward screaming that I was dying. I was placed in bed by force and given two doses of "amytal sodium" which I promptly vomited. Under the influence of the drug [amphetamine] I felt my mind was very powerful. I would not tell them [the hospital personnel] who I was. It seemed as if they were trying to figure something from the tattoos on my arms. I thought I was being very clever when I told them that the tattoos were wrong [. . .] I thought I was forcing them to transfer me to another hospital through my powerful mind. I felt that others were saying things about me and when I questioned them about it they denied talking. That evening as I lay on my bed I began to concentrate on the square that held the light and it seemed as though they had a set of mirrors made like a periscope from the office and they seemed to be watch-

ing me through it. It seemed as though the nurse would tell the rest what I was doing. [. . .] The feeling that others were talking about me lasted about a week.[4]

This paranoid adventure represents a particularly unpleasant version of the Benzedrine Inhaler experience. Euphoria was the main effect that made the habit so popular. The massive amphetamine rush transported users away from the grinding reality of life in the military or prison or wherever they did not want to be. In 1947, when Monroe and Drell's article appeared in *JAMA*, "jags from inhalers" (as *Newsweek* put it in December 1947) became a medical problem of national significance.[5] This medical report therefore marks the official beginning of amphetamine's second career as a social menace in America. But for certain subcultures, including some of the most important musicians and writers to emerge in the twentieth century, Benzedrine Inhalers meant something quite different.

The Inhaler and the Jazz Rebellion

In the 1940s, prison and the Army were not the only places where young Americans were finding escape in huge doses of Benzedrine from decongestant inhalers. The figures gathered by Monroe and Drell show that about 3.5 percent of their prison population began abusing inhalers before military service. We may never know who first discovered how to get high by cracking and eating the Benzedrine Inhaler, but the practice definitely started before the war. It can be documented earliest among people accustomed to the sharp end of the law: jazz musicians, many of whom were also into marijuana and other illicit drugs. By 1937, before he turned to heroin, the teenage saxophone prodigy Charlie Parker had picked up the inhaler habit from his musician friends in Kansas City. Around 1940, in New York, drummer Dave Tough was downing inhaler fillings in cola to prepare himself for gigs with Bunny Berigan's band. In 1942, a teenage Art Pepper was enjoying the same powerful rush of Benzedrine in Los Angeles with fellow saxophonist Dexter Gordon.[6] These jazz men all seem to have acquired the habit while playing nightclubs in the black cultural centers of large American cities. Jazz culture was the fringe of the fringe of mainstream America, doubly marginal—

first as African American and then as a musical form linked with urban vice zones.

At home on this fringe were John Birks "Dizzie" Gillespie and Charlie Parker, two of the many musicians who continued to push the limits of the genre. For a time in the early 1940s, "Diz" and "Bird" were musically inseparable, and together invented a totally new kind of jazz, first conceived as "bebop" by Gillespie in 1942. Other musicians caught on to bebop quickly, too, like drummer Kenny Clarke and pianist Thelonius Monk and trumpeter Miles Davis, all playing around the clubs in Harlem and 52nd Street during the early 1940s. Bebop was fast and free, yet cerebral and complex. It was all about spontaneity, considered essential for genuine expression. And to hear and play fresh, without being caught up in musical conventions and clichés, many of the bop artists used drugs. Benzedrine was common but so was marijuana, cocaine, and heroin. Benzedrine, even in the massive dose one would get from an entire inhaler filling soaked in coffee, was considered relatively innocuous, rather like marijuana. In early 1948, when Parker went on what he described as a "health kick" to beat his hard drug habit, he swore off everything but beer and Benzedrine Inhalers. The inhalers were a staple in Bird's diet: reportedly, after a night of playing, the floor would sometimes be covered by so many white plastic empties that it looked like snow.[7]

Bebop quickly spread during the war and gathered a following in big cities like Chicago, Los Angeles, San Francisco, and especially New York. The initial bebop crowd was intellectual, almost entirely black, and assertive in its defiance of mainstream America. Although some see in bebop the beginnings of the Civil Rights movement, it was more cynical and less political than that. Bebop was detached and "cool," and, as Lewis Macadams put it in his philosophical-historical study on the nature of coolness, cool did not fight in America's most popular war. To the beboppers, saxophonist Lester Young became "a prisoner of war" in 1944, when he was finally tracked down by a zoot-suited FBI agent with a draft notice, and ended up in uniform. Gillespie, Parker, Thelonius Monk, and Miles Davis were all happily classified 4-F. When Gillespie received his draft notice, he told the psychiatrist at the induction center that white America was as much his enemy as Nazi Germany. Gillespie and his avant-garde musician friends were not the only nonwhite Americans who felt that way. For all the wartime rhetoric of American unity and the war against Nazi racism, segregation at home was not changing and the African Americans who joined the military were still getting second-class treatment, serving mainly in menial duties like driving trucks (or worse). The greater counterculture in which bebop was situated, as an intellectual fringe, rarely appeared on the radar of mainstream American consciousness, but, when it did, it was recognized as a menace. When mobs of white sailors in Southern California went on violent rampages in Hispanic neighborhoods during 1943, police arrested the battered victims while the papers blamed these "Zoot-Suit Riots" on Mexican "gangs"—pachuco hepsters who flaunted their nonconformity in the jazz-associated fashion.[8]

Recreational amphetamine use was commonplace in the zoot suit counterculture. When 52nd Street veterans like guitarist Slim Gaillard and pianist Harry "Hipster" Gibson, experimenting with a jazz style that improvised lyrics and nonsense words, acquired a following on the West Coast at the end of the war and cut a hit record, Los Angeles radio station KMPC banned their music, because "Be-bop tends to make degenerates out of our young listeners." *Time* magazine, covering the story, told wondering readers that bebop "amounts to hot jazz overheated, with overdone lyrics full of bawdiness, references to narcotics, and doubletalk."[9] The example *Time* cited was Gaillard and Gibson's short-lived smash, "Who Put the Benzedrine in Mrs. Murphy's Ovaltine":

> She'd never, ever been so happy since she left old Ireland
> Til someone prowled her pantry—man—and tampered with her can
> (Wham!) [. . .]
> She stays up nights making all the rounds,
> Mr. Murphy claims she's getting awfully thin,
> And all she says is gimme some skin! (Mop!)

That the tune resembles ragtime more than true bebop only highlights how "bebop" had become a catch-phrase for any subversive music. And amphetamine had become associated with dangerous "bebop" music. This perceived link between Benzedrine and the jazz counterculture was not good for SKF's image as a reputable pharmaceutical firm. There were also political implications, since, as we soon shall see, a struggle over regulation of amphetamine was building in the halls of government and industry.

Poetry on Speed

Precious few white college boys would have been listening to the emerging sound in Harlem jazz clubs, but there was one named Jack Kerouac, in 1940 a confused Columbia freshman on a football scholarship. After dropping out in 1941, working in a series of odd jobs, plus two stints in the Merchant Marine and one in the Navy (ending with a psychiatric discharge), he returned to New York in late 1943—now a serious aspiring writer, looking for a radically "New Vision," a fresh form of feeling and expression beyond social conventions. His girlfriend, Edie Parker, and a sometime student named Joan Vollmer shared an apartment near Columbia, the hub of a literary circle that included one eager-eyed, gangly Columbia freshman named Allen Ginsberg. Another member of the circle was a slim and worldly thirty-year-old sporting well-pressed but unremarkable suits, who knew a lot about psychology, philosophy, and criticism. He also knew a lot about the Times Square underworld, where, as a modern literary Decadent, he was learning how to roll drunks, fence stolen goods, and buy narcotics. His name was William Burroughs, and he became something of a mentor to Ginsberg and Kerouac, while the keen youngsters inspired him to put ink to paper (Figure 16).[10]

By the end of 1944, Kerouac had split with Parker and was spending most of his time with Burroughs and Vollmer at the apartment they now shared on 115th Street, soon to be joined by Ginsberg. Vickie Russell, who roomed with one of Burroughs's junkie friends, introduced Benzedrine Inhalers to the 115th Street circle one day in 1945, when Burroughs and Kerouac dropped by her place looking for drugs. They all caught a taxi to search for heroin dealers near Times Square, and on the way she produced three inhalers, cracked them open, and fed each the contents of a whole tube. "I got so high, with her, on Benzedrine" Kerouac recalled,

> that I didn't know where I was, and I said "Are we in St. Petersburg, Russia?' [. . .] She says: 'You're buzzing, ba-by!' We get in the [subway] train [. . .] and we're all standing, holding onto the straps, talking and you know we are all buzzing and she's explaining to us what it is to be high and all the time we are digging everybody in the car, with all those bright lights, and she's telling us how to dig them.

Kerouac felt something profound that day, a new way to experience the world more immediately and less filtered by stereotypes, and a new way to experience companionship, too (it made him feel much closer to Burroughs, and he ended up spending twenty-four passionate hours in bed with Russell).[11]

Joan Vollmer, who was growing ever closer to Burroughs, acquired a heavy Benzedrine Inhaler habit. Soon the amphetamine made her mentally unbalanced so that she sometimes really did not know her friends and surroundings.[12] For Kerouac, however, the power of an amphetamine buzz to turn the familiar strange opened doors to the "New Vision" in literature that he and Ginsberg sought. Part of the inspiration was from bebop. Although the intellectual sophistication of the music seems to have been lost on Kerouac and friends, who like many white critics tended to see it as a "primitive" Africa-inspired genre, they admired the free play of spontaneous sound and wanted to emulate it in writing. As Kerouac explained, the "tenor man drawing breath and blowing a phrase on his saxophone, til he runs out of breath, and when he does, his sentence, his statement's been made . . . that's how I therefore separate my sentences, as breath separations of the mind."[13] Benzedrine was just as essential as jazz; the drug became a sacrament, the inspiration of a new, spontaneous way of writing that blasted the mind free of convention and communicated raw physical and emotional experience. Kerouac took so much amphetamine when he first discovered the inhaler high that he lost most of his hair and his legs swelled up with thrombophlebitis.[14] As he wrote to Ginsberg in November of 1945, "Benny [Benzedrine] has made me see a lot. The process of intensifying awareness naturally leads to an overflow of old notions, and voila, new material wells up like water forming its proper level, and makes itself evident at the brim of consciousness. Brand new water! The art of my past is all farce, or at least mostly."[15] Not just any drug would do. It was the particular quality of amphetamine, the acceleration of thought and feeling, that helped him plumb his unconscious and live "in the Now."

Ginsberg used Benzedrine in the same way, questing for "the ancient heavenly connection to the starry dynamo in the machinery of night," as he would put it in his brilliant poem "Howl" (although his greatest vision came from reading William Blake without benefit of drugs, in 1948).[16] But, like bebop, Benzedrine used as an instrument for experiments in consciousness was not for everyone; one needed a taste for high seriousness. As the character Hart Kennedy explains in *Go* by John Clennon Holmes—the other novelist who, with Kerouac, came to define the literary style that came to be known as "Beat"—he preferred the relaxing effects of marijuana. "When I was on benny . . . I got all mean and compulsive, you know? Always worried and hung up. Sure, I was a real big serious intellectual then, toting books around all the time, thinking in all those big psycho-logical terms and everything."[17] This was no mere recreational drug to the Beatniks.

For Kerouac especially, Benzedrine became an essential component of creativity. He wrote on amphetamine to capture raw feelings and experience, the spontaneous "fresh water" welling up from his unconscious. In April 1951, inspired by the "muscular rush" of a twenty-thousand-(plus)-word confessional letter that a friend, Neal Cassady, wrote him during a three-day Benzedrine bender, and the "factualism" of the autobiographical novel Burroughs was writing (eventually published as *Junky*), Kerouac conducted a heroic experiment with the method. He placed a continuous roll of paper into his typewriter and pounded out 120 feet of single-space stream-of-consciousness prose in less than three weeks, high on Benzedrine.[18] This was to be his greatest novel, *On the Road,* the account of a cross-country road trip he took in 1949 with Ginsberg and the manic, thrill-seeking Cassady, who was also the basis of Holmes's fictional Hart Kennedy. Cassady, Kerouac, and Ginsberg actually did use a lot of Benzedrine during their road trips, and not just for self-exploration. As in Kerouac's first experience with Vickie Russell, a powerful amphetamine buzz facilitated an especially intimate, euphoric type of sharing. In the novel, the Ginsberg character declares that he and the Cassady character "are embarked on a tremendous season together. We're trying to communicate with absolute honesty and completeness everything on our minds. We've had to take Benzedrine."[19]

Carolyn Cassady described her first experience with Benzedrine during the summer of 1947, early in her relationship with Neal. Neal Cassady and Ginsberg gave her an eighth of an inhaler with coffee, promising "eight hours of transporting delights," and vowing that the high was worth the eight hours of depression that would likely follow. Neal and Carolyn went to a hotel so as not to disturb Ginsberg, undressed, and talked for a little while. Then, she recalled:

I suddenly became aware I was prattling, and Neal was smiling and giggling, because he knew that's what the drug did. I stopped talking, embarrassed again, but then had to laugh, feeling freer than I ever could remember, less afraid each moment, but unable to control the push of a million thoughts, all of which seemed so terribly necessary to communicate at once. Neal urged me on, saying "You're so expressive!" because I made a lot of faces. [. . .]

Oh, I was having a fine time. I felt so vibrant, brilliant, witty. What fun it was to lie side by side on the cool sheet, giggling, talking, singing and watching the play of neon lights outside the open window [. . .] the two of us entirely wrapped up in the world of each other.[20]

They made an unlikely couple. But Benzedrine was a powerful way of breaking down the barriers between people, just as it broke the stereotypes of experience so as to make the familiar more real and intense. The Beatniks were using Benzedrine Inhalers rather like modern-day hipsters, in the 1990s, would come to use ecstasy as a "hug drug."

As a breaker of stereotypes, habitual perceptions, and rigid social roles, speed remained a key element of Beat sociability and community through the 1950s. In his classic study of the Beatniks, *The Holy Barbarians*, sociologist Lawrence Lipton described the Beat mind-set as a "disaffiliation" from mainstream culture, "voluntary self-alienation from the family cult, from Moneytheism and all its works and ways." As an alternative to competitive getting and spending, the Beats adopted a virtuous poverty, along with strong communalism of property. Beats would often "crash" for long periods at one another's pads, and pass furnishings and apartments on to one another when they had to leave. Apart from what conventionally would be called "property," an exchange of other valued things helped cement the subculture's identity. For instance, another less sympathetic sociologist described an amphetamine-tinged craze for stone collecting that swept through the Greenwich Village Beat community. A trumpet player claimed to have started it with his girlfriend, when, on speed, they began prospecting in parks for special rocks at all hours of the night. They would take certain stones, perceived as having magical properties, back to their apartment where they would clean them until they glistened. Soon their amphetamine-using friends caught on to the craze, and fifty or so fellow travelers, over a three-year period, became "continually engaged in a hyperactive quest for stones." Eventually, "they became confused about the ownership of the stones, and since no one was able to identify his own there began to be a regular stealing of stones when the group met at each other's homes," so that the "stones kept circulating and becoming visibly smoother in the process." Seymour Fiddle, the sociologist, perceptively described this kind of drug-affected behavior as a caricature of the mainstream "Absurd Culture" from which the Beatniks fled but failed to escape as fully as they believed: the "urban go-go," the ambitious over-work in pursuit of objects, and the "time-stuffing" people undertake to accomplish as much as possible each day. But as fuel for their alternative social life, amphetamine could be viewed as a harmless element of the distinct culture the Beats created for themselves. After all, no atom bombs were exploded as a result of the Beatnik stone exchange system.[21]

However the deadly, diabolical side of speed also showed itself to these early pioneers of high-dose amphetamine abuse, even within the circle that invented the Beat lifestyle. At 115th Street, in 1945 and early 1946, Joan Vollmer was eating a Benzedrine Inhaler a day, and taking Benzedrine tablets, too. Her skin was covered with sores, which she attributed to mutations from atomic testing. She often heard the old couple in the apartment beneath discussing her and her friends, calling her a whore and the others drug fiends. One day, she heard them having a terrible quarrel and sent Ginsberg and Kerouac downstairs to prevent the man from killing his wife. Nobody, in fact, was home.[22] In 1946, while Burroughs was on four months' probation in St. Louis, Vollmer started taking more Benzedrine and ended up in Bellevue Hospital as the institution's first female case of amphetamine psychosis, just what Monroe and Drell encountered in their mid-Western military prison. Paranoid auditory hallucinations are a typical symptom.

Burroughs came to rescue Vollmer and took her with him to a farm he had bought in Texas, where he was trying to grow marijuana. Though pregnant, she was soon back on Benzedrine, up to two inhalers a day, which she was now injecting. In August 1947, when Ginsberg and Cassady arrived for a visit, the recently born baby, William Burroughs Jr., appeared to be suffering amphetamine withdrawal. (Speed and alcohol would keep William Junior's brilliant literary career, and his life, short. As his friend John Steinbeck Jr. aptly put it, "Billy had a few strikes against him to be sure. He had tried to grow his fetal brain cells in a swirl of Benzedrine-eucalyptus amniotic fluid from her habit of shooting the soakings of nose inhalers. The first liver cell he ever owned was put to indentured servitude even as it tried to mesoderm its way into mere helpfulness.")[23]

Two summers later, in 1949, when Cassady and Kerouac came to visit Burroughs and Vollmer, now living in a suburb of New Orleans, she was using three Benzedrine Inhaler tubes a day, and her "face, once plump and Germanic and pretty, had become stony and red and gaunt," as Kerouac relates in *On the Road*. She was compulsively scrubbing their decaying shack while toddler Billy ran around naked, shitting on the floor, and at night she tried to clean lizards out of trees with a rake. Burroughs did a lot of target practice around the house, firing his handguns at the many empty inhalers.[24] Two years later, Burroughs accidentally shot Vollmer dead in a drinking game in Mexico City, where the couple had moved to escape the "drag"—the oppressive atmosphere—of the United States. If it is fair to say that drugs caused her untimely death, then Joan Vollmer was killed by amphetamine inhalers, even if Burroughs pulled the trigger. While still gaining status as a mainstream psychiatric medicine, behind the scenes amphetamine would soon be claiming many more lives, as the prevalence of its use swelled still further.

Resisting Inhaler Regulation

Although there was little notice of Benzedrine Inhaler cracking by the medical world before Monroe and Drell's 1947 paper, SKF was aware of the inhaler's potential for abuse years earlier. As noted, in 1938 a doctor published a high-profile paper describing how one can take in a powerful mind-altering dose of amphetamine just from frequent vigorous sniffs from the Benzedrine Inhaler, a piece of unwanted publicity coinciding with the "addiction" scare. In 1937, the firm actually began searching for a replacement decongestant vapor with less effect on the central nervous system, indicating that this Benzedrine Inhaler "side effect" had already been acknowledged as a problem. In June 1943, SKF learned from Canadian authorities that hundreds of drug users in British Columbia were cracking inhalers and injecting the amphetamine together with morphine, a creative twist on the cocaine-opiate "speedball." To keep the Benzedrine Inhaler off the narcotics list—and preferably available without prescription—SKF began making special inhalers with a black dye and capsaicin (the hot and stinging ingredient in chili pepper), sending an emissary to assure the Canadians that these changes made the product virtually inedible and uninjectable. At roughly the same time, SKF investigated a "rumor" that "soldier boys" were eating Benzedrine Inhalers at certain U.S. military bases. Management took the position that a taste deterrent and dye like those provided for the Canadian market should "keep away the so-called 'casual' user, if any do exist" among the soldiers.[25] There was still no evidence that the deterrent additives would work to prevent either injection or ingestion, but this move toward making the Benzedrine Inhaler less attractive seems to have forestalled restrictions on the product for the time being.

However, the inhaler abuse problem came to a boil in 1944, when Benzedrine got caught up in a California legislative initiative. The main aim of a new bill pending there was to require people buying barbiturate sedatives to obtain a fresh prescription each time, and to require pharmacists to keep special records of sales so that authorities could easily trace barbiturate supplies. Amphetamine was included almost as an afterthought, the inhalers having been recognized by law enforcement as a less widespread, though growing, problem. Other new laws like this one were springing up across the country.

Barbiturate drugs—popularly called "goofballs"—were perceived as the greatest threat because of the reckless, violent, or self-destructive behavior that came from taking the pills. They were often ingested with alcohol (for instance, in a cocktail known as the "Geronimo") or with amphetamine, either combination allowing takers to stay awake long enough to enjoy the inhibition-releasing effects of the barbiturates. Barbiturates such as phenobarbital and amobarbital, commonly prescribed as sleeping pills, easily caused death from overdose, as the American public became well aware when celebrities like Hawaiian millionaire Chris Holmes, tennis star Frank War, and radio evangelist Aimee Semple McPherson (founder and president of the Foursquare Gospel Church) all ended their lives in this way during the early 1940s. Medical experts increasingly recognized that, with frequent use, barbiturate addiction could occur, complete with high-dose tolerance and physical withdrawal symptoms. During the later war years, owing partly to the influx of thrill-seeking GIs, barbiturate-related deaths in New York City averaged twenty-one per month, a sixfold increase over the annual total of forty before the war. Estimates of national consumption rose from 2.2 million barbiturate doses per day in 1939 to triple that quantity in 1945. The press and law enforcement officials drummed up a crime wave of car thefts and armed robberies committed by "juvenile Pachuca delinquents" and similar frightening, socially marginal figures, while "jagging" on goofballs. Combined with the celebrity deaths and rumors of parental neglect, prostitution, and draft evasion all associated with barbiturates, this link with delinquents and criminals raised goofball fears to a hysterical pitch nationally (Figure 17).[26]

The abuse of pharmaceuticals like "goofballs" and amphetamines was mainly a problem for states to deal with during the 1940s, because federal government drug regulation was still weak, and the Food and Drug Administration (FDA) had already done everything within its power. As we have seen, since its establishment in 1906, the FDA had authority only over the accurate labeling of drugs; for three decades, the safety and effectiveness of drugs before marketing was regulated, when regulated at all, only by the system of voluntary AMA Council approval. But the 1938 Federal Food, Drug, and Cosmetics act gave the FDA authority to judge a drug's safety before it could be sold. The agency soon applied its new authority over safety in combination with its old authority over labeling to declare certain drugs prescription-only: unless a drug included instructions allowing any ordinary consumer to use it safely, it could not be sold without a prescription. Barbiturates immediately were declared prescription-only according to this rule.[27]

From January 1940, when the new rule took effect, SKF also chose to label its Benzedrine Sulfate tablets prescription-only, but this new labeling posed little threat to amphetamine's prospects as a psychiatric medicine. The Benzedrine Inhaler was another matter. Its brisk sales depended on its over-the-counter availability, because not many people would see a doctor to get a prescription just for a sniffle. And the Benzedrine Inhaler came with excellent instructions on how to use it safely. The product was, in fact, completely safe if people used it as directed: a sniff of the tube every hour or two as congestion required. Thus, the FDA could not touch the Benzedrine Inhaler, even though, by the late 1940s, complaints from school headmasters and senators alike were growing difficult to ignore. State governments, like California's, hoped to do more.

Gordon Alles became SKF's—and Benzedrine's—main political champion in California's political situation during late 1944 and early 1945. Working closely with the California pharmacists' trade groups, which opposed stricter regulation generally and did not want to lose sales of the popular Benzedrine Inhaler, Alles lobbied hard to alter the proposed legislation so that products not meant to be taken internally, like decongestant sprays and inhalers, would remain available without prescription. SKF instructed him to argue, with the state authorities and other concerned groups, that printing "Warning: For Inhalation Only!" on the paper filler ("pledget") inside the inhaler, together with a dye that would show in the mouth, would deter casual abusers. If state authorities did not agree, then Alles would offer to add capsicum to the pledgets, too, like those already sold in Canada, so that consuming (or injecting) the inhaler contents would cause a burning sensation. If the Board of Pharmacy and Department of Public Health were still not satisfied, as a last resort Alles was to promise to withdraw the inhalers from the California market until a stronger deterrent was available but to try to make the Department of Public Health cede authority in this decision to the friendlier Board of Pharmacy so that the firm did not have to deal with two regulatory agencies. Ultimately, the only solution was for SKF to develop a new decongestant drug for its inhaler, and, although SKF had possible replacements for amphetamine base in the pipeline, the firm wanted more time.[28]

At length, Alles prevailed, convincing the Board of Pharmacy that the Canadian-style capsicum deterrent was adequate. Alles also helped convince lawmakers and various state officials to support an amended version of the bill, which passed early in 1945. Under this California law, the Benzedrine Inhaler and other decongestants for external use were exempted from requiring a prescription. Alles also succeeded in keeping amphetamine tablets, which already required prescriptions, out of the strictest enforcement category, although refills on prescriptions would be limited. (This seemed a small sacrifice for keeping the Benzedrine Inhaler freely available, since refills accounted for only 5 percent of the sales of Benzedrine Sulfate tablets at the time.) SKF agreed to introduce a special Benzedrine Inhaler in California as soon as possible containing dye and the chemical picric acid, which tastes bad and causes nausea, making the inhaler (supposedly) "unfit for internal use." Alles personally assured the board that SKF's new deterrent would work even better than capsicum. Thus, the Benzedrine Inhaler remained available everywhere in the state without a prescription.[29]

Alles's success in California caused "great general rejoicing" at SKF, largely because amphetamine inhalers were specifically exempted from prescription-only requirements in the wording of the 1945 law, reducing the discretion of state officials to regulate the product. At that time, the firm might genuinely have believed that abuse of the Benzedrine Inhaler would go away once the war was over, when "the present misusers will be able to get something more suitable for their purposes" (presumably they meant cocaine, scarce in wartime).[30] But the inhaler "jag" issue did not go away. "The 'boys' are eating your denatured inhalers with no apparent nausea," one disappointed California state official wrote Alles in April 1945, possibly referring to pachuca "gangs." The Benzedrine Inhaler was too good and too cheap a high for a little stomach discomfort or dye to discourage its fans. Particularly after Monroe and Drell's study came out in 1947 and was picked up by the national press, FDA and state pressures on the firm to restrict the Benzedrine Inhaler mounted. By 1948, SKF was required to sell its modified California inhaler in many other states, including Alabama, Arizona, Georgia, Pennsylvania, Utah, and Washington. Meanwhile, the "improved" California inhaler with picric acid was meeting with increasing skepticism where it had been in use the longest. Physicians in the state circulated a petition to restrict amphetamine inhalers to prescription sales, because, they complained, juveniles were ignoring the deterrent and still using them to get a "cheap drunk." The critics were backed by law enforcement and by pillars of society like the state Parent-Teacher Association, and in April 1948 California regulators bent to the pressure and again moved to require prescriptions for the Benzedrine Inhaler.[31]

Thanks to Alles's lobbying and the deterrent-modified product, the Benzedrine Inhaler had remained available without prescription for an extra three years. In late 1948, SKF finally moved to introduce the new Benzedrex Inhaler, containing a different "non-amphetamine" drug (propylhexedrine). On behalf of the firm, Alles assured the California Board of Pharmacy that SKF's Benzedrex Inhaler was fully replacing the Benzedrine Inhaler in the state, and that it did not contain amphetamine or methamphetamine. To deal with mounting pressure on a national level, in early 1949 SKF assured FDA that the replacement inhaler was already being market-tested in California and would soon be introduced nationally. SKF kept its promise, moving to re-place the Benzedrine Inhaler throughout the U.S. and Canada at the end of 1949 with the "stimulation-free" Benzedrex product. The histo-rian Charles O. Jackson wrote of the episode that "the beleaguered firm had had enough" and that the product had become harmful to SKF's image as a reputable pharmaceutical firm. He might also have noted that SKF's amphetamine patents, and therefore the firm's mo-nopoly on the product, were about to expire.[32] Regulatory worries could now be left to competitors as the firm moved on.

Predictably, other manufacturers quickly filled the amphetamine void that was left when SKF's Benzedrine Inhaler was removed from drugstore shelves. Indeed, since 1944 if not earlier, other firms had been selling competing decongestant inhalers containing chemical rel-atives of amphetamine, starting with Wyeth's Wyamine (with me-phentermine), Lilly's Tuamine (with 2-aminoheptane), and Merrell's Vonedrine (with phenylpropylmethylamine). They all worked and felt much like amphetamine base; in fact, the last of these "decongestant" compounds is back on the streets today as a designer drug. During the 1950s mind-altering, over-the-counter inhalers like these proliferated. So, even though you could no longer buy a genuine Benzedrine In-haler in the United States, if you wanted "kicks" there were these and plenty of others to choose from, including (depending on the state) the Valo Inhaler with amphetamine base and the Vicks Inhaler with methamphetamine base. It became increasingly popular to extract the drugs from inhalers for injection. Finally, in 1959, the FDA, backed by some new but still uncertain authority, made amphetamine inhalers prescription-only nationally; methamphetamine inhalers were not in-cluded until 1965.[33]

Speed from inhalers thus remained a major part of the counter-culture drug scene through the first part of the 1960s. The band that would musically epitomize early 1960s youth culture, the Beatles, had their first drug experience in mid-1960 with Benzedrine Inhalers (ac-cording to John Lennon in a 1973 letter to the alternative newspaper *International Times*). The poet Royston Ellis, known as "Britain's Allen Ginsberg," showed John, George, Paul, and Stuart Sutcliffe—called the "Silver Beetles" at the time—how to crack the inhaler and eat the amphetamine-soaked wads inside in classic Beatnik style.[34]

Even the Benzedrex Inhaler had its fans, for all its purported free-dom from central nervous system "side effects." In fact, SKF management was already aware in mid-1947 that Benzedrex provided a "signifi-cant 'lift'" from the reports of test subjects trying the amphetamine de-rivative (propylhexidrine) as a diet drug. However, they might not have tested doses equivalent to eating a whole inhaler at once, like James Ell-roy did as a young degenerate in 1968. "I met a freak at the Hollywood Public Library," the mystery writer recalls in his autobiography.

> He told me about Benzedrex inhalers [. . .] They were legal. They cost 69 cents. You could buy them or boost them all over LA. [. . .] The wads [inside] were two inches long and of cigarette circumference. They were soaked in an evil-smelling amber solution. I gagged one down and fought a reflex to heave it back up. It stayed down and went to work inside half an hour. The high was gooooood. It was brain-popping and groin-grabbing. It was just as good as a pharma-ceutical-upper high.

After "eight solid hours" of the high left him feeling "dingy and schizzy," a drink of cheap wine brought "fresh euphoria." For at least five years Ellroy made it a regular habit, until the monsters he saw crawling out of toilets and a lung abscess the size of a fist made him stop.[35] Ultimately, the pleasures of cheap, easy inhaler jags lasted more than four decades, from the Benzedrine Inhaler's first introduction around 1933 into the 1970s. By the time regulatory action started mak-ing psychoactive inhalers less available, their disappearance could not have cut very much into the recreational speed supply: the nation was awash with black-market and grey-market pharmaceutical ampheta-mine tablets, easily available for people who wanted to inject, and, as we shall see, illicit "speed kitchens" were making even more.

Battling the Bootleggers

By the mid-1940s the Benzedrine Inhaler was a cash cow for SKF, an established product yielding a steady stream of income without much marketing effort. However, the product offered limited opportunities for sales expansion, because (medicinal) inhaler consumption was ef-fectively restricted by the frequency of colds and allergies, conditions people could unambiguously diagnose for themselves. Benzedrine Sulfate tablets, on the other hand, held much greater growth potential.

The sales of this product were limited only by the number of medical conditions for which doctors were willing to prescribe amphetamine, and, of course, many psychiatric conditions are open to interpretation.

In the early 1940s, Benzedrine Sulfate was AMA-approved for four medical uses (or "indications," in medical jargon): narcolepsy, a particular form of Parkinson's Disease, alcoholism, and depression. SKF advertised Benzedrine Sulfate tablets especially for "mild depression" while trying to increase recognition of the disorder among doctors, and at the same time trying to expand the definition of depression so that anhedonia (lack of pleasure) would become a key sign, as Abraham Myerson had long urged. This strategy amounts to selling the drug by marketing the disease; since amphetamine was the only available drug that had been shown to work on anhedonic depression, increased recognition and diagnosis would automatically translate into more Benzedrine Sulfate prescriptions.

The firm also arranged clinical trials to establish entirely new uses for which the drug could ultimately be marketed. But another strategy for increasing sales quickly, also crucial for long-term profits, was to block other drug manufacturers from selling amphetamine in competition with SKF. In late 1940 and early 1941, Benzedrine Sulfate sales stopped their regular quarterly growth and actually dropped, thanks to heavy competition. These rivals were not the other major drug firms but smaller companies, called "bootleggers" by SKF management, making generic amphetamine tablets in defiance of Alles's patent.[36] The leading use for "bootleg" amphetamine tablets was weight loss, and SKF was preparing the way to target weight loss as a new market for Benzedrine Sulfate, once AMA approval was secured. But first the firm had to shut down the so-called bootleggers.

Taking the bootleggers to court for patent infringement was risky for SKF. The firm perceived the New Deal courts of the thirties and early forties as unsympathetic to big business generally, and hostile to patents in particular. Moreover, in this specific case, SKF's control of amphetamine had an "odor of monopoly," as one of the firm's legal staff put it, possibly because the revenues from the medicine so outweighed the company's meager investment in its discovery. Further still, the firm's amphetamine patents covered the substance as a medicine as well as a chemical, even though the basic chemical was not actually new. Although the U.S. Patent Office had sometimes granted such "new-use" patents in the field of pharmaceuticals, this was exceptional, and patents on novel applications of old inventions had generally very questionable status in patent law. [37] (Today the American courts and patent office are much kinder to big drug companies, who routinely obtain patents on "new" uses of old drugs just before their patents are due to expire, thus keeping cheaper generic drugs off the market. "Evergreening," the perpetuation of patent protection through practices such as this, is now being exported around the world through the U.S. government's "Free Trade Agreements," to the disadvantage of health care systems everywhere, and probably also to the detriment of actual innovation in drugs.)[38] If the courts decided against SKF and ruled their patents invalid, the doors would be wide open to competition in amphetamine—and not just for weight loss.

The firm took the chance, for at least two reasons. For one, these infringers were not "gentlemen" in that they were not only selling amphetamine pills despite SKF's (Alles's) patent but were also imitating the appearance of SKF's Benzedrine Sulfate tablets. This violated laws covering trademarks and competition, quite apart from patent law.[39] For another, stakes were high: the so-called bootleggers seemed to have a large market that SKF could take if it defeated them. So, in late 1942, the SKF legal staff began to go after the bootleggers selling Benzedrine look-alikes, both for unfair competition and patent infringement. The competitors targeted by these lawsuits included a wholesale drug distributor named Lannett and a manufacturer named Rona Pharmacal, both in Pennsylvania, and also a manufacturer called Pro-Medico Laboratories in New York. The names of other amphetamine makers emerged in the course of testimony, such as Custazin Incorporated and Professional Laboratories. There apparently were many bootleggers; SKF sued the most prominent, the tip of the iceberg.

The business strategies of all the small firms were similar. They would manufacture white 10 mg amphetamine tablets that looked exactly the same as Benzedrine Sulfate: the same size, the same bevel on the edges of the pills, the same cross stamped in the top to allow quartering. These generic look-alikes, equivalent to Benzedrine medically as well as visually, were sold to pharmacists at a fraction of the price of the brand-name product. The druggists could then repackage and sell the generic substitute to doctors, or to patients with Benzedrine Sulfate prescriptions, who would often pay full price none the wiser for the substitution. Consumers broke no law buying the generic pills regardless of whether they knew that the product was not genuine

Benzedrine; the vendors did, however, if the courts judged them to have deceived buyers. Even the manufacturers were not necessarily breaking the law; that depended on the courts' decisions as to whether Alles's amphetamine patent was valid, and whether the trade practices of the generic manufacturers were really unfair.

As soon as SKF's lawyers filed suit, they clamped down on their opponents' sales directly by writing druggists to threaten them with possible lawsuits for unfair competition, fraud, or infringement if they did not stop selling the generic pills immediately. SKF placed ads in pharmacy journals with the same message. The firm also attempted to use the courts to obtain the customer lists of the generic manufacturers they were suing, and in at least one case SKF used private detectives to tail delivery trucks in order to identify customers, and followed up with (allegedly) intimidating telephone calls to the druggists. All these various actions by SKF must have cut into the generic traffic to some extent, helping Benzedrine Sulfate sales rebound a little in 1943, although the courts did not always see things SKF's way. In fact, the fight went right up to the Supreme Court. In the end, however, SKF triumphed over the whole set of challengers in an extended struggle with the Clark & Clark drug firm of Camden, New Jersey.

Clark & Clark was established by Charles Morris, an employee of the Squibb drug firm and previously a New Jersey pharmacist. A manager at Squibb had told Morris that the firm did not believe SKF's Alles patent on amphetamine salts would stand in court, but nevertheless the firm did not intend to challenge SKF in the amphetamine tablets business. (This must illustrate how the "gentlemen" players in the drug business behaved.) Morris bought a small Camden company called Standard Medical Laboratories in October 1941, started making amphetamine pills, and by April 1942 was making more than enough money to do without his job at Squibb. Like the other bootleggers, Clark & Clark manufactured a Benzedrine Sulfate look-alike—aptly called "Profetamine" to remind druggists that it might profitably be substituted for SKF's Benzedrine Sulfate product (Figure 18). The firm also did a very lively trade in diet pills called "Clark-o-Tabs," which came in six colors and several different formulas. All Clark-o-Tabs contained thyroid hormone, which boosts metabolism, and was the most popular diet drug of the day. All of them also contained amphetamine, which the quasi-medical world of weight-control doctors had already adopted for its additional slimming effects (as it turned out, largely through reduced appetite).

Profetamine tablets sold to pharmacies for prices ranging from less than $3.00 to $12.00 per thousand, a bargain compared to the $22.60 per thousand that SKF charged for Benzedrine Sulfate. SKF sent shoppers to Clark & Clark customers with Benzedrine Sulfate prescriptions, proving that druggists substituted Profetamine for the SKF product. In none of the thirty-three cases that SKF's legal team documented were significant savings passed along to the customer.[40]

SKF's case rested mainly on the argument that the similarity of Clark & Clark's Profetamine tablets to Benzedrine constituted deliberate and deceptive imitation. Stressing unfair competition was SKF's strong suit, since the pills from the two firms could hardly be distinguished, and Clark & Clark had specially ordered a tablet pressing machine to make them. Clark & Clark's defense mostly sidestepped SKF's trademark and competition claims, stressing the weakness of Alles's patent. They argued that amphetamine had been synthesized by Lazar Edeleano and other chemists long before 1930, that making the amphetamine base into a salt was obvious to any chemist, and that the medicinal uses of a chemical so similar to ephedrine were obvious to any pharmacologist. Thus, amphetamine sulfate was neither new nor non-obvious, as the law required a patentable invention to be. Clark & Clark also filed a countercharge of unfair competition against SKF, citing harassment of its customers, the druggists to whom SKF wrote threatening letters.

Expert witnesses included a chemist friendly to Clark & Clark, Alles, an SKF chemist, and Carl Schmidt, the distinguished co-"discoverer" (with K. K. Chen) of ephedrine, who impressed the court with doubts that anyone before Alles had actually produced the sulfur salt of amphetamine. Clark & Clark called the diet doctor Samuel Kalb, who basically argued that SKF's Benzedrine Sulfate was an excellent substitute for ephedrine in weight loss but was overpriced. As a medical witness on the novelty of amphetamine as a medicine, SKF called Myerson, who testified in glowing terms on the medical importance of amphetamine sulfate as the first drug to act directly on mood. In the end, the court was so impressed that the judge's opinion almost outdid Myerson in enthusiasm for Benzedrine (declaring that amphetamine "opened up a new field of medicine," because "the possibilities of the use of this drug in the therapeutic care of neuropsychiatric disorders are inexhaustible").[41]

Thus, the September 1945 ruling of the Federal District Court went entirely in SKF's favor. The court cleared SKF of unfair competition but found Clark & Clark guilty of it, particularly of encouraging druggists to palm off their generic Profetamine as SKF's Benzedrine Sulfate. Clark & Clark was ordered to cease making and selling amphetamine immediately, and for all time. They would also have to repay SKF lost profits, court costs, and damages. SKF, moreover, won a much more important and far-reaching victory than merely hobbling these generic competitors: the court upheld Alles's 1932 patent on amphetamine sulfate as a chemical ("new composition of matter") and not merely as a medicine, despite his disclaimer on this count. The reasoning here was that, although chemists like Edeleano had previously synthesized the amphetamine base, they had not unquestionably made Alles's sulfate of amphetamine, the form best suited for administering the drug as a pill. So Alles was now the indisputable legal discoverer of amphetamine sulfate, and SKF was entitled to his patent's monopoly on all uses of the chemical. This decision surprised almost everyone. In retrospect, it seemed to SKF lawyers that the firm had only won on the infringement because they were "able to mix in the case the substitution and unfair competition" with the patent issue. Probably SKF had hoped Alles's medical-use claims in the patent would hold but expected that the court would agree with Clark & Clark that no patent covered the substance itself because making amphetamine into a sulfur salt, easily accomplished simply by mixing the base with sulfuric acid, represented obvious and uncreative "kitchen chemistry."[42]

Clark & Clark ignored the court's order to cease manufacturing amphetamine, immediately appealing the infringement decision and winning temporary permission to continue business as usual. Obviously, the small firm was hoping Alles's patent would be thrown out by the higher court, but even if that did not occur, the delay in itself was beneficial to Clark & Clark. While the appeal was pending, Charles Morris, chief of Clark & Clark, had to post $25,000 bond toward any court-ordered payments to SKF. In October 1945, the day after filing his appeal, he was heard boasting at a drug industry dinner in a Philadelphia country club that $25,000 was no hardship because one month's amphetamine profits would easily make up the loss.[43] In the appeal proceedings, Clark & Clark again attacked the originality of Alles's amphetamine discovery. Meanwhile, SKF did groundwork toward getting its lost profits and damages. SKF knew that Clark & Clark produced a lot of amphetamine, since they supplied the smaller firm with the milk sugar filler used in making tablets, but they did not know exactly how much. So SKF hired a private detective named Alfred "Bill" Irby, a hardened, hard-drinking veteran of both the military

and law enforcement, who approached Morris posing as a business-
man interested in becoming the sole Clark & Clark distributor to Mexico. Talking with Irby, Morris (allegedly) claimed that Clark & Clark
were stepping up production from 1.5 to 2 million amphetamine tablets a day, most of which was (in October 1945) Profetamine—the imitation 10 mg Benzedrine Sulfate pills. Irby talked with various drug
wholesalers from across the country who (allegedly) confirmed trade
consistent with these levels of production, the largest dealers reporting sales volumes on the order of 2 million Clark & Clark tablets per
week. Based on the consumption of powdered thyroid by Clark &
Clark, used in making the colorful Clark-o-Tabs diet pills, which several sources at the plant told Irby was 200 pounds per day, SKF argued
that Clark & Clark must have been making a little more than 1 million
Clark-o-Tabs (each containing 1 grain thyroid) per day.[44] Supposing
that the diet pills accounted for half their business, this would imply
that Clark & Clark was producing 2 million amphetamine-containing
tablets a day, just as Morris (allegedly) boasted when he believed Irby
to be a drug distributor rather than a "stool-pigeon and plant."

On the other hand, under circumstances where high production
would mean stiffer penalties for the firm, Clark & Clark offered testimony that their sales of amphetamine were only about 2 million tablets
per week for the last quarter of 1945. Taking a value between these two
figures on the basis of all evidence, it might cautiously be estimated that
Clark & Clark was manufacturing one million amphetamine tablets per
day in late 1945.[45] Adding SKF's reported domestic sales of 5 million 10
mg tablets per month at the end of 1945 to 25 million Clark-o-Tabs and
Profetamines per month from Clark & Clark, the national amphetamine
consumption rate toward the end of 1945 would amount to 30 million
tablets monthly.[46] True consumption was almost certainly higher, since
apart from their conservative premises these calculations do not count 5
mg Benzedrine tablets and look-alikes, and entirely disregard amphetamine tablets made by other infringing firms—not to mention misuse of
SKF's Benzedrine Inhaler.[47] So there was more than enough speed in
circulation for half a million Americans to take the standard daily regimen of two pills, and given that most users would have been taking
amphetamines much less regularly than twice every day, the number of
medical consumers of oral amphetamines in 1945–1946 would have
stood closer to one million. Clearly, the United States already had serious national appetite for speed, and it was growing fast.

In August 1946, the Federal Circuit Court supported the lower court's decision on Alles's patent, differing only with respect to Clark & Clark's punishment by allowing that the firm could again make amphetamine once Alles's patent expired, as long as its pills did not resemble SKF's. Like the lower court, the decision generously acknowledged the novelty and significance of the drug, crediting Alles with a breakthrough discovery. His creative leap (crucial in patent law at the time) lay in purposely developing drugs to influence the mind, taking his work beyond that of Barger and Dale, back at Burroughs-Wellcome in the teens, who worked with animals whose central nervous system was deliberately inactivated so they could focus on blood pressure. Indeed, like the District Court judge, the Appellate Court judge seems to have been swept away by a vision of amphetamine as the miracle drug that for the first time allowed physicians to "affect, even create, mood."[48]

Clark & Clark appealed, but the Supreme Court denied a new hearing. Alles naturally was thrilled to have his patent upheld, and SKF must have been pleased to have its legal monopoly on amphetamine affirmed. From this point on, until the patent's expiration in 1949, it would be easy to prosecute any makers of amphetamine for patent infringement. Nevertheless, SKF did not completely control the amphetamine field, even though the firm had vanquished the bootleggers for the moment. By the end of the war, other large ethical firms had begun marketing methamphetamine—notably "Methedrine" from Burroughs-Wellcome and "Desoxyn" from Abbott Laboratories—for the same medical uses as SKF's amphetamine. Methamphetamine was too old for protection by any patent, as noted earlier. Indeed, when the courts finally stopped Clark & Clark from selling amphetamine for the remaining life of Alles's patent, the firm immediately substituted methamphetamine in its new and improved "Clark-O-Tabs Modified."[49] Thus, SKF never really held a safe monopoly on the amphetamine field after 1940, despite having in Benzedrine Sulfate the dominant brand. Smelling money in speed, competitors were circling; and with the return of peace in 1945, the drug industry as a whole was poised to build the consumption of amphetamines to massive levels.[50]

5

A Bromide for the Atomic Age

IN THE 1940s and 1950s the world of the American family doctor, where amphetamine found its largest market, differed little in essence from that of general practitioners a generation before. Contrary to romantic notions we might now have about the "good old days," the average doctor has always been too busy. From the late 1800s through the first half of the twentieth century, general practitioners were seeing as many as forty patients a day, often sixty, and not uncommonly eighty. Then as now, the overworked physician did not have much time to serve as a friend and counselor. However, a counselor was exactly what many patients needed. Although data from around 1930 found that doctors typically devoted only 2–2.5 percent of their time to "nervous complaints," this number refers only to the official, explicit reason for the patient's visit. Doctors were well aware that many if not most patient visits were actually psychosomatic, that is, prompted by physical complaints that doctors could only explain as "imaginary" or caused by mental distress. (The situation has not changed much since; current estimates place psychosomatic complaints at 38–60 percent of doctor visits, the same or perhaps up a little since the 1960s).[1]

In the early twentieth century, general practitioners dealt with their nervous patients by prescribing them tonics or sugar pills to quell the mystery symptoms. These prescriptions relied on the placebo effect: the patients' faith in a doctor's wisdom, their expectations that medicine would help, and the psychological reassurance that both provided. As time advanced the pills changed, but the management of psychosomatic complaints with prescriptions did not. Studies in the 1950s found that 60–95 percent of doctor visits culminated in a prescription, and the most commonly prescribed drugs were barbiturates and bromides to restore calm and sleep. Yes, this was the age of wonder drugs like penicillin, often used as a placebo itself. Nevertheless, the use of old-fashioned drugs like bromides in this old-fashioned

way reflects a continuation of traditional doctoring practices. Eskay
Neurophosphates and similar stimulating tonics, whose value by the
standards of scientific medicine was always doubtful, remained on the
market well into the 1960s (and in two formulas, red and green!).[2]

The main postwar change in the management of psychosomatic
complaints was not the number of cryptic psychiatric problems encountered in general practice but rather public attitudes toward mental health. Nowhere was the shift in perceptions of psychiatry more
dramatic than in the United States. As we saw in the previous chapter, psychiatrists were involved intimately in the American war effort,
both in screening recruits and treating mental health casualties, and
the specialty emerged from the war with a greatly improved image.
Both government institutions and the general public suddenly became
concerned with psychiatric illnesses—now pronounced by experts to
affect 10 percent, 25 percent, or even 50 percent of the population.[3]

Patients became much more willing to accept a psychiatric diagnosis, and a matching prescription for psychiatric medication. With
the postwar rise in the profile of mental illness, the field of psychosomatic medicine became fashionable in medical schools and journals.
The eternal facts of life for family doctors finally received official scientific recognition, when careful studies in the 1950s found that at
least a quarter of patient visits were driven by a concealed mental
health problem. General practitioners began hearing from all sides
that they needed to recognize psychiatric disorders, read up on psychiatric theory, and follow up-to-date psychiatric practice. These developments added up to a golden opportunity for SKF: in amphetamine the firm owned not just the only recognized antidepressant on
the market in the late 1940s but the only psychiatric drug with real scientific credibility.[4]

So right after the war, from late 1945 through 1947, SKF renewed
the Benzedrine marketing push with a fresh ad campaign to capitalize
on the new prominence of psychiatric disorders. Compared to wartime Benzedrine advertising, the postwar campaign was more focused
on general practitioners and was also less technical. For instance, each
ad in one postwar series stressed a particular patient type that would
commonly present depressive symptoms to family doctors, with the
apparent goal of making a Benzedrine Sulfate prescription routine in
such cases. Each of these full-page ads also carried a distinctive, over-
sized "b" logo, building on the Benzedrine brand identity (Figure 19).

One featured a big blue "b" together with photos of an elderly man changing from sad to smiling, illustrating how the drug helps "when persistent depression settles upon the aged patient." Another showed a big green "b" below a drawing of Saint George slaying a dragon, illustrating how Benzedrine serves "to combat depression associated with persistent pain" (for instance, in arthritis or cancer). A third showed a big pink "b," with photos of a baby and a housewife changing from frowning to smiling, illustrating results when Benzedrine is used "to alleviate prolonged postpartum depression." This postwar push boosted prescriptions significantly: in 1947, SKF's sales of Benzedrine Sulfate tablets reached their all-time peak at about $2.2 million, up from about $1.3 million for 1945.[5]

Competition from similar products was the main reason why SKF's postwar Benzedrine advertising campaign did not make greater headway. Apart from methamphetamine pills made by other pharmaceutical firms, and whatever amphetamine the so-called bootleggers were still selling despite the lawsuits, Benzedrine Sulfate's postwar competitors included a new amphetamine product from SKF itself. As already mentioned, like many chemicals the amphetamine molecule is asymmetrical, and therefore comes in two or more versions (or "optical isomers"). Benzedrine was an equal ("racemic") blend of both right-handed and left-handed amphetamine molecules. In 1938, Alles and SKF chemists had isolated and tested each isomer of amphetamine separately, finding that dextroamphetamine, the right-handed form, gave a greater mood lift and less jitters than Benzedrine. The left-handed form, or levoamphetamine, had little effect on mood, but it raised the blood pressure and caused headaches, along with most of amphetamine's other unpleasant side effects. Thus amphetamine's desirable effects on the brain could largely be separated from the rest, because the desirable ones are all caused by the right-handed form.

In early 1939, SKF chemists found a commercially practical way to separate the twin left- and right-handed amphetamine molecules, and proceeded to file patent applications on the method. They also filed patents on both optical isomers of amphetamine, although they expected rejection on the grounds that both isomers were fundamentally the same chemical and were thus covered under Alles's original patent. In 1942, SKF's Fred Nabenhauer was granted a patent on his separation method, good for seventeen years, although there was no telling when another chemist might discover an even better method for making dextroamphetamine. Then, in 1944, after several rebuffs and appeals, the courts upheld the Patent Office's final rejection of the patent application for dextroamphetamine as a new chemical.[6] This left the drug protected only by Alles's original 1932 amphetamine patent. The year 1949, when that patent expired, would be the witching hour for SKF: competitors, jealous of SKF's monopoly, would surely flood the market with a multitude of new amphetamine products. SKF's limited future control of dextroamphetamine helps explain why management decided to launch the drug on the market in 1943—despite Benzedrine's still promising sales, and the dampening effect of the war on civilian business.

Dexedrine, SKF's brand name for dextroamphetamine, did not enjoy the same advertising fanfare for its launch that Benzedrine tablets received before, during, and immediately after the war. Early Dexedrine advertisements, the few that can be found at all, appear largely in specialty psychiatric journals and do not highlight any of the product's distinctive features. For instance, one ad promised that Dexedrine would "brighten the outlook in Menstrual Dysfunction," specifically by relieving "depressive symptoms . . . associated with primary dysmenorrhea," and "apathy, depression of mood, and psychogenic fatigue" generally. Another promised that Dexedrine would help "when mild depression develops . . . during convalescence, in dysmenorrhea . . . following childbirth . . . at the onset of menopause . . . following bereavement or misfortune . . . in old age."[7] High-profile Benzedrine ads of the time made the same claims. The Dexedrine ads, moreover, never mentioned dextroamphetamine's biggest advantage, fewer jitters than its racemic counterpart, Benzedrine. The newer product must have been viewed by SKF management as a direct, cannibalistic threat to their profitable older drug: any boost in Dexedrine sales might be at the expense of Benzedrine. But despite this less than full commitment to Dexedrine, sales of the new drug already began to take off in 1945, rising much more quickly than Benzedrine sales, and for an unexpected reason.[8]

Diet Pill Breakthrough

By 1946 Dexedrine was selling itself, and the main use making it popular was probably weight control, even though it was not advertised for that purpose in mainstream medical journals. At least since 1941, SKF had quietly been preparing to market amphetamine products for weight loss, arranging and funding experiments to prove the drug's effectiveness. The firm had long known that the drug might make a good diet medicine, ever since the early, surprising reports of weight loss by Nathanson and Myerson in 1937 and 1938. Diet doctors discovered amphetamine for themselves by the end of the 1930s, and the booming business in patent-infringing diet pills during the war confirmed amphetamine's commercial promise for weight control. Standard medical texts had noted amphetamine's use for weight loss as early as 1938 but discouraged it as "probably undesirable" on safety grounds. To overcome this cautious opinion and convince large numbers of doctors to prescribe amphetamine for overweight patients, SKF would have to advertise in medical journals. Thus, the firm needed impressive scientific studies to win AMA approval to advertise and to fight suspicion of their product. In July 1942, while Alles and SKF were pressing forward with their unlikely patent application on dextroamphetamine as a new substance, and were about to file suit against Clark & Clark, the firm was already gathering information from their collaborating doctors on the advantages of dextroamphetamine over regular, racemic amphetamine in weight reduction. These studies, some of them published in 1942 and 1943, indicated that both forms of amphetamine reduced patients' appetites. What prevented the AMA from granting approval was not a lack of evidence that people lose weight on amphetamine but a worry that they did so because of toxic effects.[9] After all, when people are poisoned, they tend to stop eating.

It seems that a couple of years then passed without SKF taking much action on weight loss. Perhaps the firm was waiting for peacetime in order to make a bigger splash with its weight-loss products; possibly it was also waiting for the patent infringement litigation to be resolved, lest the firm pay for clinical research and for advertising that mostly benefited competitors like Clark & Clark. But with the generic bootleggers and the Axis armies both in retreat in early 1945, SKF moved forward again, organizing a detailed study by A. C. Ivy—perhaps the leading American expert on the physiological effects of amphetamine at the time, thanks to his wartime research.

Ivy talked with both the sales and research departments at SKF and drew up a plan to test the theory that appetite reduction represented a toxic side effect. A small group of otherwise healthy obese patients would be studied in an extraordinary live-in experiment covering two eight-week periods, along with a couple of normal-weight subjects as controls. The first eight weeks would be divided between four weeks of taking a placebo followed by four weeks of Benzedrine taken before each meal, and the second, after a vacation, divided between four weeks with placebo and four weeks with Dexedrine. Participants could eat all the food they wanted, but every bit was prepared and measured by Ivy's team. They were subject to regular blood and urine tests for signs of toxicity, as well as measurements of their metabolic rates, an uncomfortable procedure at the time. The technical aspects of the study were elaborate, and the design was also sophisticated for its day (an early approximation to the "cross-over"–type trial). Still, in the end, its sponsors must have been pleased. Ivy concluded that amphetamine caused no detectable toxic effects in the normal dose range, that it worked for weight loss simply by reducing food consumption, and that the drug did this by acting on one of the brain's higher centers (and not, for instance, affecting the stomach or the nerves linking it to the brain).[10] The drug basically altered the appetite, an individual's attitude toward food.

This idea that weight problems could be remedied with a psychiatric medication fit beautifully with the shifting understanding of fatness at the time. Although endocrinologists were still widely consulted about weight loss, by the late 1940s medical science had rejected the old notion that a hormonal "slow metabolism" caused obesity and that correcting it by speeding it up with thyroid hormone made sense. Now obesity and overweight were explained simply as psychosomatic problems of overeating, that is, signs of mental illness with emotional causes—very commonly, depression. According to the new view, all overweight people could benefit from seeing a psychiatrist, but since this was not always possible, it was up to the general practitioner to intervene. And intervention was essential, the medical profession was now hearing in increasingly strident tones, as pathbreaking population research from the insurance industry brought to light the health consequences of obesity, particularly its statistical contribution to heart disease. With the needed evidence of amphetamine's safety and efficacy in hand from Ivy's study, and with only two years left of Alles's amphetamine patent, SKF had no time to lose in making the most of the opportune situation. In late 1947, SKF won AMA approval to advertise Benzedrine and Dexedrine tablets for weight control and began marketing both products for that use. Many of the firm's advertisements urged not only that obesity was a serious medical problem and that fat people were often emotionally disturbed (Figure 20) but also that the "best time to check obesity is while your patient is still in the marginally overweight class—before he becomes grossly obese." Thus people even a few pounds overweight ought to be prescribed amphetamine because they were at risk of obesity, and obesity put them at risk of heart disease and other serious illnesses. Essentially, this advertising constructed any degree of fatness as an amphetamine-treatable, incipient illness that today we might describe as "pre-obesity."[11]

In 1947 sales of Benzedrine rose by a third to $2.2 million compared to the sales in 1946, and Dexedrine sales leaped 260 percent to $3.6 million, far outstripping the older product. In 1948, Dexedrine sales rose another 45 percent to $5.2 million, and Benzedrine began declining despite heavy advertising for weight loss (Figure 21). Obviously, consumers approved of Dexedrine for weight loss, and would continue to do so for almost three decades more. Between 1947 and 1949, sales of Dexedrine Sulfate tablets had nearly doubled to $5.9 million, but the product's future was uncertain. SKF was energetically searching for new diet drugs to replace Benzedrine and Dexedrine, but neither Benzedrex nor anything else worked as well.[12] To retain the weight-loss market when Alles's amphetamine patent expired, SKF had no new drug to offer, only its established brands and its marketing prowess.

And, as expected, with the expiration of Alles's patent, a flood of competing amphetamine-based products exploded into the marketplace—many from smaller, more specialized firms such as Strasenburgh and Irwin-Neisler (Figure 22). Total U.S. amphetamine production nearly quadrupled between 1949 and 1952, virtually all of the increase coming from SKF's competitors. Dexedrine annual sales stayed at the $5–$6 million plateau in those years, while sales of Benzedrine Sulfate tablets slumped, falling below $1 million in 1951.[13] With sales consistent with daily consumption by several million Americans, Dexedrine remained a success for SKF. But the best was yet to come. Thanks to brilliant product repackaging and marketing, SKF would break out of their doldrums, doubling the firm's amphetamine sales between 1950 and 1955, and taking the nation's affair with amphetamine to another level.

Reconceiving Amphetamine

Two main innovations put SKF back in the forefront of the amphetamine trade, despite the stiff competition the firm faced in the early
1950s. Both could be described as old wine in new bottles, as is so often the case when pharmaceutical firms require a new product for
business reasons but their research fails to find a genuinely new and
better medicine. They were clever innovations just the same. The first
was a new kind of capsule called the "Spansule," which released the
contents evenly over up to twelve hours, leveling the initial rush of
drug into the bloodstream. The time-release Spansule was introduced
in 1952, and the Dexedrine Spansule was SKF's first product offered in
that form, giving the firm's amphetamine a unique claim to superiority (all the firm's amphetamine products would soon be offered in
Spansule form). Dexedrine sales, flat from 1949 to 1952, doubled in the
next two years to $11 million. Obviously many doctors and ampheta-
mine users liked it, whether for weight loss or depression. Dexedrine
was probably used more for dieting, judging by the information manual SKF distributed for doctors prescribing the drug (which gave the
most space to weight loss). If so, it may seem surprising that SKF
chose to advertise the product at least as heavily for depression in
general medicine journals during the early 1950s, stressing how Dexedrine was "the antidepressant of choice" and the best way to "lift your
patient from depression and help restore him to an effective place in
society."[14] An explanation for this focus may lie in the fact that the majority of prescription amphetamine pills that flooded the market when
Alles's patents expired in 1949 targeted weight loss—once-famous
products like Obedrin, Biphetamine, and AmPlus (with added vitamins) (Figure 23). Since competitors ruled much of the obesity territory whereas SKF had a greater edge on the competition in psychiatric
amphetamine use from a decade of carefully cultivating this market
segment, mental health–oriented marketing efforts might have been a
more efficient use of resources for increasing SKF's sales of Dexedrine
and other amphetamine products after 1949.

There was plenty of room for amphetamine's psychiatric prescription uses to develop further, but the drug's pharmacology presented a
basic problem in the anxiety and agitation it often causes.[15] The other
new product that put SKF back on top of the speed business after 1950
overcame this obstacle, though it, too, was not a new amphetamine,

chemically speaking. The product was Myerson's brainchild. Back in the mid-1930s, Myerson had tested Benzedrine in combination with sedatives on "cooperative and passive" schizophrenics at Boston State psychopathic hospital. The amphetamine would wake patients heavily sedated with barbiturates, just as it woke sedated guinea pigs. More surprising, some of Myerson's patients became more talkative and rational under the combined influence of the two drugs, as if they briefly woke from their deep mental illness as well as their sleep. The effect seemed strongest when the particular sedative used was amobarbital, best-known as a sleeping pill sold by Lilly under the brand name Amytal. So the two opposing drugs apparently did not cancel each other out altogether, even though Benzedrine stimulation did reverse the sleep-inducing effect of the barbiturate. Alongside the mood-elevating effect of amphetamine, there remained amobarbital's inhibition-loosening effect (the very effect that made barbiturate abuse so popular with everyone from GIs to juvenile delinquents).[16]

Myerson quickly followed up with a placebo-controlled trial of amphetamine-amobarbital combination therapy on various less hopeless cases, including some of his own depressed clients and moderately to seriously depressed inpatients at Boston's elite Mclean Hospital. Results on the symptoms of depression surpassed those from amphetamine alone, claimed Myerson, and the combination therapy was safe and broadly effective when carefully supervised. Thanks to the synergy of the drugs in combination, patients could have the best of both worlds—the calming effects of barbiturates without grogginess or heavy sedation, and the mood-elevating effects of amphetamine without jitters and sleeplessness.[17] Perhaps the idea of a single pill to treat both generalized anxiety and lack of "energy feeling" excited Myerson because it fit his theories so well: both symptoms were manifestations of anhedonia, he believed. Myerson promoted this discovery in the scientific literature before the war, convincing a few other psychiatrists to try the "mutually correcting" amphetamine/barbiturate combined therapy. Myerson also tried to interest SKF, but for nearly a decade the firm remained cautious about marketing the two drugs in combination as a product.[18]

Meyerson's idea of a calming antidepressant was only slightly ahead of its time. With the end of the war, the amobarbital-amphetamine combination was starting to look like a profitable product to SKF management. The experiences and attitudes of the thousands of psychiatrists who served in the U.S. Army represent one key reason why its prospects had changed. After initial skepticism, the military had come to regard psychiatry as highly valuable, and during the war psychiatrists of all stripes were drafted to staunch the massive loss of manpower to combat fatigue. A therapeutic approach that distinguished itself on the front was the use of barbiturates, together with hypnosis, to help shocked soldiers recall the terrible battlefield experiences that lay at the root of their incapacity. After breaking through patients' self-censorship with the sedatives, the psychiatrists could use talking therapies to restore the men to some degree of sanity—and then return them to their units. For this "narcosynthesis" or "narcoanalysis" technique, amobarbital was the most popular barbiturate drug.[19] Entering the prime of their careers immediately after the war, this generation of American psychiatrists was more strongly influenced by Sigmund Freud's ideas than any generation before or since. Freud's basic concept was that virtually all mental illnesses result from suppression of traumatic experiences, especially those of childhood, and inappropriate channeling of sexual drives. Many of the young psychiatrists perceived no great conflict between narcosynthesis and Freudian theory; indeed, the two could be nicely harmonized. Talk was the cure for all neurotic conditions, "neuroses" being defined (for Freudians) as unconscious conflicts. Therefore, anything—even drugs—that sufficiently loosened up patients to talk about their inner conflicts was good for psychoanalysis. Still part of the eclectic and pragmatic American tradition, many psychiatrists in the late 1940s were not afraid to mix narcotherapy and psychoanalysis, pills and penis envy. Pharmaceuticals for psychoanalysis could not have represented a very large market, but some drug firms did market amphetamines explicitly for this purpose, perhaps for prestige value (Figure 24).[20]

A second key change was the transformed general perception of psychiatry. In postwar United States, psychiatry was not just a medical specialty enjoying newly improved status but a national obsession. As noted, medical authorities pronounced that at least "one in ten Americans is now mentally ill or will become so during his lifetime," and, still worse, the trend was accelerating.[21] People flocked to psychiatrists, and many Americans experienced Freudian psychoanalysis firsthand. The unconscious mind and the various ways in which

Freud's theories described its actions—anal retention, oral fixation, the Oedipus complex, the Ego and the Id—all became household words. Alternative psychological theories also shared the limelight with Freud in America's fascination with mental instability, triggering therapeutic fads like the "orgone accumulators" of Wilhelm Reich, with which Burroughs was much enamored. Neuroses now seemed to be everywhere, but the more serious, psychotic mental disorders represented a public threat of even greater urgency. Quite simply, mental illness was crushing the American hospital system. More than half the nation's hospital beds were already occupied by mental patients, and since psychotics usually remained hospitalized for the rest of their lives once admitted, they would soon leave no room for anyone else. The wish to do something about these permanent residents of the back wards and asylums motivated a surge in lobotomy, or "psychosurgery," during the late 1940s. On the national level, politicians responded to the twin crises of psychosis and neurosis by creating the National Institute of Mental Health (NIMH) to investigate and cure psychological problems from schizophrenia to juvenile delinquency. The anxieties created by the Cold War, well under way by the end of the 1940s and threatening everyone everywhere with sudden unnatural destruction (as symbolized, perhaps, by the rampaging giant ants and radioactive rabbits of B-grade films), only amplified the sense of rising madness.[22]

A third factor boosting the commercial potential of Myerson's product idea after 1945 was the situation of general practitioners. Now that tens of millions of Americans needed to see a psychiatrist, according to the experts, there were not nearly enough psychiatrists to go around. General practitioners heard from every corner that they should take up the slack by paying more attention to their patients' neurotic conditions and address these with a simple form of talking therapy. But whatever general practitioners may have thought about the causes of neurotic conditions and the Freudian approach to treatment, they never abandoned their way of dealing with psychosomatic complaints using bromides and tonics. As noted above, the great majority of physician visits in the 1940s and 1950s ended with a prescription, and barbiturate and bromide sedatives were still the drugs most commonly prescribed. After all, a good placebo makes a patient feel that her doctor is doing something, and a patient so convinced may heal herself or put up with symptoms until they go away on their own. [23] Writing a prescription takes less time than listening to a patient's life story.

Thus, psychiatric experts were telling general practitioners that even more of their patients had psychosomatic problems than they already suspected, general practitioners were still sending patients home with prescriptions, and patients were still benefiting from the magic of the placebo effect. If, in this postwar era of psychiatric sophistication, antique bromides remained best sellers, so much the better if family doctors could prescribe a pill that (experts agreed) would actually relieve depression and anxiety, "scientifically" doing the job of a tonic and a bromide in one. No wonder a barbiturate- and amphetamine-based drug to treat a broad range of neurotic conditions began to look like a good business prospect in the late 1940s.

A fourth factor changing SKF's position was that, at some point in 1945, the firm adopted distinctive amphetamine combination drugs as a commercial and legal strategy for dealing with the impending expiration of Alles's patent. "SKF would have stronger sales position after Benzedrine patent expires if it could introduce as many 'combination products' as possible," or so the thinking in the sales department went; a "good combination has far greater stick." It was important to make new products as distinctive as possible, both in composition and appearance, so as not to be easily imitated by the new amphetamine pills expected from competitors.[24] (One might cynically suggest that combination drugs could be expected to "stick" best when both ingredients are addictive, but the addictiveness of amphetamine was not yet widely accepted).

As a final overarching factor one could cite, albeit speculatively, the new cultural climate around getting and spending prevailing in the United States ever since the wartime boom abruptly replaced the Great Depression in 1940–41. As one Philadelphia jeweler summed up the atmosphere created by full employment, ready cash, and pent-up consumer demand that he encountered in 1942, "people are crazy with money . . . they don't care what they buy . . . they purchase things just for the fun of spending." This vibrant wartime consumerism evolved into a postwar era of insecure, almost desperate, material aspiration as masses moved to new suburban homes with the new cars and refrigerators they had dreamed about in their foxholes and munitions factories.[25] Compared to the austere Depression years, the new climate would offer circumstances more favorable to Myerson's amphetamine-friendly anhedonia concept of depression, in which insufficiently vigorous pursuit of pleasure and material reward counted as mental illness. After all, only against a background of affluence could failure to enjoy oneself become a plausible standard of "abnormal" conduct.

Thus, for a complex set of reasons probably typical of what drives the introduction of new pharmaceuticals—considerations ranging from therapeutic promise to trends in medicine to legal problems to commercial expedience to cultural climate—SKF began to move forward with Myerson's combination amphetamine idea in 1946 and 1947. In early 1947, top SKF management asked Myerson for a detailed account of what he envisioned for the possible new product and, in particular, why amobarbital had to be the barbiturate in the combination since it did not seem special in animal experiments. Myerson pointed out that he and other psychiatrists found amobarbital best for releasing inhibitions and increasing "tranquility" and "communicativeness" in their patients, effects that cannot be measured in animals. Myerson could not have been more enthusiastic that SKF was finally taking seriously the idea he had been pushing since 1940. How common were the neuroses and other psychiatric conditions that might be treated with the combination therapy? The "sky is the limit," replied Myerson; the proposed product perfectly suited the anxiety and depressive conditions that had become "the most common diseases of the human being." Myerson also assured the firm that, with the rising general awareness of psychiatric problems, general practitioners as well as psychiatrists would prescribe the new combination.[26]

Some of the scientific staff within the firm, and likewise Alles, harbored misgivings because this combination drug idea seemed to come from "clinical trial and error" alone. Not only did it seem impossible to conduct animal experiments showing how amobarbital increased "communicativeness," but the animal evidence they did have indicated that the stimulating effects of the amphetamine and amobarbital's sedative effects would peak at different times when taken in combination. Alles thought he might be able to invent a new barbiturate drug with the same duration of action as amphetamine, as well as a greater relaxing effect without inducing sleep. He continued trying well into 1949, but the best relaxant drug candidate he found in more than a year of research caused severe itching. Time was too short to wait for more science: SKF needed a next-generation antidepressant to sell when the amphetamine patent expired in 1949, so in 1948 the development of "DEXAM" (as the dextroamphetamine-amobarbital combination became known within the firm) moved into high gear.[27]

These feverish efforts took place even as SKF was preparing to introduce a separate amphetamine-barbiturate combination, one that did not employ amobarbital. This product's life began with market research data around 1940 indicating that a lot of prescriptions were being written for amphetamine—to SKF's alarm not specifying "Benzedrine"—plus phenobarbital, another barbiturate sedative to reduce the insomnia and jitters, but with a long duration of action closer to amphetamine's. The marketing people at SKF proposed a combination that would capture the business from these prescriptions, some of which must have gone to the generic bootleggers as they proliferated during the war. SKF tested the waters with a phenobarbital-amphetamine combination pill in 1941 but found it difficult to recruit doctors to do clinical research with the experimental product. Noting also that each patient seemed to need a different dosage of the two drugs, the firm soon abandoned the idea.[28] (This way of trying out a new drug idea nicely illustrates how sponsorship of medical research not only helps companies generate studies proving effectiveness, but also helps them conduct preliminary market research about the likely popularity of potential products.) After the war, SKF revived the idea and launched this combination product in 1949 as "Benzebar." Marketed as an antidepressant suitable for relieving the agitation of menopause and restoring "emotional equilibrium for the geriatric patient," Benzebar was purely a stopgap measure.[29] Its replacement already waited in the wings, almost ready to launch.

The firm confidently expected market acceptance of DEXAM, based not just on Myerson's opinion. SKF's procedure for planning the new product reflects the transitional nature of the drug business in the late 1940s, when companies were growing more bureaucratic and federal regulation more demanding. After a high-level policy committee in the firm decided that DEXAM held both commercial and medical promise, in mid-1947 SKF moved to the next stage, a combined exercise in preliminary marketing and clinical research. For this, SKF prepared a promotional circular announcing that it would soon introduce an experimental dextroamphetamine-amobarbital combination "for treatment of the psychoneuroses," citing Myerson's research articles as the scientific rationale, and both offering sample tablets and asking for reactions. Sent to fifty-five selected doctors this "mail hawk"—the informal term revealing how closely related such research was to "hawking"—netted fifty-one responses, none of them negative. Based largely on this feedback, the medical department then approved preliminary clinical trials. Research managers arranged for doctors, some familiar and some new to collaboration with SKF, to try the drug out in studies of varying formality. The work of these clinical experimenters was closely monitored by the firm, and it was the continuing positive signals from them that kept DEXAM moving toward the drugstore shelves.[30]

In April 1948, SKF already had half a dozen doctors at work on clinical trials with DEXAM. There was one obesity expert, as well as four general practitioners and psychiatrists trying it for mental health problems of various types. Myerson, too, appears to have been experimenting with it on his own for neuroses, and also for epilepsy with a colleague at Boston State. In these clinical trials, the doctors addressed questions that were marketing issues as much as medical issues. For instance, the DEXAM development team wanted the medical department to recruit enough psychiatrists and general practitioners to obtain a reasonable sample of opinion from both on whether one dosage form would be sufficient. (Initially, pills were prepared with 5 mg dextroamphetamine combined with either a low 0.5 grain or a high 1.5 grain dose of amobarbital). Toward the end of the year many results were available.[31] Charles Burn, a University of Pennsylvania psychiatrist, thought DEXAM was better for mild depression than Dexedrine alone, because it improved "communicativeness" in both hospital and private outpatients. Herbert Gaskill, from the Penn psychiatry clinic, reported that DEXAM appeared to help twenty-seven of thirty-seven assorted inpatients, mostly seriously depressed manic-depressives as well as some involutional melancholics (a type of major depression rarely reported today). Surprisingly, in Gaskill's hands, the mildly depressed neurotic patients seemed to benefit less than more severe cases. This finding did not fit SKF's general practice plans for the drug, and received no response from the firm. Much more welcome were results reported by Philadelphia general practitioner Henry Grahn, from thirty-five of his patients given DEXAM for conditions other than obesity. He found the drug extremely valuable for all forms of distress among his patients, and he particularly appreciated the effect it had in cheering up terminal cancer patients, judging DEXAM a miracle drug even more important than penicillin.[32] By the beginning of 1949, SKF had ample evidence to submit for both AMA and FDA approval to market the new combination drug for neurotic depressions.

The obesity results looked good, too. A close look at the history of this particular company-sponsored trial provides insight into how major drug firms interacted at the time with typical clinical researchers— as opposed to superstars like Myerson—in order to generate the kind of medical science they could use. Ella Roberts, a metabolic specialist and faculty member at the University of Pennsylvania, was one of the fifty-five doctors targeted in SKF's 1947 "mail hawk." Although the original SKF circular had emphasized DEXAM for psychiatric uses, she had tried the sample tablets on anxious, obese patients for whom the stimulation of Benzedrine and Dexedrine alone was undesirable. Her patients liked the drug, and they lost weight. In November 1947, Roberts contacted Charles Killen of SKF's medical staff proposing a study that the firm might like to sponsor. Roberts suggested that, since obesity is often connected to anxiety and other neurotic conditions, a drug that helps reduce appetite, depression, and anxiety all at once would be better than any diet drug that neglected mood. This idea must have sounded promising to SKF, because after talking it over with Killen, Roberts drew up plans. The firm's medical staff thus tactfully acted as a go-between for management; outside doctors would mainly negotiate with physicians working for SKF, whom they would have seen as collaborators in clinical science rather than businessmen issuing orders.

According to the study planned with Killen, Roberts would compare a standard reducing diet to this diet plus DEXAM on patients at Philadelphia Woman's Hospital. Patients from the Diabetic Clinic, which she managed, would be compared to similar non-diabetic patients, and the sugar tolerance and metabolic rates of all patients would be monitored (to determine if DEXAM made a difference to either). SKF would cover the cost of the patients' laboratory tests (estimated at $300 for six months), and reimburse the hospital for extra clerical and nursing labor to record the data (estimated at only $130 for six months). Roberts's own efforts would earn her a $450 "physician's service fee." She would use special forms from SKF for recording data for each patient. Furthermore, according to the bargain, neither SKF nor Roberts could publish the results except by mutual agreement, and, after three months, all the preliminary data would be sent to the firm for evaluation. If SKF did not like the results, it could discontinue the study at that point. Since $880 seemed a reasonable price, and SKF could prevent publication if they decided not to market DEXAM or if the outcome was unfavorable, and since the trial might well produce a favorable result, the arrangements satisfied the firm.[33] If there ever was a golden age in which doctors conducting clinical research with drug company funding could expect to pursue and publish the truth without corporate interference, it was clearly not the late 1940s (which, as we have seen, were no better than the 1930s for academic freedom or for the full reporting of patient outcomes in clinical trials).

Roberts's study yielded weight-loss results good enough to use for advertising, and also to publish. From her trial, Grahn's, and others', SKF management concluded in January 1949 that DEXAM would sell. The product seemed "acceptable to psychiatrists in spite of the fact that they try to minimize the use of and dependence on drugs," and, second, the product "should be accepted by the G.P. [general practitioner] for a wide variety of conditions if our copy is carefully directed to them." SKF went ahead with plans for submission to the FDA, for a possible national launch onto the market late that year.[34]

Some serious product design issues still had to be resolved. One was whether a single strength of the drug combination would do. SKF decided to go with the low-strength barbiturate version only, much more popular among the doctors who had tried the experimental product. Another issue was the use of Lilly's trade name "Amytal" for the amobarbital, since this was the name most recognized by doctors. Lilly proved easy to persuade; they allowed SKF use of their brand name in exchange for a small share of royalties and, furthermore, SKF would buy the amobarbital from Lilly. After some concern that "Dexam" would not be a good name because it too closely resembled that of another trademarked drug, SKF chose "Dexamyl" as the brand name for the new product, evoking the powerful brands Dexedrine and Amytal together.[35]

Another key issue was what the new tablet should look like. Looks mattered immensely. Not only might the shape and color of a pill affect its perceived potency among both doctors and patients, but appearance was a crucial defensive weapon against the competition. This thinking came from the legal department: SKF spent considerable time and money fighting court cases against firms infringing on Alles's patent. As we have seen with the cases of Clark & Clark, SKF had prevailed against the so-called bootleggers largely because the infringers' products were designed to look like SKF amphetamine tablets, making this a matter of unfair competition and not just patent law. A triangular, blue tablet with a groove down the center, resembling a heart, was chosen as distinctive enough to protect the new Dexamyl product—or, rather, to make it easier to challenge the imitators that would inevitably come. Dexedrine, too, was changed to a yellow heart-shaped tablet for the same reason, and Benzedrine to a pink heart-shaped tablet.[36]

Out of fear that competition would destroy Dexedrine's lucrative sales once Alles's patent expired, SKF's strategy called for switching as much Dexedrine business to Dexamyl as possible, both because of the product's inherent appeal (less jitters thanks to the barbiturate) and "stick," and also because of its greater legal defensibility against imitators as a novel and distinctive (though not patentable) product. The only worries the firm had about "pushing hard" to move all amphetamine customers to Dexamyl were the danger of narcotics regulations and the growing medical resistance to routine use of barbiturates. As we saw in the "goofball" control measures that grew increasingly widespread during the 1940s, barbiturates were now recognized as addictive and were subject to special constraints, so marketing approaches would have to remain mindful that this component of Dexamyl was not considered harmless. Thus, like any modern industrial product, the new drug was engineered not just for its pharmacological action but also for its entire social context, positioning both the user and the maker advantageously within it.[37] Dexamyl went much further than most products, however, in altering the user's state.

A General Practitioner's Answer to the Cold War

SKF launched Dexamyl on the national market in late 1950 with heavy promotion and full-page advertisements in the largest medical journals (Figure 25). The campaign's key message was that the "balanced combination of 'Dexedrine' and 'Amytal'" constituted a "remarkable new preparation for relieving mental and emotional distress," and was "widely useful in everyday practice." The direct-mail campaign consisted of letters addressed to "Dear Doctor," explaining how the "smooth and profound antidepressant action" of Dexedrine combined with the unsurpassed "calming action" of Amytal would relieve all sorts of "mental and emotional distress." The letter also urged doctors to try the enclosed bright blue, heart-shaped tablets; whether the Dexamyl samples should be tried by the doctor or his patients it does not say.[38]

And, of course, the sales force of SKF "detail men" distributed plenty of glossy brochures. One brochure, for example, displayed on its cover a frayed rope and the legend "for the management of everyday mental and emotional distress . . . Dexamyl tablets." The second page pictured the rope binding two hands, with the legend "anxiety and depression are usually tied together." Inside one finds a lengthy description of why the combination of amobarbital, "the sedative that improves mood," and Dexedrine, "the antidepressant of choice," is the best possible drug for managing "everyday" psychological problems encountered by the general practitioner (as in cases of family strife, financial crisis, menstrual distress, obesity, and old age). It goes on to urge Dexamyl as the right remedy for emotional distress whether or not accompanied by any identifiable medical condition (beyond distress itself), because the "unique normalizing effect" stemming from the "synergy" between the barbiturate and the amphetamine relieves the anxieties that cause all psychosomatic complaints. Little explicit theory justifies all these claims for Dexamyl, but the references to anxiety as the root cause strike a Freudian note, and the brochure cites a 1947 article by Myerson on how anxiety and depression both stem from anhedonia.[39]

Dexamyl essentially was positioned as the drug for the family doctor to prescribe whenever there was little else he could do. The confluence of cultural trends perfectly set the stage for Dexamyl's explosion onto the medical scene. Now that it was authoritatively recognized that general practitioners had to deal with vast numbers of emotionally driven complaints every day, and now that these were considered real medical problems even if psychosomatic, the door had been opened for drug companies to sell new drugs for psychosomatic distress with the full authorization of science. Dexamyl's potential was virtually boundless, and for five years the product would dominate this rich market almost unchallenged.

Grahn's study on treating everyday distress targeted the general practitioner with the concept in the popular *American Practitioner*. Published almost in perfect synchrony with Dexamyl's launch, the article described Dexamyl's use with eighty-five of his patients suffering neurotic anxiety or depression, reporting that the drug "in almost every case" brought excellent or very good results. Grahn offered no statistics or quantitative analyses, but he detailed three typical cases helped by Dexamyl. One was a fifty-five-year-old telephone lineman who became depressed after abdominal surgery. Another was a forty-seven-year-old "white American female of a high type" approaching menopause. The third patient was a thirty-three-year-old welder who dealt with his long-standing depression through alcoholic binges every weekend, and whose life was sliding downhill until he turned around his marriage and work problems after a few months on Dexamyl. Almost an old-fashioned testimonial, Grahn's report suggested no limits to the drug's value for patients suffering "emotional distress," whether based in depressive personality or triggered by life events (like surgery or menopause). "This is a Dexamyl age," Grahn pronounced in his conclusion, "an age of unrest; probably no other period in history has been dominated by a mood of uncertainty and disquiet."[40] Perhaps he had a point. A sedative antidepressant could well have been just the right prescription in 1950 for a postwar United States craving civilian comfort but unable to barricade itself completely against the monsters of atomic war, communism, and domestic disharmony.

Roberts's much more formal and quantitative article on Dexamyl soon followed Grahn's into print. In the prestigious *Annals of Internal Medicine,* she reported how the drug helped sixty-four patients (sixty of them women) previously unable to lose weight on a diet alone. Almost all of them lost weight on Dexamyl, saying enthusiastic things like "I can follow my diet now that I don't get starving hungry." Furthermore, Roberts reported no problems using Dexamyl with diabetics, nor did she observe tolerance or addiction in the three months covered by the study. Notably the paper did not report the second three months planned for the study. If Roberts's findings with amphetamine were typical, she would have found that weight loss did not continue after the first months and that patients were taking increasing doses just to stave off hunger—that is, patients were developing tolerance.[41]

The paper as published also showed another interesting deviation from initial plans. Although Roberts herself considered the psychiatric effects of the drug just as important as its appetite-suppressing action for helping overweight people with their emotional difficulties surrounding food, the publication only described weight loss and said nothing about mental health. Probably SKF preferred a simple result supporting Dexamyl's use for weight loss no matter what the patient's mental state, just as Grahn's omission of obese patients in his paper reflected the firm's wish for a sharp focus on everyday neuroses. Nevertheless, Dexamyl advertisements were soon extolling the drug's effectiveness for obesity especially when psychological distress figured among the causes. In other words, according to the ads, the drug reduced food intake directly by its action on appetite, and indirectly by improving the neurotic conditions that drive overeating, much as Roberts had thought.[42]

It is impossible for the historian to recapture the private experience of those who received Dexamyl prescriptions from their family doctor during the 1950s. However, we can get a sense of who got the drug for what complaints from the illustrative cases in early Dexamyl marketing material, since these must have rung true with the many doctors who prescribed it for everyday "mental and emotional distress." One glossy brochure presented five "Dexamyl case histories—with thirty photographs" of supposedly real patients "from the files of a Philadelphia General Practitioner" (likely Grahn). One patient was a "sensitive and reflective" thirty-eight-year-old mother of two teenagers, prone to anxiety and irritability. Dexamyl cheered and "soothed her" so much that it has "thus far given her family a two months' vacation." The second was a seventy-five-year-old man who worked two or three times harder than anybody else in his accounting firm, giving himself ulcers and palpitations in the process, for fear he might be replaced by a younger man. Dexamyl relieved the anxieties of this elderly workaholic. A third was an emotionally volatile, fifty-two-year-old "menopausal matron" of the sort "found in every physician's practice," obese from eating just to fill the empty hours. "Dexamyl brought this feminine dynamo under control . . . raised her from despair, and eliminated her nervous overeating," and made domestic life "safe again for her husband." A fourth was an overweight, thirty-six-year-old unmarried woman, a secretary in an insurance firm whose "whole life revolves about that job." On Dexamyl she lost forty-seven pounds, felt less of her perpetual fatigue and palpitations, and much less "nervousness." Finally, there was a twenty-four-year-old, "easily upset" and nervous "newlywed" man, whose rocky marriage was making him an insomniac, error-prone at work, and highly irritable. Dexamyl "provided a poultice for the wound of nervous uncertainty," helping to "elevate his ego and debunk his feeling of inferiority" so that he could sleep regularly once again and perform well at work. Alone among the five, this man was able to stop taking Dexamyl; the pseudo-Freudian jargon suggests that this case aimed to appeal to psychoanalytically inclined doctors who saw insight rather than pills as the main game.[43]

Evidently, Dexamyl was suitable for patients young and old, male and female, single and married, of all dispositions and classes. The most prominent Dexamyl journal ads in 1951–53 followed the same theme, depicting patients in "un-posed photographs" during an "actual interview" with their physician, again said to be a Philadelphia general practitioner. Like the "real-life examples" in the marketing brochures, these advertisements promised that Dexamyl could help doctors ease their patients' marital strife, their difficulties in the workplace, even their objectionable hygiene and habits.[44] By the same token, the pill promised to help people live up to the demands of their social circumstances and families.

Especially after 1954, when Dexamyl came out in Spansule form, sales of the product rose dramatically and began to rival Dexedrine's despite its later start. Paying the ultimate compliment to Dexamyl's prospects and to its creators, SKF's competitors soon offered copycat versions of Dexamyl, like Abbot's Desbutal (methamphetamine with pentobarbital) and Ambar from Robins (methamphetamine with phenobarbital). Amphetamine prescribing patterns during the 1950s in the United States are hard to determine, but better information is available for Britain thanks to some key research done there around 1960. Though all such extrapolations are imperfect, the British findings are probably a fair guide to contemporary medical amphetamine use in America, given the similarities in culture and in medical practice, and given that amphetamines accounted for about 3 percent of all prescriptions at pharmacies in both countries at the time. (If anything, numbers derived from British surveys are likely to underestimate American medical amphetamine consumption, because prescribing rates were a little higher and also for reasons discussed more fully later).[45]

In 1960, enough prescriptions for amphetamines were filled to keep 1.5 percent of the population of the Newcastle area on two tablets daily. These numbers only speak to how much drug was prescribed in that city, not how many or what kind of people were getting amphetamines. A British follow-up study based in the same time and place surveyed general practitioners to gain information on the prevalence of amphetamine use and the characteristics of amphetamine patients. Two tablets containing 5 mg amphetamine daily was the typical prescription, and Dexamyl (called Drinamyl in Britain) was the most prescribed amphetamine product. About a third of the amphetamine prescriptions were for weight loss, another third for clear-cut psychiatric disorders (depression, anxiety), and the remaining third for ambiguous, mostly psychiatric and psychosomatic complaints (lack of confidence, tiredness, nonspecific pain). Thirty-six- to forty-five-year-olds dominated, and 85 percent of all amphetamine patients were women. Therefore, even setting aside weight-loss prescriptions on the simplifying assumption that they were entirely for women, doctors were giving women more than three times as many psychiatric amphetamine prescriptions as men.[46]

This means that around 1960 women were twice as likely as men to get an amphetamine prescription to adjust their mental state *per doctor visit*, even taking into account that women seek medical attention more often. (Female patients accounted for up to 1.5 times as many general practitioner office visits as men at the time.) As British investigators put it, the typical user was indeed a "middle-aged housewife"—also the main consumer of tranquilizers in the United States, as feminist critics of American medicine would point out in the 1970s.[47] The predominant feminist explanation at that time, that a largely male medical profession in a male-dominated society treats unhappiness with the female social role as a medical condition, and thus keeps women in their place, still has a lot to recommend it. (Dexamyl advertising at least cannot be blamed for the imbalance, since it often urged prescription of the drug to men.) However, we must remember patient initiative: people unable to escape their social roles might well prefer chemical relief to nothing. And unlike tranquilizers with their tendency to promote passivity, amphetamines would if anything increase chances that a woman might take action to change her oppressing and depressing circumstances. Indeed, heavy amphetamine users tended to break free of social constraints in extreme ways, as we soon will see.

Among all amphetamine products, by 1960 Dexamyl had achieved a commanding position in the general practice psychiatric market, despite a host of competitors. [48] In addition to the way its barbiturate component took the edge off amphetamine and achieved more desirable effects with anxious patients, Dexamyl's phenomenal success in the 1950s must also have stemmed from the way the product's marketing tapped into trends in primary care. As already noted, one of the most significant trends in postwar medicine was recognition that milder (neurotic) psychiatric conditions drove a huge number of doctor visits, and that anxiety was an essential aspect of neurosis. Primary-care authorities in the 1950s, for instance, the textbook authors John Fry and Watts and Watts, commonly endorsed barbiturates, amphetamine, or amphetamine-barbiturate combinations for relief of the symptoms of mild depression or other emotional disturbances. Psychiatric specialists writing on general practice also endorsed these drug approaches, such as Frederick Lemere of the University of Washington. In a high-profile 1957 review in *JAMA*, Lemere described amphetamine along with methamphetamine and methyphenidate (Ritalin), then classed as a new amphetamine, as "the most helpful" medicines for depression—most of all in combinations like Dexamyl.[49]

Not that the psychiatric experts viewed amphetamine therapy as a true cure for mood disorders. Rather, the physician's sympathy and reassuring concern were understood as the main therapy for all neuroses and neurosis-driven complaints in family practice. But the amphetamine prescriptions did relieve symptoms of mild depression and thus alleviated many psychosomatic complaints, and also allowed for the placebo effect; that is, the pills bought time and communicated comfort, in the tradition of bromides. As the medical historians German Berrios and Christopher Callahan recently summed up the situation during the 1950s, then as now patients frequently saw doctors for emotional distress, and patients expected pills rather than just counseling (again, then as now). Instead of the bromides or tonics that general practitioners gave such patients in the 1920s, in the 1950s they gave them barbiturates and amphetamines. Today the same kind of patient gets the latest antidepressants.[50]

Grappling with the Dark Side of Speed

In the United States, Canada, the United Kingdom, and other nations where Benzedrine, Dexedrine, Dexamyl (or Drinamyl), and their imitators were marketed as a general practitioner's answer to both obesity and psychological distress, millions of patients probably did benefit in something like the advertised way. Dexamyl "worked" beautifully, satisfying patients and doctors alike, fulfilling amphetamine's psychiatric potential in the 1950s, and helping make SKF the industry leader in mental health drugs. During that decade, however, evidence for the harmful effects of amphetamine began to accumulate, as is so often the case after a pharmaceutical becomes popular and millions of patients use it. And as usual, when a onetime miracle drug enters the declining phase of its life, there was some delay before the negative effects began to be widely admitted by medicine.

The British studies of around 1960 already found strong evidence for a hard core of heavy and constant users of prescription amphetamines supplied by unwitting doctors and pharmacists. One Newcastle woman was using Drinamyl prescriptions for herself and three relatives simultaneously. Another brought her druggist a bottle full of white pills labeled with the Drinamyl prescription she had filled the night before, claiming that the man who filled her order gave her the wrong medicine. Naturally, she wanted the white pills replaced with heart-shaped blue Drinamyls. Some of these heavy users had been taking amphetamines for years; many had started with a normal prescription and worked themselves up to enormous daily doses.[51]

Data from the family doctors participating in the Newcastle studies indicated that 0.8 percent of the population they served received an amphetamine prescription during a three-month survey period, and that (in their doctors' judgments) up to a quarter of these mostly middle-aged amphetamine patients were "habituated or addicted"— in today's terms, dependent to some degree. The investigators calculated that about 0.2 percent of the total population was "habituated or addicted" at the time. They did not directly determine how many patients in the total population received amphetamine prescriptions in a year, but based on their data that figure almost certainly lies between 2 percent and 3 percent. If we assume that a total of about 2 percent of the total population received amphetamines by prescription in a year, then about 10 percent of those were dependent. If we assume the high but still plausible figure of 3 percent of the entire population instead of 2 percent receiving amphetamines in a given year, then their rate of dependency would be 6.7 percent.[52]

Another northern British study in the early 1960s experimentally investigated amphetamine dependency in this type of patient, trying to separate physical dependence or addiction from mere psychological dependence and the placebo effect (which the investigators treated as identical). Substituting look-alike placebo Dexamyl/Drinamyl tablets for this most popular of pills, or plain white tablets containing the same amobarbital and dextroamphetamine doses, it turned out that about one-third of these "habituated or addicted" Dexamyl patients were in fact "addicted" or physically dependent. This finding suggests extensive iatrogenic (i.e., medically caused) amphetamine addiction in the general population at the time: 2.2–3.3 percent of all patients receiving amphetamine prescriptions in a given year, or one-third of the 6.7–10 percent that were dependent. The estimate may be slightly high, to the extent that amphetamine and methamphetamine alone were less addictive as prescribed than Dexamyl. On the other hand, a very high proportion of amphetamines prescribed in general practice were combination products like Dexamyl—over 50 percent were Dexamyl itself in one of the Newcastle studies.[53] This rate of addiction to prescribed amphetamines can be extrapolated to the United States circa 1960 fairly safely, for the same reasons noted above: the similarities in retail prescribing rates at the time, and of medical practice and culture. So, between one in ten and one in fifteen Americans receiving a prescription for an amphetamine product from their family doctor must have been getting hooked, a third of them addicted physically.

While suspicions surrounding amphetamine's addictiveness started to build at the start of the 1960s, reports had long been mounting of a new mental disorder, known as "amphetamine psychosis." This terrifying illness did not confine itself just to the marginal populations who liked to eat inhalers. The alarming stories had begun as a trickle. By 1938, three of the first patients to take large and regular doses of Benzedrine, for their narcolepsy, had already developed psychological problems. One man went to the police for protection, believing that mysterious enemies were poisoning him and were conspiring against his family. In the mental ward, he went through a phase where he believed that snakes and alligators were in his bed, but after a few weeks without amphetamine he returned to normal. Another individual thought that he was constantly being watched, that people were plotting against him and saying things about him "with homosexual content." At first, psychiatrists mostly supposed that these narcoleptic patients were already suffering a hidden paranoid schizophrenia, which amphetamine merely "unmasked" or amplified.[54]

This explanation was becoming increasingly questionable by the end of the 1940s, as the trickle of these cases swelled into a steady stream. One forty-nine-year-old lawyer turned up in a Massachusetts mental facility in 1945 insisting that six cars regularly trailed him, that his son (who was serving in the military) communicated with him from an invisible helicopter overhead, and that the government was spying on him and testing his loyalty for a top-secret mission. The man had started taking Benzedrine tablets five years earlier in a successful effort to quit drinking, but he had gradually increased his intake to twenty-five of the tablets (250 mg) daily. A thirty-four-year-old bacteriologist from California, with both an M.D. and a Ph.D. and an important research job at a major drug company, sought help for his speed problem at a Boston hospital in the early 1950s. Several years earlier he had begun taking Benzedrine tablets to keep up with an increasing workload, to manage stress at home and in the office, and to stave off depression. His intake gradually increased, and he changed from Benzedrine to Dexedrine until, by the time he was admitted to the hospital, he was taking more than 200 mg each day (forty pills, a month's prescription for some), as well as barbiturates. The drugs changed his personality from quiet to aggressive and volatile, as when he once deflated his neighbors' tires to retaliate for some trivial slight. One thirty-two-year-old man turned up in a Kansas City hospital in the early 1950s complaining that his thoughts were being controlled telepathically and that he had been overhearing several of his acquaintances plotting against him. When he eventually calmed down, it emerged that he been taking amphetamine by prescription since 1945, for narcolepsy.[55] Joan Vollmer, with her theory that radioactive fallout was infecting her skin, and Monroe and Drell's patient at the Midwestern military prison, who thought the nurses were watching him through a periscope, had plenty of company now. The same attacks of paranoia and the belief that people were saying bad things about you ("ideas of reference," in technical psychiatric language) were springing up among long-term prescription amphetamine patients, just as they did among recreational consumers of Benzedrine Inhalers.

In 1958, British psychiatrist Philip Connell confronted the medical community with the inconvenient truth, in the form of a detailed study of amphetamine psychosis based on more than forty patients institutionalized for the condition. Although many were recreational users, more than a third of the patients Connell investigated had originally been prescribed amphetamine tablets by a doctor; thus, it could not be argued that the condition occurred only in deviant thrill seekers. The psychosis generally took time to develop, as patients took more and more of the drug, which in itself implied that amphetamine was not merely unmasking an existing madness. Although different people could withstand varying amounts before they cracked, too much amphetamine eventually resulted in the characteristic paranoid delusions of sinister voices emanating from toilet bowls, mysterious forces hatching evil plots, and spies following one's every move. The same kind of psychotic delusions afflicting a wide variety of personality types implied that they did not stem from a shared flaw or feature of the patients' characters. Instead, Connell argued, amphetamine psychosis could happen to anyone—the drug's doing, not the victim's fault. Further, virtually all the victims of amphetamine psychosis fully recovered a week or two after they stopped taking the drug, proving they had not been concealed schizophrenics all along.[56]

The drug's defenders were resilient, however, and could still argue that a character flaw caused most victims to start taking so much amphetamine in the first place, even if, as Connell showed, too much amphetamine can cause psychosis in anyone. As one Freud-influenced psychiatrist, Peter Knapp from Boston University, theorized in the early 1950s: activity is preferable to "annihilation" for the orally fixated, emotionally needy patient whose cravings for something to soothe a perpetual sense of inadequacy drove him or her to habitual amphetamine use. Abusers' brains might be biologically normal before they started taking too much amphetamine, but childhood had given them weak personalities. That neediness drove them to drug habituation and addiction, whether via prescriptions or inhaler cracking, which in turn drove them to consequences like amphetamine psychosis. With theories like this, which explained addiction by stigmatizing the victim, doctors could still cling to the idea that amphetamine was safe for most people.

Henry Grahn, the Philadelphia general practitioner who had so enthusiastically helped SKF launch Dexamyl, put the view well in a

1958 article: "It is truly remarkable that there are so few reports of amphetamine addiction," given how pleasant and frequently prescribed the drug then was. In thirty-two of his patients who had been given amphetamine over long periods, he only knew of one that developed symptoms of excessive use, but she was a former asylum patient who had already had extensive shock therapy. Grahn admitted that a few others had become dependent on the drug, or "habituated," but he claimed that amphetamine kept them healthy and productive. A heavy amphetamine habit is "caused by a factor in the individual's psychologic make-up that leads him to abuse the drugs rather than by any pharmacologic action of the drugs themselves," Grahn reasoned, echoing Knapp.[57] It would be a shame if medicine were deprived of so valuable a remedy just because a few weaklings and closet "psychopaths" could not handle it. The American medical community was not ready to give up amphetamines at the end of the 1950s, and would still not be ready a decade later. The drug remained the most convenient and effective way for family doctors to help distressed patients get on with their lives, and cheerfully.

Still, the mounting numbers of amphetamine users flowing into the emergency rooms and mental wards made a significant impression on medical science in the late 1950s. As researchers found that many psychosis victims had started on doctors' orders, and ended up taking ever greater doses of their prescription amphetamines just to maintain the same effects, amphetamine psychosis reopened the question of the drug's addictiveness. Two decades earlier, in 1938, shortly after SKF first marketed Benzedrine tablets, the firm had narrowly escaped having its new product's addictive qualities recognized. As we saw, they were saved thanks to the hardening of a distinction between drugs that were properly "addictive," in showing measurable physical withdrawal symptoms in the same way as heroin, versus those that were merely psychologically habit-forming. SKF had already done what it could to shore up this addiction-habituation distinction in the medical literature at the time.

Now, in the 1950s, a new definition of drug addiction was emerging, and one factor driving the change was that the old concept of "addiction" did not fit stimulants well. A broader concept of "drug dependency" was starting to replace it, backed by authorities in influential positions such as the World Health Organization (WHO) and the Clinical Research Center in Lexington, Kentucky, the former federal narcotics prison hospital. These experts considered that "dependency," the term that should be used instead of "addiction," was any "state of periodic or chronic intoxication" "detrimental to the individual and to society," characterized by "compulsion to continue taking the drug"; the common tendency "to increase the dose" suggested "physical dependence" on the drug in addition to "psychic dependence." The new concept was behavioral and hinged on impairment of function in a social context. Physical withdrawal symptoms, like the opiate addict's experience of tremors and sweating (which could be reproduced in lab animals), no longer defined the condition of "drug dependency" that had taken the place of "addiction." What mattered was a person's inability to stop using a substance that became central to his or her life. The WHO made the new view official in 1964–65.[58]

Although the medical profession was slow to absorb the message, by this newer definition amphetamines definitely counted as addictive —or, in the new terminology, "dependency-producing." Craving and tolerance to high amphetamine doses had actually long been reported in the medical literature but had been largely ignored by authorities who strictly adhered to the older idea of addiction modeled on heroin. As far back as 1940, two doctors had published letters in *JAMA* about patients who had become addicted to the Benzedrine they were prescribed for weight loss in one case, and for quitting drinking in the other. A dozen years and many published cases of addiction later, Knapp, who had also reported the case of the overworked Dexedrine-crazed microbiologist, described an insurance salesman who had been taking amphetamine for fifteen years. The man began taking Benzedrine after surgery to speed recovery, prescribed as suggested by SKF, and then over the years gradually worked his way up twenty to forty Dexedrines (100–200 mg) per day. Though he sometimes stopped taking the drug on weekends, he always resumed for the working week, because this salesman could not "meet the public" at work without amphetamine, and besides felt lethargic, insecure, and very "melancholic."[59] Again, we catch a glimpse of how social demands—of cheerful and outgoing salesmanship, of shapeliness, of superhuman productivity—played a role in making amphetamine popular among patients. However they may have started, people ended up stuffing down handfuls of pills or else switched to eating the cheaper inhalers, just to make it through their day. Depression was evidently a common withdrawal symptom from this antidepressant, creating a vicious cycle of dependency that, for many, ended in psychosis.

In the second half of the 1950s, then, there was abundant evidence that amphetamines were harmful; indeed, amphetamine displayed every feature of a dangerously dependency-producing substance, and the drug certainly could cause a paranoid psychosis. But even after the WHO and Connell, amphetamine still had staunch defenders, including general practitioners like Grahn and experts like Chauncey Leake, whose 1958 book *The Amphetamines* maintained that amphetamine and methamphetamine were not genuinely addictive, that negative psychiatric side effects were rare, and that amphetamines were tremendously versatile remedies. Speed remained "one of the fundamental drugs in medicine," as one Benzedrine advertising campaign put it, right through the 1950s and 1960s.[60] By 1960, at least 2 percent of the total population were actively taking the drugs on prescription, if we very conservatively extrapolate the British data to the United States. As physicians turned a blind eye to the illness they were creating and continued to feed the national appetite for amphetamines, that figure in the United States would reach 5 percent by the end of the decade.

Why did the growing evidence for the dependency-producing (or addictive) and "psychotoxic" (mind-poisoning) effects of amphetamines not cause American doctors to reject them as prescription medicines? One reason was that the old concept of addiction as defined by heroin-like withdrawal faded slowly, in the thinking of practicing physicians, causing them to underestimate the harms of amphetamine dependency. Another was that doctors saw the amphetamines as excellent pills to help patients cope with everyday depression and psychological distress, as we have seen, making the perceived benefits of amphetamines weigh heavily against the perceived risks and harms. And then there was pure expediency. No better antidepressant than amphetamine would become available until the 1960s, and none that would prove popular until much later. As for weight loss, it can be argued, no more effective drug would ever be found. Liking their pills, most patients went away satisfied customers, and so doctors were very reluctant to give up amphetamines. Nevertheless, the medical novelty and glamour was wearing off, as newer drugs became trendy —particularly in the psychiatric branch of medicine.

Riding High on Psychotropics

Alles's amphetamine products (including the decongestant hydroxy-amphetamine, never popular compared to amphetamine itself) accounted for about 30 percent of SKF's annual sales from 1949 to 1954 (Figure 26). Competition grew fierce after his patent expired, but through the 1950s the firm retained dominance of the amphetamine business in the U.S. and many other countries thanks to its powerful "Dexedrine" and "Benzedrine" brand names, its "Spansule" sustained-release capsule, and its combination products like Dexamyl and Edrisal (an amphetamine-codeine painkiller). SKF's marketing experience in psychiatric drugs was unmatched, because of the trail the firm had blazed with amphetamine beginning in the late 1930s.

In 1952 an opportunity to build on that success came when the French firm Rhone-Poulenc approached SKF with a new drug. Called chlorpromazine, it was an antihistamine, but it also produced strong effects on the central nervous system such as calmness and drowsiness. Rhone-Poulenc planned to sell it in Europe at the end of 1952 for three main uses: surgery, where it supposedly improved anesthesia and reduced post-surgical shock; nausea, especially among pregnant women; and psychiatry, since it seemed to soothe agitated mental patients. Lacking the means to market chlorpromazine in North America, Rhone-Poulenc sought a U.S. partner to handle it, in exchange for a percentage of sales. Boyer, who had just succeeded C. Mahlon Kline as SKF's president, saw promise; SKF was already seeking non-barbiturate sedatives that could be used as sleeping pills or as anti-anxiety drugs (perhaps to replace the amobarbital in Dexamyl), and chlorpromazine seemed a likely candidate. So SKF struck a bargain with Rhone-Poulenc and distributed the drug for clinical testing among the firm's network of collaborators in 1953, especially its testing for psychiatry.[61]

By early 1954, SKF started to see results from its chlorpromazine trials, and they looked good. Some reports were nothing short of amazing. In one mental institution trial on agitated psychotics, frenzied manic-depressives settled down and even catatonic schizophrenics relaxed. Both became much more cooperative and open to conversation, and, furthermore, they made more sense; that is, the patients actually appeared saner, not just subdued. Another study looked specifically at schizophrenic inpatients, finding that only a tenth failed to improve at all, and two-thirds got so much better that they were sent home. This result was revolutionary, since psychotic patients like these were just the sort overloading the state hospitals, and for whom little could be done (other than "psychosurgery," or lobotomy, a procedure then in its heyday). Chlorpromazine, moreover, showed promise outside the mental ward, in office psychiatry and general practice for quelling neurotic anxiety and obsessive tendencies. The FDA swiftly approved chlorpromazine, and SKF launched it on the market in 1954, under the brand name Thorazine.[62] Psychiatrists could hardly believe that a drug could turn an asylum from a prison into something much more like a real hospital; within a year, however, many did become believers as their worst cases seemed to wake from raving madness. Inmates were discharged in droves. Newspapers and magazines all hailed the miracle drug that was solving America's mental health crisis, and SKF's total sales jumped 40 percent from $65 million in 1954 to $92 million in 1955. At least $20 million of that gain must have come from Thorazine sales, about the same as prescription amphetamines. By 1956, 70 percent of SKF's sales came from drugs for mental conditions, with Thorazine now well ahead of amphetamine products. Basking in revenue and acclaim, in 1957 SKF became the second most profitable U.S. corporation in the *Fortune* 500.[63]

Amphetamine was no longer unique. Chlorpromazine was only the first of a new wave of "psychotropic" medications—drugs to alter the mind in specific ways—that transformed the medical landscape in the 1950s. America's obsession with mental health in the early Cold War years fueled not only an infatuation with Freud and psychoanalysis but also enormous enthusiasm for drugs to heal the mind. The period marks a high point in America's faith in science, thanks to world-changing novelties such as penicillin and atomic weapons; "better living through chemistry" was a motto more likely to be heard with hope than irony. This faith in the ability of science to remake the world no doubt explains the readiness with which chlorpromazine was welcomed as a miracle cure for schizophrenia. And there seemed no reason why the pharmaceutical chemists of America's drug industry should not soon cure every other mental illness. The boundless market for "mind drugs" signaled by Thorazine's success quickly launched a mad scramble among the other drug firms to catch up with SKF in this field. Merck decided to launch a crash program to find its own antipsychotic "major tranquilizers" (a drug category created to fit chlorpromazine) and other psychiatric drugs as early as June 1954 (more on this later).[64]

However, the best-selling new psychotropic medications of the later 1950s were not antipsychotics but "minor tranquilizers," calming drugs less powerful than chlorpromazine and purportedly more suitable for commonplace anxieties. In 1955 the first minor tranquilizer, Miltown, took America by storm, at roughly the same time that chlorpromazine was making headlines. Pharmacies had to ration the drug as demand outstripped supply. Daily tranquilizers to quell anxiety became a normal aspect of middle-class American culture, and soon all the drug firms had one for sale. As a number of historians have noted, the runaway success of the tranquilizers in the late 1950s has much to do with the way the drugs could be made to fit with the dominant Freudian psychiatric theory of the day. These drugs claimed to reduce anxiety, and, in Freudian theory, anxiety was not a distinct psychiatric condition but the universal sign of inner conflict. Therefore, anxiety-reducing tranquilizers could be suitable for any patient afflicted with neuroses, no matter what the nature of their particular psychological distress. (Amphetamines, as we shall soon see, were often viewed by psychiatrists as drive enhancers suitable for particularly repressed patients but certainly not for everyone.) Even psychoanalysts embraced the minor tranquilizers as an aid to talking therapies, much as they had embraced amphetamine a very few years before—but even more so. The main prescribers of the minor tranquilizers, however, were not psychiatrists but general practitioners and other primary care providers, who accounted for more than two-thirds of all psychotropic drug prescribing in the 1960s (a figure that has only declined since the 1980s). The same marketing strategies and trends in general practice that favored Dexamyl's success did the same for tranquilizers, making them the family doctor's new drug of choice for psychosomatic complaints.[65]

Three of the top ten most frequently prescribed drugs in the United States in 1955 were tranquilizers, major and minor.[66] In 1956, SKF felt the shock from this new trend toward tranquilization that it had helped create, as the firm's overall sales of amphetamine products plunged 40 percent from the previous year (Figure 26). Sales of minor tranquilizers continued booming right through the 1960s and beyond, even after Miltown was recognized as addictive and replaced with the benzodiazepenes (like Librium and Valium). Dexamyl had paved the way for Miltown, but by the second half of the 1950s amphetamines were left out of the limelight, as medicine focused on calming the anxious, conflicted soul, and less on lifting the spirits. That Dexamyl sales still rose and did not decline until the later 1960s (and remained a best seller until after 1975) testifies volumes to its tremendous "sticking power," the way it had become an indispensable part of the lives of hundreds of thousands of Americans.[67]

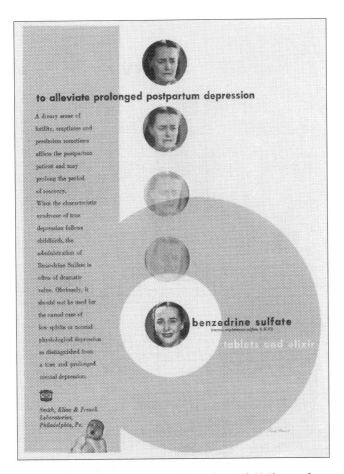

FIG. 19. Benzedrine advertising from the mid-1940s emphasized the many types of patient in general practice that could benefit from amphetamine's antidepressant action. Source: *JAMA*, June 6, 1945.

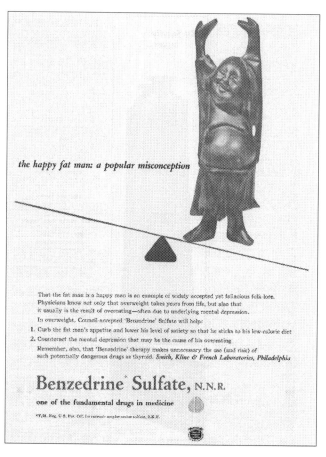

FIG. 20. Amphetamine became an officially approved diet medication in the late 1940s. Some advertising stressed the psychiatric causes of overeating as well as the dangers of even slight overweight. Source: *JAMA*, February 7, 1951.

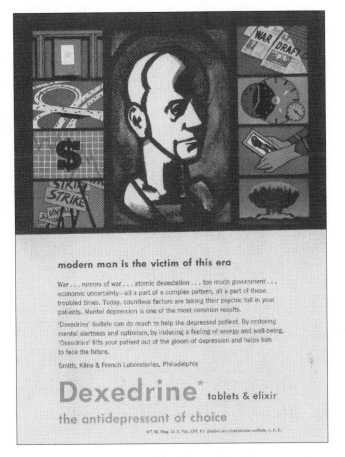

FIG. 21. In the mid-1940s sales of Dexedrine (dextroamphetamine) quickly outstripped sales of Benzedrine, despite less
intensive advertising both for weight loss and depression.
Source: *California Medicine*, September 1952

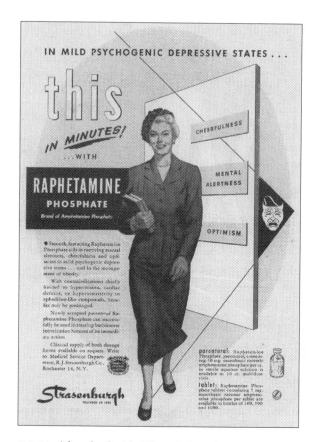

FIG. 22. After the Smith, Kline & French patents on amphetamine expired in 1949, other manufacturers produced competing antidepressants based on the drug. Source: *JAMA*, February 19, 1951.

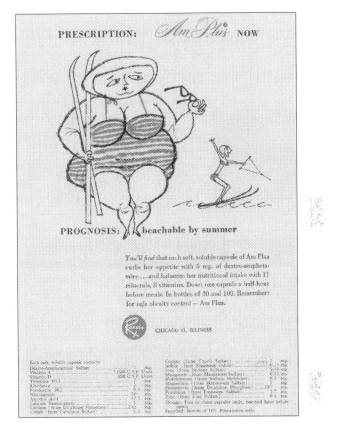

FIG. 23. After the expiration of Smith, Kline & French's patents on amphetamine, many other manufacturers entered the market with weight loss pills based on the drug, few of which stressed the psychiatric angle. Source: *California Medicine*, May 1955.

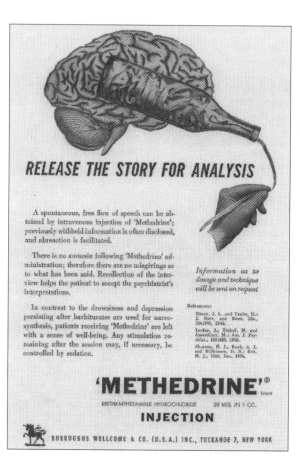

FIG. 24. Methamphetamine was marketed for both weight loss and depression in much the same ways as amphetamine was. Using the drugs to elevate mood and encourage talking was compatible with psychoanalysis, at least in the United States. Source: *American Journal of Psychiatry*, June 1952.

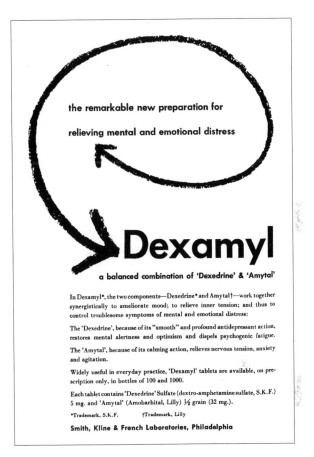

FIG. 25. In 1950, Smith, Kline & French released Dexamyl, a combination of dextroamphetamine and amobarbital, as an anxiety-reducing alternative to amphetamine for both depression and weight loss. Source: *American Journal of Medical Science*, December 1950.

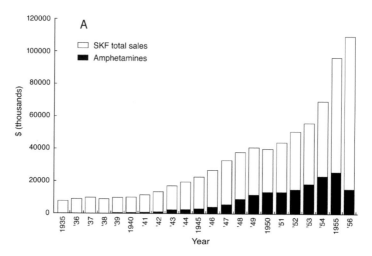

FIG. 26a. Smith, Kline & French total annual sales and annual sales of amphetamine products, excluding inhalers, but including all Benzedrine, Dexedrine, and Paradrine or hydroxyamphetamine products (hydroxyamphetamine products were never more than a minor fraction of amphetamine product sales). Source: *SKF vs. Alles* records, Smith, Kline & French's Answers to Defendant's Interrogatories, First Set, filed 26 February 1968, Exhibit 32.

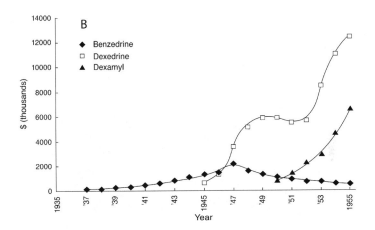

FIG. 26b. Smith, Kline & French annual domestic sales (excluding government sales) of Benzedrine tablets and spansules, Dexedrine tablets and spansules, and Dexamyl tablets and spansules. 1955 annual sales obtained by doubling sum of Q1 and Q2 sales. Sources: Anon., "Sales Record of 1-Phenyl-2-aminopropane Sulfate in Tablets" [1950?], GAP Box 11, folder: "SKF Accounting to Alles on Products 1936 to Date"; and Anon., "Summary of Royalties Payable and Amounts Paid" 1948–1955" [1955?], GAP Box 2, folder: "SKF vs. Alles Documents Received from Alles Office."

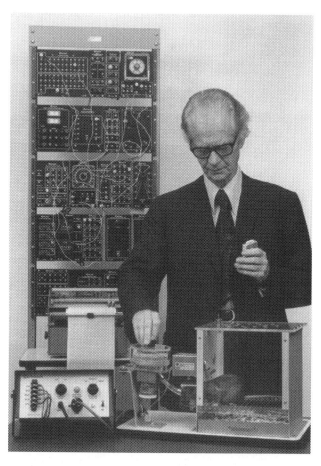

FIG. 27. The Harvard psychologist B. F. Skinner with a "Skinner Box" device, which he helped adapt for the drug industry's search for new antidepressants in the late 1950s. Courtesy of the B. F. Skinner Foundation.

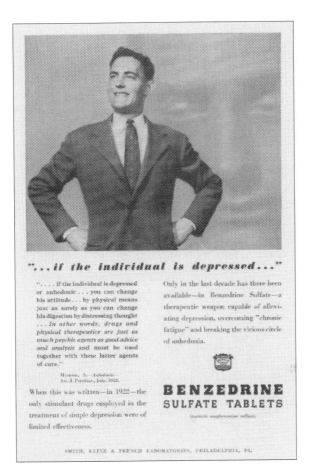

FIG. 28. In the 1940s and 1950s, amphetamine advertisements like this one emphasized and promoted Myerson's anhedonia concept of depression. Source: *California and Western Medicine*, April 1945.

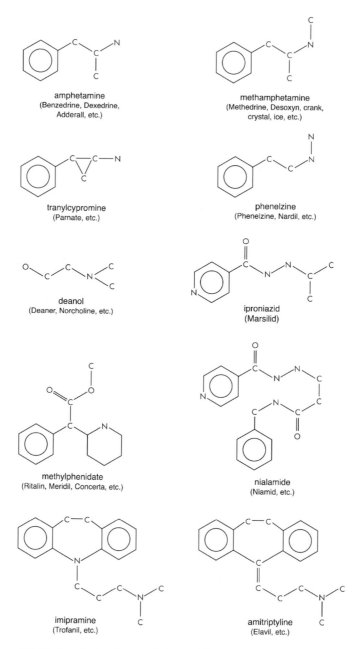

amphetamine
(Benzedrine, Dexedrine,
Adderall, etc.)

methamphetamine
(Methedrine, Desoxyn, crank,
crystal, ice, etc.)

tranylcypromine
(Parnate, etc.)

phenelzine
(Phenelzine, Nardil, etc.)

deanol
(Deaner, Norcholine, etc.)

iproniazid
(Marsilid)

methylphenidate
(Ritalin, Meridil, Concerta, etc.)

nialamide
(Niamid, etc.)

imipramine
(Trofanil, etc.)

amitriptyline
(Elavil, etc.)

FIG. 29. Amphetamines and the antidepressant drugs that began to replace them in the late 1950s and 1960s.

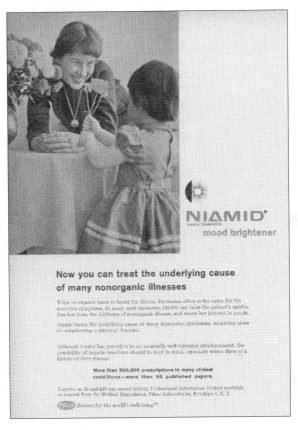

FIG. 30. Newer antidepressants such as monoamine oxidase inhibitors were advertised to general medical audiences for the same uses as amphetamine antidepressants such as Dexamyl. Source: *California Medicine*, June 1960.

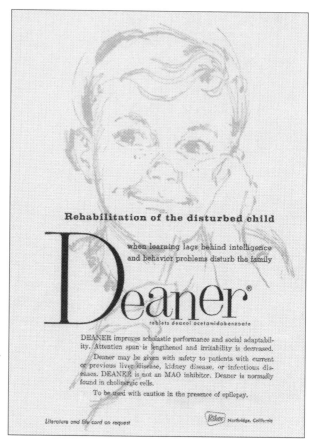

FIG. 31. In the late 1950s and early 1960s, some of the less successful new antidepressants targeted the minor niche of childhood hyperkinesis (today's Attention Deficit Disorder). Source: *Journal of the American Medical Women's Association*, July 1960.

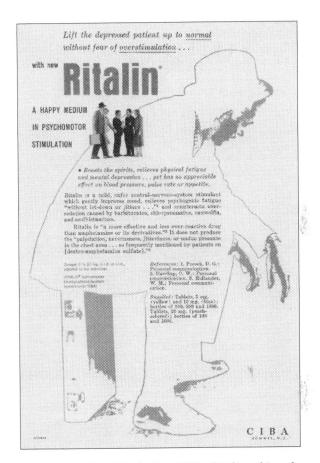

FIG. 32. Introduced in the late 1950s, Ritalin achieved limited success as an antidepressant. Source: *California Medicine*, March 1956.

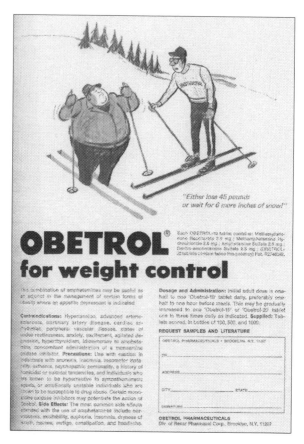

FIG. 33. One of many methamphetamine-containing diet pills popular in the 1950s and 1960s, this particular blend was favored by Andy Warhol. Source: *California Medicine,* February 1970.

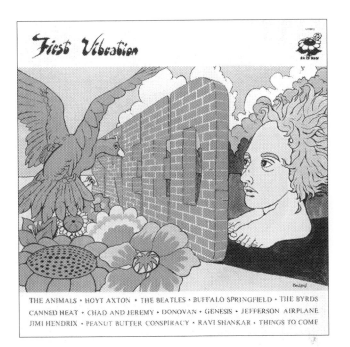

First Vibration

THE ANIMALS · HOYT AXTON · THE BEATLES · BUFFALO SPRINGFIELD · THE BYRDS
CANNED HEAT · CHAD AND JEREMY · DONOVAN · GENESIS · JEFFERSON AIRPLANE
JIMI HENDRIX · PEANUT BUTTER CONSPIRACY · RAVI SHANKAR · THINGS TO COME

FIG. 34. Major recording artists such as Jefferson Airplane and the Grateful Dead participated in the "Speed Kills" anti-amphetamine campaign, and many produced anti-amphetamine radio announcements urging users to "Put Speed Down—Do it Now." This compilation album raised money for the Haight Ashbury Free Clinic. Courtesy DoItNow Foundation.

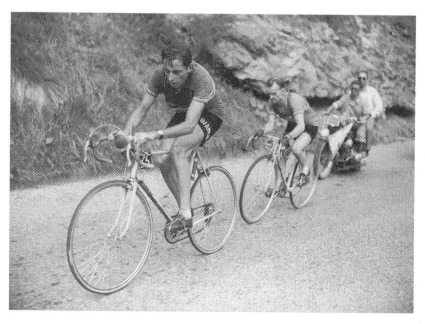

FIG. 35. Fausto Coppi, Europe's greatest postwar cycling champion, relied
heavily on amphetamines, as did many other cyclists. Courtesy Bettmann/
Corbis.

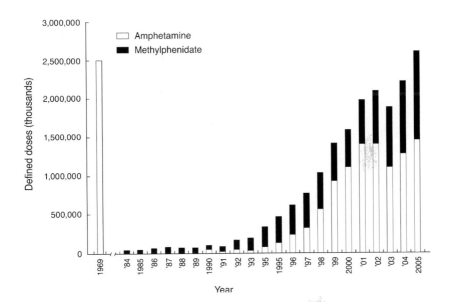

FIG. 36. In the U.S., pharmaceutical amphetamine consumption for Attention Deficit Disorder has recently reached levels similar to *medical* amphetamine consumption at the height of the first amphetamine epidemic, when federal regulation finally placed meaningful restrictions on the drug industry. Graph shows federally reported and authorized production of the Attention Deficit medications amphetamine (e.g., Adderall) and methylphenidate (e.g., Ritalin), expressed in terms of standardized units: 10 mg amphetamine base and 30 mg methylphenidate base, roughly equivalent doses at least for recreational purposes. Sources: Drug Enforcement Administration, final production quotas of amphetamine and methylphenidate for years specified.

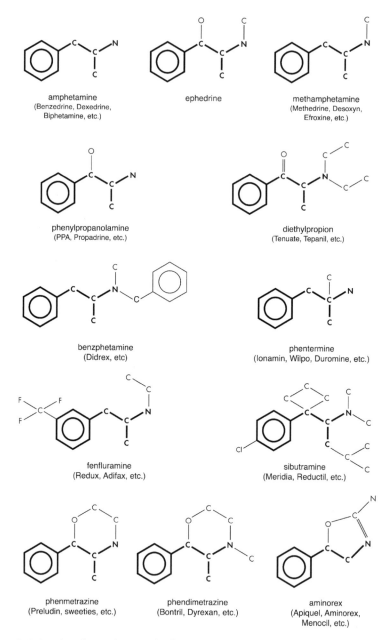

FIG. 37. Amphetamines and other major diet drugs, showing the chemical relationship to amphetamine (amphetamine structure in bold).

6

Amphetamine and the Go-Go Years

HISTORICAL ACCOUNTS TYPICALLY treat tranquilizers as beginning the widespread medication of everyday psychological distress. The drug industry's interest in antidepressants supposedly came later.[1] Mistaken though this perspective certainly is, in overlooking the two previous decades during which amphetamine-based antidepressants paved the way as psychiatric medications in general practice, it remains true that in the late 1950s anxiety overshadowed depression as America's most fashionable neurotic complaint. With tranquilizer sales booming and both popular and medical attention on anxiety, a naïve observer then or now might suppose that amphetamines were on their way out, at least for psychiatric uses.

However, out of the limelight though unvanquished, the medical use of amphetamines for depression continued to flourish, and their use for other purposes also proliferated. (One might even wonder if the continuing popularity of amphetamines, especially among women for weight loss, might have driven the quick uptake and massive demand for tranquilizers because they offered relief from amphetamine side effects such as tension and insomnia.) But in the late 1950s and 1960s, with old amphetamine-based drugs no longer protected by patents, competition in this market was fierce. Therefore, because the greatest profits come from new, unique, and patentable pharmaceutical products, the industry's leading firms poured energy and resources into the search for novel antidepressant drugs to replace the old standby amphetamines—amphetamine and methamphetamine.

Searching for the Next Antidepressant

Commercial research into new antidepressants in the late 1950s deserves a short detour in our story of amphetamine, for several reasons. First and most obvious, the effort devoted to this research emphasizes that ever since amphetamine became a big seller in the 1940s, antidepressants have been important to pharmaceutical firms, even in the heyday of the tranquilizers. Second, simply describing the research of the drug firms in their quest for antidepressants offers inherent interest, because much of what the industry did has never been disclosed except in technical conferences, and even there only in general terms because trade secrets were at stake. Third, the details of the search for novel antidepressants reveal that the drug effects sought by pharmaceutical firms were profoundly shaped by amphetamine. That is, as the founder of the drug category, amphetamine established much of what it meant to be an antidepressant, fixing criteria that subsequent antidepressants had to meet in both laboratory and clinic. Fourth, the elaborate drug discovery efforts described here did not in fact lead to the next breakthrough drugs for depression. The disconnection between the laboratory approaches used to search for the next antidepressants and the way the next generation drugs were actually discovered offers important insights into the flaws of the postwar pharmaceutical research and development enterprise—the same basic system of medical innovation that today generates so much controversy. Fifth, and finally, by looking at the failure of these new drugs in the 1960s to dislodge amphetamines as the most common antidepressants, we can learn much about what made amphetamine so popular as a prescription drug in the first place.

In the 1950s, the American pharmaceutical industry was learning to discover drugs in a new way. Whereas important new drugs used to come mainly from scientists outside the industry—at universities, in government bureaus, or, more rarely (as in Alles's case), independent inventors—after the Second World War American firms established ambitious internal systems to discover new products through a drug development assembly line, or "pipeline." Routinely, endless new compounds created by chemists would flow onward to a biological testing department, which would conduct tests not just for toxicity but also for several kinds of biological action. The most promising would flow on to clinical investigations at large hospitals managed by the medical department, then to test marketing, and then, if still promising according to market analyses, at last to the sales force and prescribing doctors. Advanced life science still played a role in these corporate mechanisms of drug discovery, but it was built into "screening" experiments (or assays), standardized tests of biological action applied

to large sets of new chemicals. Each screening assay, designed to identify compounds with a particular commercially desirable effect, added
knowledge about what the chemicals did inside living things. Compounds with the desired characteristics would be screened further and
studied in other tests, at ever greater expense from one stage to the
next. The more potential drugs that could be tried at early stages, and
if faulty "screened out" or removed from the pipeline, the quicker and
more efficient the hunt for new drugs became. Screening made the latest science a matter of mass production, or so the thinking went, and
the drug industry demonstrated the method's productivity with a
long string of new (but not necessarily better) antibiotics to replace
penicillin in the 1950s.[2]

The antidepressants were another class of drug to which the new
assembly-line screening strategy was applied in the mid-1950s. To discover novel antidepressants, drug firms devised two main types of
screening assays: biochemical and behavioral. Both were efforts to find
chemicals with effects similar to amphetamine. Biochemical screening
for new antidepressants depended on reproducing some of amphetamine's chemical effects in brain tissue, even though the particular biochemical action by which amphetamine "brightened" mood remained
a mystery.

One common biochemical approach depended on the observa-
tion that amphetamine interferes with the action of a certain enzyme
present in the body, called monoamine oxidase, which, among other
things, breaks down adrenaline in nerve endings once the hormone
has delivered its signal. As Alles and others speculated in the mid-
1950s, this interference with the enzyme increased levels of adrenaline
in the brain circuits controlling mood and thus could explain why amphetamine worked as an antidepressant. However, adrenaline was no
longer the whole story in biochemical thinking about depression.
Physiologists in the 1950s were discovering that the brain used more
hormones, or "neurotransmitters" (so-called because the hormones
transmit signals between nerve cells), beyond the adrenaline and acetylcholine about which Myerson had theorized in the 1930s. One of
the newly recognized neurotransmitters was the hormone serotonin,
and, to many scientists, serotonin seemed to play a key role in depression. Like adrenaline, however, serotonin was also broken down in the
nerves by the same enzyme.[3] Thus, regardless of which neurotransmitter was more important, a viable new approach was to look for a

"monoamine oxidase inhibitor" (MAOI), as the blocking agents were called, by screening chemicals for their ability to reduce this enzyme activity in a test tube, on the belief that they would increase adrenaline or serotonin, or both, in the brain. Countless thousands of chemicals passed through the hands of researchers looking for new antidepressants using enzyme inhibition screens during the late 1950s, both in large drug firms and in government institutions like the Walter Reed Army Medical Center and the National Institute of Mental Health.[4]

The alternative, behavioral screening strategy for discovering new antidepressant drugs has been discussed very little in historical accounts. This strategy depended even less on understanding why amphetamine worked. In fact, the most prominent American school of experimental psychology in the 1950s, Behaviorism, prided itself on not even caring about the actual mechanisms of brain and mind. The leader of Behaviorism for many years, the controversial Harvard professor B. F. Skinner, believed that psychology should be limited to the study of how predictable behavioral patterns are created and altered (Figure 27). Behavioral patterns could be tested experimentally, whereas states of mind could never be directly observed, Skinner argued.[5] One might suppose that this pragmatic, deliberately superficial perspective ruled out the study of emotional states. However, despite refusing to look inside the black box of the brain, the resourceful Skinner found ways to define and study emotions strictly in terms of measurable patterns of behavior. And, like the biochemists, the way he approached depression and antidepressant drugs depended crucially on looking for the same sort of effects on the organism that amphetamine produced; that is, Behaviorists sought chemicals that did what amphetamine did to behavior.

Skinner actually became interested in amphetamine soon after the drug was first introduced. In 1937, he compared the effect of Benzedrine and caffeine on "extinction"—the gradual disappearance of a conditioned behavior once it was no longer rewarded—using his famous "Skinner box." This device was a sound- and light-proof animal cage with a lever connected to a counting device and a "reward" or food dispenser, as well as lights and buzzers to provide "stimulus." With a Skinner box one measured mental states simply as the rate of lever pressing, recorded by a counter tape. Skinner found that, even more than caffeine, amphetamine made conditioned rats press their levers more aggressively after this behavior ceased to win a reward.

This could mean that amphetamine either retards learning or causes the persistence of inappropriate behavior. However, Skinner's initial interpretation was that the drug raised the energy output of the animal, what he called "drive."[6]

In the 1940s, Skinner expanded his box experiments to the emotions. For example, he measured anxiety as the effect of anticipated punishment on the work of a conditioned rat. Skinner trained his rats to expect food rewards from pressing a lever, and also taught them to expect electric shocks when a tone was sounded; the decrease in lever pressing caused by that warning tone represented "anxiety." Amphetamine increased anxiety as measured by this kind of experiment, causing a greater decline in lever pressing after the warning stimulus. This work by Skinner gave drug companies some major leads. First and foremost, it suggested that to search for psychiatric drugs you could use Skinner boxes, instead of more labor- and skill-intensive methods. As Skinner put it at a psychiatric drug conference in 1956, his "equipment doesn't need to sleep"; a few technicians could keep rooms full of Skinner boxes operating around the clock without even looking at the animals inside.[7]

In 1955, Skinner entered into an intimate collaboration with the Merck drug firm, and the program he helped establish there illustrates how amphetamine shaped the behavioral search for new antidepressants. When the firm recruited Skinner, Merck was struggling, despite a brilliant scientific reputation and recent successes like the introduction of cortisone. A disruptive merger was under way with the marketing-savvy firm Sharp and Dohme, and the newly enlarged company desperately needed new products. To management, the "mental drug field" seemed especially attractive, so in 1955 Merck launched a three-pronged strategy for discovering tranquilizers and antidepressants: a biochemical screening program, a "neuropharmacology" program (which looked for new drugs based on changes in the electrical activity of animal brains), and also a behavior-based "psychopharmacology" screening program. To help Merck set up the psychopharmacology program, research managers brought in Skinner as a consultant, along with Joseph Brady, another behavior-oriented drug researcher based at the Army's Walter Reed research center. Using tests designed by the two scientists, by mid-1956 the Merck unit was able to screen seventeen new chemicals in three months, with a series of Skinner box tests using half a dozen trained rats each. At the end of the year, the program was scaled up to screen forty chemicals per month.

To detect tranquilizing effects, the Merck psychopharmacology unit chiefly looked for a reduction of the "anxiety" effect already described—the decrease in work output caused by an anticipated electric shock. They also used a test in which animals learned to avoid a shock through a particular pattern of lever pressing. Any chemical that kept the rats working hard despite inevitable punishment as well as chlorpromazine, but which did not also reduce this "appropriate" avoidance behavior where the shock could be prevented, was considered a promising candidate for human testing. The hope was that it would become an antipsychotic major tranquilizer as effective as chlorpromazine, only without creating as much zombie-like detachment, or perhaps a less powerful minor tranquilizer suitable for everyday anxiety.[8]

To screen for new antidepressants, the Merck psychopharmacologists used tests for intensified reward-driven behavior, like the increase in lever pressing shown by rats on speed, but with less of amphetamine's drawbacks. Skinner and Brady again helped Merck design two kinds of tests, some for amphetamine's positive effects and others for its undesirable effects. The screening tests for amphetamine's desirable, antidepressant effect essentially measured increased work output under very poorly rewarding conditions, discussed in more detail below. The screening tests for amphetamine's drawbacks measured agitation and impairment of judgment, as well as anxiety. For instance, the agitation caused by amphetamine was measured as increased random movement, easily gauged with an electric eye that counted how often a rat moved past a particular point. Impairment of judgment was measured by an experimental setup that periodically changed the rules, after a warning bell or light, so that the rat would be rewarded with food only with slow, rather than rapid, lever pressing. Results with each new chemical were compared to those obtained using dextroamphetamine, using the same rats and tests.

Four years and hundreds of chemicals later, Merck's behavioral psychopharmacology screening program finally identified one highly promising new antidepressant. Code named MK-202, the chemical increased lever-pressing work output under a range of conditions, in seemingly more adaptive ways than amphetamine. For instance, in the "strained fixed-ratio" test, designed to measure "an animal's ability to handle an overly large workload with inadequate motivation," MK-202 performed better than dextroamphetamine. Here, hungry rats were given a drop of condensed milk only after pressing a lever two hundred times in response to a light signal. However, in the middle of their heavy and under-rewarded task a second light would turn on intermittently, and if they immediately responded by pressing a second lever they would get a milk drop instantly. Thus, this experiment measured both willingness to do "a particularly long and tedious job" as well as "alertness" to a second stimulus, according to Merck researchers. The rats on amphetamine performed well on the repetitive task but tended to miss the second stimulus; not so the rats on MK-202. Given the similarity between the rat's situation and the repetitive work that most people must endure to make a living, a drug that increased lever pressing without producing unresponsiveness would seem a likely antidepressant—provided we accept that inefficiency in unrewarding jobs indicates psychiatric depression.

This implicit identification of impaired work efficiency with depressive illness, inscribed in the use of amphetamine-boosted lever pressing as the benchmark that subsequent antidepressants had to meet, applied to the highest level executive type of work also. (The business world is called a "rat race" with reason!) This is evident from another test, designed to measure a rat's capacity to perform complex tasks. Here, to get a reward, rats had to press a lever rapidly when a white light was on, slowly when a red light was on, and not at all when both lights were on. The rats on amphetamine pressed their levers fast no matter what lights were on, but the rats on MK-202 only pressed fast when high speed was rewarded. In these and a half a dozen other experiments with trained rats subject to diabolically ingenious "reinforcement schedules" (that is, particular programs of reward and punishment), MK-202 outperformed amphetamine for boosting work output, maximizing reward, and minimizing punishment, particularly when tasks were both difficult and unrewarding. A more promising antidepressant drug candidate could hardly be imagined, and in January 1960 the behavioral psychopharmacology unit passed it on for human testing as an antidepressant, with its highest recommendation.[9]

Merck did launch a new antidepressant brand-named Elavil on the market in 1961, with moderate success. But Elavil was not MK-202. Whatever happened to this once promising drug candidate? The only reference to it in medical journals I have found describes use of the drug, now renamed "methastyridone," on withdrawn, immobile depressives at a mental hospital. In a few of the patients, the drug seemed to increase activity slightly and make behavior less abnormal.[10] Presumably, since the drug was expected to be useful as an antidepressant, it must also have been tested in common, milder forms of depression—and failed, the results never published. No different from thousands of other drugs we have never heard about, the failure of methastyridone in clinical testing bespeaks the particular inefficiency of mass screening approaches to drug discovery developed by large pharmaceutical firms, as well the yawning gap between bedside and laboratory bench that still afflicts drug discovery half a century later.

Despite five years of intensive effort and several thousand chemicals screened, by 1960 Merck's behavioral psychopharmacology program had yielded no marketable products. In 1958, Skinner had proposed ambitious new refinements, more ingenious ways to screen for specific "anti-discouragement," "anti-fatigue" and, intriguingly, "anti-guilt" drugs (these last defined as chemicals improving appetite-satisfying and penalty-avoiding task performance during anticipated punishment). Each one of these drug types imagined by Skinner would be distinct from ordinary antidepressants, now understood as nonspecific "energizers." But there is no indication that Merck's psychopharmacology program was scaled up to accommodate Skinner's dreams. Rather, by the beginning of the 1960s, corporate leaders were talking about shutting it down because of the poor correlation between rat lever-pressing and mood effects on patients.[11]

As for Elavil (amitriptyline), the new antidepressant, it had also been tested in the rat behavior program: the psychopharmacologists rejected it as an antidepressant and gave it a mediocre mark as a possible tranquilizer. Only after word reached Merck of the success of another firm's related compound (Geigy's imipramine) was the drug reevaluated as an antidepressant, this time using humans. So Elavil had been rescued from the trash bin, and its effects on depression discovered, by luck and by the oldest method of all—physicians playing their hunches and experimenting on their patients.[12]

Internalizing and routinizing the drug discovery process turned out to be harder for big drug companies than they had anticipated. Within a few years, the behavioral screening programs and Skinner boxes were not eliminated, but they were overshadowed by a suc-

cession of newer approaches, and became just one of the many av-
enues to new drug discovery used by the drug firms. The biochemical
screening approaches of the companies proved no better than the behavioral screening approaches at making the initial breakthrough—although once the breakthrough was made, biochemical screening lent
itself to the invention of new and possibly improved chemical variations, "me-too" or "copycat" drugs as they are disparagingly called.
Some insider critics today contend that the pharmaceutical industry
has never mastered fundamental drug discovery research, despite a
huge investment in building up internal scientific capacity for half a
century, and is today as dependent as ever for truly significant contributions to medicine on the publicly funded research of university biologists or the accidents and hunches of doctors.[13]

Next Generation Drugs Arrive

Accidental observations and clinical hunches, and not the "pipeline,"
certainly played the lead role in discovering the major new antidepressants introduced around 1960. One of the new types of antidepressant started as a potential antihistamine in 1950, or as a potential
sedative since it seemed to make animals drowsy; this made sense, because its chemical structure was closely related to chlorpromazine,
which has both kinds of effects. The Swiss company that invented it,
Geigy, tested their three-ringed (or "tricyclic") compound on people
for both purposes, but it went nowhere. In 1954, Geigy became aware
of chlorpromazine's success in psychiatry and made a new series of
tricyclic compounds closely related to their first one. Hoping to find a
better antipsychotic major tranquilizer, a me-too chlorpromazine, the
firm induced a number of psychiatrists with patients on chlorpromazine to switch their medication to one of the new compounds. Most
of the patients did badly, but a few of the doctors happened to notice
an improvement in mood, alongside the worsening delusions and
other psychotic symptoms. The Swiss asylum psychiatrist Roland
Kuhn, who had noted this effect with one of the new compounds, became enthusiastic and conducted studies, in 1956 and 1957, showing
its effectiveness specifically for depression. In 1958, Geigy launched
the new drug, called imipramine and trademarked Trofanil, as an antidepressant in Europe, and soon after in North America.[14]

The way in which clinical researchers evaluated the new antidepressants shows that, as in the realm of animal behavior research, two decades of amphetamine's use as an antidepressant had informed medicine's understanding of depression. From the start, as we have seen, the anhedonia concept of depression had been promoted in SKF's marketing of amphetamine for psychiatry (Figure 28).[15] Over time, anhedonia's status in thinking about depression advanced in step with accumulating experience with amphetamine's use in depression, along with exposure to such marketing. At the end of the 1950s anhedonia and apathy appear in Max Hamilton's highly influential rating scale for depressive disorder severity, under the rubric "work and loss of interests," and anhedonia has remained a key feature of depression-measuring instruments used in psychiatric research ever since.[16] In this sense, in the clinic as in the lab, amphetamine has been built into the definition of neurotic depression. Amphetamine and its action on anhedonia helped cement the notion that reduced pursuit of pleasure in itself represents a mental illness, even though later antidepressants differed from amphetamine in ways not anticipated by systematic drug screening programs.

Since amphetamine was what an antidepressant looked like, the American psychiatrists who first tested imipramine for depression in the late 1950s expected a "super-amphetamine." This means they would have anticipated a positive effect on anhedonia (or pep), elevated activity in the patients who were passive and retarded, undesirable effects on those who were agitated, and generally less beneficial effects the worse the patient's depression. However, the new drug's actual effects differed in ways that demanded new thinking about anhedonia. Before treatment, most of the seriously depressed patients on whom the psychiatrists tested imipramine lacked appetite, had severe insomnia, and were either very agitated or very passive. Unlike amphetamine, imipramine improved appetite and sleep, and actually calmed agitated individuals, thus helping a wider range of patients. Like amphetamine, it made many patients feel more cheerful, more outgoing and interested, and more active. In other words, the drug reduced apathy and restored pep without agitation. This is what usually happened, but not in every case. A minority did not get peppier with imipramine, even though they slept and ate better, but adding amphetamine to their imipramine treatment restored their pep. (Today, some doctors still find the same thing, that certain depressed people who do not respond fully to the current antidepressants do better when given amphetamines.) These exceptions suggested that amphetamine and imipramine work differently and, furthermore, that there are at least two basic sides to depression, as indicated by two kinds of anhedonia. Pep and the physical appetites for sex and food were usually impaired at the same time, but not always.[17]

Furthermore, there was an unusual, "atypical" kind of seriously depressed patient suffering apathy and disinterest in life, but no great disturbance in sleep or appetite. These patients did not improve much with the tricyclics, but they did respond to amphetamine. The psychiatrist who noticed this difference between "atypical" and "typical" depression when testing imipramine, Donald Klein, explained it in this way: two reward systems exist in the brain, and two forms of anhedonia correspond to their failure. Pleasures from food, sex, and sleep come from satisfaction of bodily needs, and typical major depressions impair this reward mechanism. Tricyclics reinforce the mechanism and help reverse this kind of anhedonia. But there was also a kind of satisfaction from exciting action in the world, the "pleasures of the hunt," as Klein put it. In atypical major depressions this was the reward mechanism that failed, resulting in patients who ate and slept normally but still lacked initiative and drive. Tricyclics did not help these patients but amphetamine did. So, from this perspective, Myerson got it largely right, except that he confused two kinds of anhedonia: amphetamine only helps one kind, restoring the pleasures of the hunt and building the "energy feeling."

Klein's thinking on anhedonia and the action of antidepressants commands more respect today than in the early 1960s, since it fit poorly with the then dominant Freudian theory that all depressions are equally self-punishment driven by unconscious guilt. However, Freudian psychiatrists of the day still left room for antidepressants, such as New York psychoanalyst Nathan Kline, who saw all such drugs as energizers of the unconscious drives, or Id, allowing greater expression of animal urges against the repressive forces of the conscious Ego and Superego (or conscience).[18] That made all anhedonia the sign of an oppressed Id, an idea very like Myerson's notion of disconnected, frustrated drives. Regardless, just as in the 1940s, the diversity of psychiatric theory presented no great obstacle to drug marketing, and by the beginning of the 1960s Trofanil and Elavil were heavily advertised to doctors in North America.

Another new type of antidepressant was starting to make an impression on the market around the same time as the tricyclics, although the initial discovery dates slightly earlier. Doctors trying out two new tuberculosis antibiotics called isoniazid and iproniazid at the beginning of the 1950s noticed that they seemed to elevate mood as a side effect. Tales of one-lunged, barely living consumptives dancing in hospital corridors caught the attention of psychiatrists, and by 1953 a few were prescribing the antibiotics for depression. When biochemists found that iproniazid inhibited the monoamine oxidase enzyme, just like amphetamine, it suddenly made complete sense, chemically speaking. Drugs that inhibited this enzyme had antidepressant action. Therefore, in the brain, monoamine oxidase inhibitor (MAOI) drugs like iproniazid, and also amphetamine, must raise levels of adrenaline —and serotonin—by preventing the enzyme's breakdown of the neurotransmitters. Iproniazid thus triggered the search for new antidepressants that inhibited monoamine oxidase, as already mentioned.

By 1960, new MAOIs came on the market, less toxic than iproniazid, and these improved versions like phenelzine (brand-named Nardil) and tranylcypromine (branded Parnate) were very close chemical relatives of amphetamine (Figure 29). Unlike tricyclics, they increased "pep" and helped Klein's atypical depressives, while they also helped typical depressives. Indeed, they resembled amphetamine enough both chemically and pharmacologically that they could easily have been called new and improved amphetamines, had that been a good marketing strategy.[19] However, it was not.

By the end of the 1950s amphetamine was out of fashion in depression, and psychiatrists wanted something different. There were now several new drugs that seemed to work better for anhedonia than amphetamine, and experts generally endorsed tricyclics like imipramine as the best antidepressants, mainly on the grounds that they were safer than MAOIs. Amphetamine now held "a very doubtful place in the treatment of depression."[20] Presumably, the basis of this judgment among psychiatrists was their clinical experience with seriously depressed patients in the mental ward, in that expert opinion seems to have run ahead of supporting evidence from any randomized controlled trial (RCT)—fast becoming the gold standard of clinical science around 1960 (discussed in more detail below).[21] But whatever their grounds, the psychiatric experts embraced the tricyclics in the early 1960s and wasted no time in urging general practitioners to prescribe them instead of amphetamine.[22]

At this point, with new antidepressants available and marketed by the leading pharmaceutical firms, and expert opinion entirely on their side, one would expect that amphetamine would quickly fade to obscurity as a psychiatric medication. But despite the urging of both experts and advertising, the new antidepressants never fully caught on with primary-care physicians like general practitioners, the main prescribers of psychotropic medications. The reasons behind this curious turn of events can tell us much about why amphetamine became so popular for depression in the first place.

Family doctors mainly encounter mild depressions triggered by unhappy life events (so-called reactive depressions), and they treat them in the context of the patient's overall health and well-being. For these transitory bouts of mental distress, the placebo effect is crucial, buying time for the patients to get through the rough patch and recover spontaneously. Any sensation of drug action amplifies the placebo effect, since patients are convinced the medicine is working (even if all they notice are the nonspecific side effects). And if the pills also relieve emotional symptoms or otherwise make patients optimistic, so much the better. Amphetamine meets these criteria. The last thing you want from a medicine intended for psychosomatic complaints and mild depression would be a serious toxic reaction, worries about toxic reactions, or any unpleasant side effect, all of which might make patients stop taking their pills. The MAOIs never shook an early reputation for toxicity, when some patients on the drugs died from eating the wrong cheese, and many doctors feared prescribing them. The tricyclics, on the other hand, cause side effects like dry mouth, constipation, and lethargy—the opposite of pep. Patients often disliked them and would stop taking their pills. To avoid this, many doctors prescribed tricyclics at doses so low that they would have no side effects —nor any effects on brain chemistry either. Used as a placebo to tide patients over their difficulties, amphetamines worked better, since they gave a pleasant boost in energy and patients kept taking them. So, by the mid-1960s, a large number of general practitioners had gone "back to the old standbys, amphetamine and amphetamine-barbiturate combinations" for depression, as one psychiatrist's 1965 review lamented.[23]

In an early 1970 letter to the editor of the *New England Journal of Medicine,* one general practitioner spelled out and defended this aspect of amphetamine's enormous and stubborn appeal. Replying to an earlier letter from a specialist criticizing doctors who still prescribed amphetamines, despite the large body of scientific evidence in favor of the newer antidepressants that had by then accumulated (based mainly on testing with seriously depressed mental hospital patients), the irate GP retorted:

> This attitude toward amphetamines is one . . . held by numerous hospital-based physicians of many disciplines, for they are often functioning as specialized technicians removed from the world of ordinary illness and medical problems. These common problems are not life-threatening, but merely debilitating, illnesses or complaints that diminish the possibility for the pleasurable enjoyment of, or even adequate coping with, the everyday routine stresses of their lives. I have several patients for whom fatigue or mild despondency is a chronic problem. No organic illness other than "the tired-housewife" syndrome can be found for their complaints. Small, regular doses of amphetamines, often taken only during the working week when the demands upon their energies and psyches are the highest, keep them functioning, coping, capable of performing or even enjoying their duties.[24]

For the bulk of men and women receiving medical care through a family doctor rather than a specialist "technician," amphetamines would remain the antidepressant of choice right through the 1960s into the 1970s. Psychiatrists even stopped calling amphetamine an antidepressant, reclassifying it as a "psychostimulant" to reflect its nonspecific action on the mind, but to no avail. Whatever experts might call it, amphetamine beautifully suited the interaction between general practitioners and their distressed patients, the needs and expectations each brought to the short office visit. Nothing else seemed to satisfy vast numbers of unhappy people needing a little help to "perform and enjoy their duties." Development and marketing teams at major drug companies beat their head against this wall, promoting one new (and patented) drug after another throughout the 1960s as the next big office-practice antidepressant, the one that could finally fill amphetamine's shoes. In the meantime, though, most drug companies saw no compelling reason to stop selling their own amphetamine-based medicines.

Amphetamine Saturation, Mind and Body

The 1960s are rightly remembered as the golden era of mind-altering drugs, on the street as well as in legitimate medicine, where optimism ran high about finding magic chemical bullets for every type of mental ill. Though by now old and out of fashion scientifically, medical amphetamine use proliferated in this environment. The mental heath drug market had exploded, with some 30 million Americans, 15 percent of the total population, on prescription drugs for psychiatric complaints in 1963. That year, according to the Census Bureau, U.S. manufacturer sales of minor tranquilizers that year were $109 million, amphetamines $48 million, and non-amphetamine antidepressants $19 million. (SKF's Dexamyl annual sales at this point were running at about $12 million, evidently a quarter of the domestic amphetamine market.) With manufacturers selling another $86 million in major tranquilizers like chlorpromazine in 1963, mental health drugs altogether accounted for over $250 million, or about one-tenth of the entire U.S. prescription drug market. Surveys later in the decade found that about twice as many adult Americans used tranquilizers as antidepressants (including—indeed mainly—amphetamines).[25] This two-to-one ratio in sales and consumption also roughly fits with the ratio of advertising effort devoted to prescription tranquilizers versus antidepressants that I found in one-month samples of full-page drug ads in 1960 and 1963. Unsurprisingly, the newer antidepressants still protected by patents and therefore most profitable, received virtually all the prominent advertising, even though amphetamine was still more popular as an antidepressant among patients and doctors.[26]

Although all the newer antidepressant drugs in the early 1960s claimed to be different and unique, they were still amphetamine replacements. That is, despite their acclaimed superiority in psychiatry, they struggled to capture amphetamine's market appeal, to emulate amphetamine's usefulness in primary care especially for psychosomatic complaints. Their advertising could just as well have been selling Dexamyl, except for the fine print. When Pfizer advertised its MAOI antidepressant nialamide (brand named Niamid) that same year, it urged that the product would help patients like one mother in her thirties whose "many imaginary ills" were psychosomatic (Figure 30), and likewise one older man whose "chronic fatigue" had only emotional causes.[27] And Merck marketed Elavil simultaneously for all three main psychiatric uses that SKF had targeted during the initial campaign for Dexamyl more than a decade earlier. According to one 1963 advertisement, doctors should prescribe Elavil "when DEPRESSION underlies physical complaints," "when DEPRESSION is complicated by concurrent anxiety and tension," and "when DEPRESSION accompanies somatic disease."[28] This is just the combination of indications that made Dexamyl the perfect drug for general practitioners to give to any emotionally distressed patient, regardless of whether their physical complaints were imaginary.

Advertising for the new antidepressants focused on markets already established for amphetamine, the commercial model for them all. This generalization also applies to a small niche market in the 1960s: children's misbehavior. As noted earlier, during the initial clinical testing of amphetamine in the 1930s, SKF had explored the possibilities of marketing the drug to improve school performance in children but had chosen against doing so for various reasons including bad publicity.[29] In the absence of advertising, the idea of using amphetamine in this way did not catch on among family doctors or psychiatrists.

By the 1950s, however, the idea was taking hold that "hyperkinetic" misbehavior in children (especially boys) was often caused by a distinct and treatable form of "emotional disturbance." Psychoanalytically inclined child psychiatrists attributed it to toxic motherhood, whereas the biologically inclined attributed it to "minimal brain damage."[30] Either way, a market was emerging for amphetamines and other drugs to treat hyperkinetic misbehavior. For instance, one called "Deaner" (deanol), made by the small Riker firm, had begun life during the early 1950s as a potential tranquilizer or sedative, based on its biochemical profile as an antagonist to adrenaline action. By 1958, the drug was restyled as a stimulant effective for chronic fatigue, mild depression, difficulty in concentrating, and behavioral problems in children (Figure 31). "Do not confuse it with tranquilizers," one 1959 ad urged, "Deaner is a gentle, slow-acting antidepressant—a totally new molecule," without amphetamine side effects like irritability and appetite loss. Another 1959 ad claimed that "psychonormalizing

Deaner" was effective "in the adjustment of school-age problem children," and a different ad proposed the drug "for emotionally disturbed children whose intelligence is masked by behavior problems." Deaner stayed on the U.S. pharmaceutical market, particularly as a treatment for childhood hyperkinesis, until it finally succumbed to failure in randomized controlled trials in 1983.[31]

Another next-generation antidepressant, this one a closer chemical relative of amphetamine, fared much better as a medication for the same childhood problems. In the mid-1950s, the Swiss firm CIBA discovered that a compound called methylphenidate relieved fatigue and elevated mood. By 1956, the firm was marketing it for depression under the brand name "Ritalin," the "happy medium in psychomotor stimulation," to "lift the patient up to normal without fear of overstimulation" (Figure 32). As an antidepressant, Ritalin's chief selling point was as a "mild, safer central nervous system stimulant" without amphetamine's side effects. However, complaints of anxiety and even rare "schizophrenic manifestations" (essentially, amphetamine psychosis) soon surfaced. The drug did not do particularly well as an antidepressant, but since 1961, when it followed Deaner in targeting the market for "normalization" of disturbed children, Ritalin has proved extremely successful. It remains to this day a hugely popular drug for Attention Deficit Hyperactivity Disorder (ADHD), the label psychiatrists now apply to the pattern they used to call "childhood hyperkinesis," "emotional disturbance," and "minimal brain dysfunction." And, as we shall later see, the other most common drug for Attention Deficit today is, remarkably enough, amphetamine itself.[32]

Amphetamine was losing some ground to new psychiatric drugs in the early 1960s, but it remained a big money pharmaceutical, and for purposes beyond mental health, too. A physician survey in 1962 found that about half of amphetamine prescriptions were written for mental distress and half for weight loss, while other sources indicate that closer to two-thirds of amphetamine prescriptions were for weight loss.[33] Unsurprisingly, plenty of drug firms wanted a share of the prescription diet pill market. In my one-month sample of full-page ads in *JAMA* in 1960, eight ads for seven different slimming pills appeared, twice the advertising effort going to antidepressants in the same pages. Four of the seven advertised weight-loss drugs were newer amphetamine derivatives, and three of these seven were just old amphetamines.

Abbot was still marketing its "Desoxyn" brand of methamphetamine, now in sustained release form, and the overweight middle-aged man depicted in the ad appears to have had a little less trouble touching his toes with the drug's help. Patients like him also enjoyed an "increased sense of well-being and more pep or energy" on 10 to 15 mg daily, claimed the ad. The smaller drug firms Robins and Strasenburgh also followed a well-worn marketing formula with their speed-based weight-loss products. "Ambar" from Robins was a combination of methamphetamine and phenobarbital, the barbiturate said to prevent possible nervous system "overstimulation" while it enhanced the mood-elevating amphetamine effect, helping patients stick to their diets in combination with the appetite-suppressing effect. Advertisements for Dexamyl in weight loss had been making the same claims in the same pages not long before. And Strasenburg's "Biphetamine" was nothing but ordinary amphetamine in sustained release form (enriched with dextroamphetamine, like a combination of Benzedrine and Dexedrine, or like the currently popular Attention Deficit medication Adderall).[34]

These were some of the more respectable amphetamine weight-loss medicines. Out of sight, beyond the mainstream journals and largely sold direct from weight-loss clinics, the 1960s also saw a booming trade in colorful thyroid hormone and amphetamine combination pills. These were just like the Clarkotabs of the 1940s—despite the fact that medical science had by this time completely rejected thyroid hormone as an obesity treatment. According to the FDA historian John Swann, approximately five thousand American doctors specialized in the weight-loss business in 1967. These "fat doctors" typically made huge profits on the diet pills they dispensed directly, cutting out the pharmacist; for example, one paid $71 for one hundred thousand amphetamine-containing tablets and sold them for $12,000. The practice must have been widespread, since patients were estimated to be spending about $120 million annually on the products, implying pills by the billion.

Many of the diet clinics these physicians ran were effectively created by large-scale, shady manufacturers of the thyroid-amphetamine pills. For instance, Lanpar Pharmaceuticals of Dallas ran a nationwide network of educational meetings to recruit new doctors. At these seminars, Lanpar's paid "experts," who received a commission on sales, advanced unconventional theories about weight loss that flew in the face of medical science, explaining how obesity was a form of hormone-controlled heart failure and thus could be treated by the firm's thyroid-amphetamine formulations. Lanpar could supply any doctors who wanted to open a weight-loss clinic with a complete kit of products and services, including laboratory tests for the patients. Because licensed doctors can practice medicine as they see fit, so long as the drugs they proffer are legal, the federal government lacked authority to stop the wholesale prescription of speed by weight-loss clinics—even when the FDA had proof that the pills were killing patients.[35]

The top medical journals in the early 1960s also featured ads for newer appetite-suppressant drugs alongside the old amphetamine products, and they were all closely related to amphetamine. Strasenburgh offered "Ionamin" (phentermine) for the overweight patient "if she's active" and might dislike amphetamine's extra stimulation. National Drug Company advertised "Tepanil" (diethylpropion) as a lifesaving remedy for deadly obesity, only without amphetamine's risk of nervousness and excess "psychic stimulation," and with the bonus that it could be taken in the evenings without preventing sleep. Merrell's advertising for its "Tenuate" brand of the same chemical (diethylpropion) laid greater stress on its safety for heart patients compared to amphetamines, which often raise blood pressure. And one of the main selling points of Geigy's "Preludin" (phenmetrazine), along with the promises that uncomfortable "side reactions" were rare and "central stimulation" negligible, was that the drug elevated mood and thus helped patients stick to their diets. Again, this is essentially the same marketing strategy adopted by makers of a host of amphetamine-based diet pills beginning with Benzedrine, casting the mood "side effects" as a virtue.[36]

Although ads stressed the opposite, there was abundant evidence that the new "non-amphetamine" diet drugs could cause all the less desirable mental effects of amphetamine: the AMA's drug guide for 1962 already lists agitation, insomnia, euphoria, and anxiety as typical side effects to be expected of all three (phenmetrazine, diethylpropion, and phentermine). Furthermore, by 1962, reports of full-blown addiction and amphetamine psychosis, along with recreational abuse of new diet drugs, were already appearing, especially with phenmetrazine.[37] Thus, the newer weight-loss drugs worked the same way as amphetamine and had much the same dangerous effects and recreational potential. This should come as no surprise, of course, since structurally they were mostly minor variations on the amphetamine molecule. But since they were newer, their drawbacks were less well known in the early 1960s. Until prescribing doctors caught up, and the mounting anecdotes and case reports reached a point beyond plausible deniability, the ads could claim amphetamine-like side effects to be rare or absent.

Speed on the Medical Fringe

Amphetamine use swelled and spread in the 1960s, beyond the boundaries of mainstream medicine as well as within them. This ubiquity of amphetamines created little stir for the greater part of the decade, as few saw much to worry about in the familiar (if slightly naughty) pharmaceutical. Even the president of the United States was a heavy user. More than any other leader, John F. Kennedy symbolized the cultural sea change that came over the world in the 1960s, so it seems suitable that he also represent the new generation's familiarity with psychotropic drugs. Kennedy made a point of projecting an image of youthful vibrancy and easy vigor, but behind the facade was a driven man, whose massive effort to appear relaxed and healthy historians are only now beginning to appreciate. Since childhood he suffered from Addison's Disease, an adrenal insufficiency, and had regularly been treated with experimental injections of adrenal hormones at the Mayo Clinic to overcome chronic exhaustion. The condition did not stop him from becoming football captain in school or from fighting in the Second World War, where he served as a torpedo boat captain. By the time he reached the White House, however, Kennedy suffered from an astonishing range of health problems, the most painful of which was his injured back. He swam laps in a super-heated pool in the middle of most working days, and took five hot showers to relieve the back pain that remained despite constant anaesthetic injections from White House physician Janet Travell.

Kennedy also saw many other physicians, coming to rely on one named Max Jacobson, beginning with the president's winning 1960 campaign. Jacobson's signature therapy was an injection of vitamins, steroids, placenta, and amphetamines (trained in Germany before the war, Jacobson used methamphetamine), a potion that earned him the nickname of "Dr. Feelgood" from grateful patients. Jacobson injected

Kennedy on the occasion of his first television debate with Nixon, traveled with the Kennedys through Europe in 1961, and injected the president during his first summit talk with Russian premier Khrushchev in Vienna. Jacobson paid at least thirty-four calls on the president in 1961 and 1962, and helped Kennedy face down Khrushchev when the Cuban missile crisis brought the world to the brink of nuclear war. According to Jacobson's son, the good doctor gave Kennedy shots containing 10–15 mg of amphetamines up to twice a week. When people close to him expressed concern, Kennedy snapped back, "I don't care if it's horse piss . . . it's the only thing that works."[38]

In the back room laboratory of his Manhattan office, Jacobson prepared the injections using what was described by a visitor as boiling "cauldrons and masses of rocks [and] . . . colored lights," supposedly with the help of uranium, "ultrasonic bombardment," and a "strong magnetic field" as well. Like many old-time doctors, Jacobson often kept the ingredients of his medicines to himself so as to enhance their mystery and thus their placebo power, but these shots were strong enough not to require the placebo effect. One patient reported that when he received his "vitamin" shots "it felt like the top of my head was coming off," and another described "this fantastic feeling, this rush . . . this fantastic energy." Patients usually started with one visit a month, but eventually they graduated to more frequent injections, without which they became too depressed to function. Some patients took home vials of pure methamphetamine containing thirty hefty doses, so that they could inject themselves for a month. A few died and a larger number became paranoid and psychotic from the drugs, but the majority (including some of the psychotic) remained fiercely loyal to their doctor, including many New York and Hollywood celebrities. According to filmmaker Billy Wilder, Jacobson accompanied Cecil B. DeMille to Egypt for his filming of the acclaimed 1956 epic *Ten Commandments*, where regular injections helped the seventy-four-year-old director climb ladders and shout instructions with his usual energy, despite a heart attack during the shooting. Jacobson also cared for the Broadway songwriter Alan Jay Lerner, Congressman Claude Pepper of Florida, the writer Truman Capote, the playwright Tennessee Williams, and the avant-garde filmmaker Maya Deren. When the Rolling Stones came on tour to New York in 1966, Jacobson treated manager Andrew Oldham's herpes and, while he was at it, gave both Oldham and guitarist Brian Jones high-voltage "vitamin" injections.

Jacobson is also rumored to have treated Spiro Agnew, Nixon's vice president.[39]

In mid-1971, Jacobson was dispensing eighty grams of amphetamines a month, or enough for one hundred 25 mg methamphetamine injections per day, which is a lot of speed. He was already under investigation by the New York attorney general, and after the *New York Times* began following his story in late 1972, also by the New York Medical Society. Post-1970 legal restrictions on speed brought unwanted attention to amphetamine prescribing habits, and revealed that Jacobson was not alone. By 1973, many "speed doctors" around New York fell afoul of the law, like Robert Freymann, Alois Peter Warren, Jack Cohen, and John Bishop, now prosecuted for prescribing practices they had been engaged in throughout the 1960s. Some patients, it emerged, were seeing several of the doctors at once; "if you wanted to make a big night of it," one reported, "you'd go over to Max's and get a shot, and then over to Freymann's and then down to Bishop's." (Bishop, physician to Timothy Leary and many filmmakers and entertainers, treated the whole cast of the hit musical *Hair* while it was playing on Broadway). These cases raised important questions about the autonomy of the profession: the limits of physician authority to decide appropriate treatment, physician duties toward patients, and society's right to interfere with doctor-patient relationships. What crime, after all, were the speed doctors committing? As Warren's lawyer pointed out, patients "knew what they were getting," so nobody could accuse the physicians of fraud. Amphetamines were, and still are, legal pharmaceuticals. If the crime was too freely dispensing an addictive substance, then their guilt depended on the claim that medical science knew amphetamines to be addictive. But Jacobson insisted that amphetamines are not genuinely addictive drugs, merely habituating, and many doctors still agreed. Thus, we can appreciate why the issue of amphetamine addiction remained controversial beyond 1970, that is, why the American medical profession refused to acknowledge it for so long, notwithstanding repeated pronouncements from the World Health Organization and plenty of damning evidence.[40] Jacobson represents an extreme example, but in a smaller way, vast numbers of physicians also needed amphetamine every day, to deal with their patients' psychosomatic complaints and distress caused by problems of living. In this sense, the American medical profession was itself addicted to amphetamine.

The media circus around Jacobson virtually forced the medical profession to sacrifice a few especially embarrassing members, much as it had sacrificed physicians who continued to prescribe heroin maintenance therapy for addicts in the 1920s.[41] Jacobson himself eventually lost his medical license in 1975; by then, however, he probably would have retired because of old age and federal regulations that finally made it really difficult to prescribe amphetamines. But this is getting ahead of our story; until the end of the 1960s, amphetamine bore nothing of the stigma that it eventually came to share with heroin. Throughout the decade, millions received amphetamine prescriptions and took their pills without a second thought. Compounding the situation, massive quantities of pharmaceutical amphetamines found their way to recreational users. According to FDA estimates, only half of the billions of amphetamine pills produced by drug firms each year during the 1960s were dispensed by prescription. Indeed, a stream of speed roughly equivalent to a month's supply of Dexedrine (about sixty 5 mg tablets of dextroamphetamine) per adult American per year was flowing directly from the drug companies to the public without any intervention of medical judgment—without even passing through the hands of a "Dr. Feelgood."[42] Some was bought from manufacturers by bogus drug wholesalers for resale on the street, some disappeared during shipment, and some simply could not be accounted for. America was amphetamine saturated, and medicine had lost control.

Speeding, Beyond the Fringe

"I could never finally figure out if more things happened in the sixties because there was much more awake time for them to happen in (since so many people were on amphetamine), or if people started taking amphetamine because there were so many things to do." The man who later made this quip was moving into a large new studio loft on 47th Street in November 1963, the month President Kennedy was assassinated, and he was a rising star in New York's fickle modern art scene. With his trademark silver wigs and paintings of commercial icons like Coca-Cola bottles and Marilyn Monroe, Andy Warhol made this studio—The Factory, he called it—the hub of a frivolous bohemian scene quite different from the earnest Beatnik culture still flourishing in Greenwich Village. Warhol soon drew visits from Max

Jacobson's patients Truman Capote and Tennessee Williams, and another less illustrious crowd as well. One faction of Factory regulars was known as the "Mole People" because of their underground lifestyle and the dark glasses they wore night and day—on their rare daylight appearances, that is. These larger-than-life deviants, including Warhol film "stars" like Freddie Herko, Diane DiPalma, Ondine, Brigid Berlin, Edie Sedgwick, and Rene Ricard, also called themselves the "amphetamine rapture group" after their favorite drug. Warhol himself became a habitual amphetamine user before founding the Factory, initially using a low dose by prescription to keep weight off.[43] But he took to the drug immediately, no surprise given his anxieties about sleep. (His friend Henry Geldzahler recalled that Warhol "was very much a night creature and literally afraid to go to sleep at night. He wouldn't fall asleep until dawn cracked because sleep equals death and night is fearsome.")[44]

Warhol's first major film *Sleep* (1963) actually addressed this issue, with eight hours of deadly dull footage of his lover John Giorno sleeping. Later, Warhol recalled that amphetamine itself inspired him: "seeing everybody so up all the time [on speed] made me think that sleep was becoming obsolete, so I figured I'd better quickly do a picture of a person sleeping." His favorite kind evidently was a powerful diet tablet named Obetrol (containing up to 10 mg of methamphetamine, 5 mg of dextroamphetamine, and 5 mg of original Benzedrine-style amphetamine, adding subjective "buzz") (Figure 33). He reportedly enjoyed Dexamyl as well. The morning one of his crazed former actors shot him in 1968, he was filling his Obetrol prescription, and he continued taking amphetamine until the day he died in 1987.[45] Without his speed, Warhol would not fully have been Warhol—and being Andy Warhol was a constant work of performance art.

Neither would Britain of the swinging sixties have been the same without speed. During the early 1960s, the growing British amphetamine habit began alarming physicians in that country—and no wonder, when about 3 percent of all prescriptions were for amphetamines (just as in the U.S. at the time, though without triggering alarm among many American doctors). Apart from the supposedly typical "tired housewives" who badgered family doctors for extra prescriptions, and apart from that other major group of speed abusers whom doctors had to watch out for, "physicians, pharmacists, nurses or musicians who present with tension anxiety," another common type of amphetamine abuser emerged in urban Britain during the early 1960s: teen-agers and young adults showing "aggression to parents . . . changes of mood . . . staying out late," and frequent "attendance at coffee bars and clubs."

Like the "housewives," these young abusers preferred Drinamyl (Dexamyl), but they differed in deliberately taking too much, just for fun. Psychiatrist Philip Connell, who earlier wrote the definitive study on amphetamine psychosis, noticed this usage pattern at his clinic in London's Maudsley Hospital. Generally, as part of their social scene at nightspots in Liverpool, Brighton, and London's Soho, some of his teenage patients were taking fifty or more "purple heart" tablets (tri-angular blue Dexamyls) in a single session, a walloping dose of am-phetamine even greater than one could get from an entire inhaler. When young users like this came to the clinic, it was usually with a bad case of "the Horrors," paranoia and other symptoms of ampheta-mine psychosis. Otherwise, they had no interest in medical attention for their habits.[46]

By 1964–65, the issue was generating worried headlines in Britain; for instance, one newspaper story entitled "My Pep Pill Soho Trip" describes "tireless, sleep-free, talkative super-teenagers drifting from club to cafe with strange, sterile energy," and another story in the weekly magazine *New Society* relates how, on purple hearts, "you can talk like a genius. Everything is beneath you and under control. Sleep is unnecessary so you go to the all-night sessions in Soho and stay high the whole weekend [. . . talking] brittle, flashy gibberish with your friends."[47] The popularity of Dexamyl on the street in 1960s Brit-ain owes a lot to the sacramental status it attained among the Mods youth subculture, whose flashy suits, Italian scooters, and clashes with the Rockers subculture were musically immortalized by the Who in their operatic album *Quadrophenia*—whose main character seems to suffer an attack of amphetamine psychosis at the story's turning point. (And, in Frank Roddam's 1979 film version, he takes a handful of pur-ple hearts at a party beforehand.)

Not only was high society, swinging Soho, and avant-garde New York making amphetamine a deliberate lifestyle choice, but ampheta-mine, as a recreational drug, had grown so common in the mid-1960s that it had become an issue among the general public. In a 1966 issue of the *Atlantic Monthly*, one reporter, Bruce Jackson, recounted having been taken by a Chicago friend to a "white-collar pill party"; there he marveled at the way colorful pills were being politely passed around like canapés and discussed with all the elements of connoisseurship, at the civilized manners of the participants despite their sleep deprivation, and at the gossip about various doctors and pharmacists who made it easy for those in the know to get the drugs. Guests helped themselves from a five-pound box of Dexedrine, and from candy dishes filled with Dexedrine, Dexamyl, Eskatrol (an SKF weight-loss drug containing dextroamphetamine and the chlorpromazine-related tranquilizer prochlorperazine), and other pills he could not identify. Nearby stood "The Book"—the *Physicians Desk Reference,* a medical publication describing all prescription drugs—for those who wanted to compare and discuss ingredients. Jackson watched "a distractingly pretty girl" carefully sawing blue and yellow tablets in half for hours. His friend explained that these were Desbutal Gradumets made by Abbot Labs, a Dexamyl-like combination of methamphetamine and the barbiturate Nembutal. The young woman was collecting the blue amphetamine halves in one jar for immediate consumption, and the yellow barbiturate halves to use later if she wanted to sleep. Noting that she took half an hour to split one pill, whereas it took him half a minute, his friend pronounced it "a sign of a fairly confirmed head when they reach the ritual stage."

Pharmaceutical amphetamines as recreational drugs certainly penetrated blue-collar circles, too. The medical anthropologist Seymour Fiddle, who studied the problem, described a nineteen-year-old, working-class white man, "John," from a large family in the New York suburbs. He did not associate with the "wierdos" of Greenwich Village, or with any particular counterculture, and he saw himself as normal and mainstream. He began taking Dexedrine to get high, about ten 5 mg tablets at a time. John enjoyed the buoyant mood and the lively talk it encouraged with his speed-using friends, as well as the energy it gave him. He did not mind that the drug took away all interest in food and girls, and he quickly became a regular user. After a few months he was taking about thirty (5 mg) Dexedrines at a time, but even this huge dose now left him tired, so he switched to about thirty-five (10 mg) Benzedrine tablets, which he mistakenly believed were stronger. (This is only a marginal increase, since, by weight, ordinary racemic amphetamine is actually about half as powerful a brain stimulant as dextroamphetamine, but it is easy to see why John thought Benzedrine more powerful, since it produces a greater subjective "buzz" by raising blood pressure and has other side effects as well.) John found very soon that amphetamine brings unpleasant effects along with the pleasant, if you use it every day: "a guy comes up behind and touches you—you jump out of your skin . . . you can feel your heart beat . . . it enlarges your eyes, y'know, and they start to hurt." John ended up spending three months in a psychiatric ward, but, after discharge, he immediately returned to amphetamine. He became a successful small-time dealer, thanks to a relationship he developed with a local druggist, and at one point he was distributing about a thousand amphetamine pills a week to other young people in his neighborhood. Clearly, amphetamines were easy to get by the mid-1960s, even for those who could not afford a Park Avenue "Dr. Feelgood."[48]

Fiddle's anthropological studies, like Jackson's journalism, reflected America's mounting anxiety about its relationship with drugs in general, both legal and illegal. On the one hand, illegal drugs moved from the shadows into the spotlight, as experimentation with forbidden drugs like marijuana blossomed among middle-class youth on university campuses everywhere. To American parents, drug abuse no longer seemed confined to a fringe of degenerate "junkies," a move to the mainstream that might well have made the topic seem more worthy of study by medical anthropology and sociology. Furthermore, with the way people actually use drugs under the microscope, the myth of a sharp divide between medical and nonmedical "recreational" drug use began to weaken. Some of the pharmaceuticals that people get from our modern medicine men suddenly started looking a lot like the illegal drugs that people take in alternative manners; perhaps some street "abusers" were actually self-medicating, and some legitimate patients were merely junkies hooked by the doctors and drug firms.[49]

This new ambiguity helps explain the opinion shifts discovered by the historian Susan Speaker, in tracing the journalistic treatment of psychiatric pharmaceuticals in the American press over time. As problems with the originally miraculous "mind drugs" began emerging in the 1960s, Speaker found two major trends in interpretation, one blaming the medical system for their abuse and the other blaming the user.[50] For instance, a prominent 1966 article in the New York Times attributed our "Addicted Society" to the way, in modern culture, we all expect to be happy, industrious, thin, calm, and well rested, simply through the technological fix of a prescription. Jackson's "Pill Party" story partly resonates with this social critique category: our pill-using society as a whole is cast into the old role of the psychologically defective junkie. In this perspective, which can verge into "pharmacological Calvinism," when pill-using individuals rather than society as a whole are chiefly blamed, overdependence on medications represents a symptom of underlying moral weakness, not a cause.[51]

But whereas some critics puritanically blamed unhealthy, hedonistic consumer culture for drug problems, others, associated with the rising "consumer's movement," blamed the medical system and specifically the pharmaceutical industry (as Jackson did, too). Journalist Morton Mintz, who wrote a hard-hitting series of articles in the early 1960s and the 1965 bestseller *Therapeutic Nightmare,* cast an especially harsh light on the scale of harms to patients caused by drug companies and their products, which, according to him, were mostly shoddy and dangerous. At a more intellectually refined level, the same anticorporate reformism that fueled the consumer's movement in 1960s America also manifested itself in what is often called the "antipsychiatry movement," a direct attack on mental health drugs. This perspective, associated especially with the libertarian medical sociologist Thomas Szasz, suggested that mental illness is nothing more than those traits and behaviors considered undesirable by the powers that be. That is, psychiatric clinics are today's sanitized version of the dungeons once used to neutralize disruptive noncomformists, and the tranquilizers—especially the antipsychotic major tranquilizers used in mental wards—are just "chemical straightjackets" of conformity. Thus medicine's authority, particularly in the matter of psychiatric prescription drugs, came under siege from journalists without and dissidents within.[52]

In retrospect, both sides clearly had a valid point: the medical profession and drug industry started the American public on its prescription psychotropic drug habit, thanks to the profit motive, professional convenience, and more subtle factors such as the need to demonstrate medicine's power over the newly terrifying realm of mental illness. At some point, however, a consumer "pull" began to outstrip the supply "push" from the medical system, as high rates of nonmedical amphetamine use testify. Both supply and demand sides must figure in any adequate analysis of the social forces behind the enormous consumption levels of amphetamines reached in the 1960s (see below). In any case, by the late 1960s the over-medication of the American public had become a major political issue. And well it might, given that the rate of consumption of psychiatric drugs then was considerably higher than the rates condemned by critics of antidepressant overuse today. (In the mid-1960s Americans consumed, on average, as many amphetamines and minor tranquilizers as all kinds of psychotropic prescription drugs consumed in 2000, and indeed, depending on definitions, up to twice as much psychotropic medication. Thus, although there may be more users of psychotropic drugs today, they are taking on average less drugs than in the 1960s.)[53] Even though amphetamine consumption was actually greater in volume, the trendier tranquilizers took the brunt of the late-1960s critiques, for the quick fix of emotional challenges they promised. But speed shared in the punishment, as we can see from "Addicted Society's" disdain for the American quest for easy slimness, industriousness, and happiness—all promised by amphetamines (if "happiness" is the opposite of depression). In such a climate, where psychiatric drugs had become so problematic and no traditional authority remained unquestioned, the pharmaceutical industry could only delay but ultimately not escape controls on its mind-altering offerings.

The national amphetamine problem had indeed reached daunting proportions by the time the voices of concern grew loud. Estimating precisely how many Americans were taking how much amphetamine in the late 1960s is tricky, since it requires accounting for volume and prevalence of consumption, both medical and recreational, as gauged by several un-standardized methods and sources. At a time when the bulk of pharmaceutical amphetamines were being dispensed not by pharmacists filling ordinary prescriptions but on the black market and the grey market by dispensing physicians and diet clinics, production figures rather than retail prescribing audits are the most reliable index of overall consumption. The FDA's manufacturer survey in 1962 arrived at a figure of 8 billion standard 10 mg tablets of amphetamine salts, based on production reports amounting to 4.5 billion typical pills plus a rough estimate of the additional output of the two largest manufacturers, who did not cooperate. In 1969, that figure (or perhaps somewhat higher, 10 billion typical pills) was still the best estimate FDA could offer Congress, and the stability of this number fits with the stability of retail amphetamine prescription rates over most of the decade.[54]

How many of those 8–10 billion 10 mg amphetamine pills were medically dispensed is a harder question to answer. As a conservative estimate we might adopt the figure of 4 billion 10 mg pills in 1969, the production for that year as later reported by drug firms submitting applications to the FDA and narcotics authorities for permission to produce more, after amphetamine had become a controlled substance.[55] Even 4 billion tablets, representing twenty 10 mg amphetamine doses per year for every man, woman, and child in the United States, seems a lot of speed for doctors to be prescribing. And that figure only accounts for around half the amphetamines Americans were actually consuming.

How many people were taking all this medical and nonmedical amphetamine is a different and entirely independent question. The only large national survey on drug consumption in that period found that, in 1970, 5 percent of the adult population had used amphetamines and related stimulants in the previous year, or about 7 million people, considering only those taking prescription drugs obtained through medical channels.[56] Although many users may not have endured any great harm, these massive numbers point to a large underlying subpopulation of people suffering the damaging effects of medical amphetamine dependency. The British studies of the early 1960s had indicated on the order of 6.6–10 percent of the population receiving amphetamine prescriptions from family doctors in a given year were habituated or addicted—that is, dependent to some extent. Experiments with such dependent patients showed that a third of them were, in fact, "addicted" or physically dependent on their prescribed amphetamines (although they might not all have met current standards of "addiction"). As argued above, these British data imply a medical addiction rate of roughly 2.2–3.3 percent; in other words, in Newcastle, around 1961, from one in fifty to one in thirty patients receiving an amphetamine prescription each year were physically dependent. Applying this proportion to the 7 million adult medical users of amphetamine in the late 1960s yields the conclusion that the United States contained half a million dependent amphetamine patients and, of these, 175,000–230,000 were physically dependent addicts.[57] All these addicts were supplied by doctors and the pharmaceutical industry.

Many speed users were also supplied indirectly by the pharmaceutical industry through the extra billions of amphetamine tablets "diverted" annually from medical channels. A more thorough 1970 study in New York state explored both nonmedical and medical amphetamine use. In this survey, 6.5 percent of the state's 13.8 million residents over fourteen years old had used amphetamines in the past six months. Counting only those using pharmaceutical amphetamines, 39 percent used them nonmedically and 22 percent "abused" them, defined by obtaining amphetamines without prescription and using them for social occasions. More than half the regular users of the psychiatric-type amphetamines obtained at least some of their pills without a prescription, as did a smaller (but still large) proportion of amphetamine diet pill users.[58] There must also have been many thousands of people we would now count as abusers who obtained their amphetamines entirely by prescription. Thus the boundary between medical use and illicit use was highly porous, to say the least.

Given that the New York rate of adult medical amphetamine use (i.e., with a prescription) was consistent with the national survey, there is no reason we might not cautiously extrapolate the rest of the state figures to the whole United States at the time.[59] Doing so would indicate that, in 1970, 10.6 million Americans used amphetamines in the past year medically and nonmedically, 4.1 million of them used the drugs nonmedically at least some of the time, and 2.3 million "abused" the drugs by the New York definition.[60] (These are surely underestimates of the epidemic's peak around 1969, because by late 1970, when the surveys took place, consumption was declining; also, high-dose methamphetamine users were excluded from these calculations.)[61] Again applying our northern British dependency rates to our estimated 10.6 million users of pharmaceutical amphetamines in the United States, we would conclude that, in 1970, 710,000 to 1,060,000 Americans were amphetamine-dependent, and 240,000 to 350,000 physically were addicted, the higher number being more likely.[62] With more than 10 million users in America, close to 1 million dependent and some 300,000 addicted, speed had undeniably become a man-made plague.

This epidemic was produced by the medical system itself. Still, we cannot blame the medical system alone for this first amphetamine epidemic—however aggressively the drug industry marketed loose definitions of neurotic depression and obesity, and however much it suited some physicians to prescribe amphetamine as a scientifically authorized remedy for problems of living. Not all pharmaceutical marketing campaigns succeed, after all. The broader culture, as well as the medical profession, must be predisposed to accept a new pharmaceutical. What cultural predisposition or "latent demand," then, can account for the enthusiastic reception of amphetamine as a medicine, and thus explain why the amphetamine epidemic took root so deeply in postwar America? The social theorist Nikolas Rose, building on Michel Foucault's insight that political change depends on shifting norms of personal conduct and the institutions that shape conduct, has observed that the late twentieth century has seen the rise of a new concept of citizen and subject as "consumer"—insatiable, yet responsible and self-regulating. Furthermore, for Rose, the institutions of mental health (psychology and psychiatry) have been mainly responsible for instilling the required, uneasy mixture of an avid striving for wealth and pleasure with the quest for personal fulfillment.

Many historians have noted that a new and intense, almost frantic consumerism took hold during the war and especially in the postwar years (partly driven by the fear of a return to the Depression). American citizens were encouraged to move into new suburban tract housing en masse, furnish their newly spacious homes with domestic "conveniences" to occupy women freshly removed from the workforce, and buy new cars regularly in order to service life in these dispersed communities. Versions of this way of life spread throughout the Western developed countries as postwar economic expansion made the deprivations of Depression and war a distant, bad memory.[63] Enjoying consumption (and consuming "enjoyment" via the leisure industries) became as much an ethical imperative as working hard. The new consumerism brought with it a materialistic new "fun morality," as social theorists have aptly put it.[64]

These insights go a long way toward explaining society's vulnerability to the amphetamine epidemic. In America of the 1940s and 1950s, avid consumption, achievement, and enjoyment became important new social norms. This change in values promoted the wider recognition of apathy and mild anhedonia, the failure of consumerist avidity, as diagnostic criteria for neurotic depression. In this context, amphetamine represented an obvious remedy because of its enhancement of pep and "zest," and in turn the apparent effectiveness of amphetamine in boosting drive and enjoyment naturally reinforced the apathy-anhedonia concept of depression. Thus, eager pursuit of consumption, advancement, and enjoyment became not simply new standards of behavior but medically enforced requirements. Of course, "healthy" appetites for achievement and consumption have their limits, being bounded by manic excess (and grandiose shopping sprees are regarded as a key sign of mania) at the opposite extreme from depressive deficiency.

The same insights also help explain amphetamine's popularity for weight loss. To the extent that overeating was understood as driven by underlying emotional illness, as was maintained by much although not all marketing for amphetamine diet pills, the drug was also an obvious remedy for the faulty self-control behind obesity.[65] (However, since the vast majority of amphetamine users for weight loss were women, a full account of the drug's popularity would also require discussion of postwar femininity.) By helping people meet these new norms of acquisition and self-fulfillment, like so many millions of rats eagerly pressing their levers no matter how meager the rewards, amphetamine became a crucial "technology of the self" for constituting the healthy postwar consumer. As our previously quoted amphetamine prescriber declared in 1970, no other therapy helped keep her distressed patients "functioning, coping, capable of performing or even enjoying their duties" nearly so well.[66] For two decades, the use of amphetamine to meet such social demands raised few questions in America. Only in the anti-materialistic cultural rebellion of the later 1960s would this medicated consumerism begin to seem problematic.

7

Amphetamine's Decline

From Mental Medicine to Social Disease

HOW WAS THE 1960s amphetamine epidemic ever brought to an end? This question is critical if we wish to apply the lessons of history to the drug problems of today. Some of the events that finally led the American public to view amphetamines as a seductive monster, and to bring sufficient force to bear in controlling the drugs, were unique to the late 1960s. This makes the task of drawing general lessons difficult. Still, for purposes of generalization, we might break down the changes that stopped this original epidemic into three main categories.

First, public opinion shifted across different sectors from the youth counterculture to political authorities, wherein what had been viewed as an ordinary medicine, or an innocuous recreational drug, began to be seen as deadly and diabolical. Second, developing scientific knowledge, and, to a lesser extent, medical opinion, supported the emerging popular perception of amphetamines as sinister. Finally, strong government agencies had to be in place, with leadership willing to take advantage of public sentiment in order to justify unusually aggressive action against entrenched business interests. Eventually, in what can fairly be portrayed as a triumph of both public health and popular will, these three factors converged to turn the amphetamine taps with sufficient force that consumption was reduced to less dangerous levels. But it would take time.

Amphetamine versus Love

While Congress was only taking its first ineffectual actions, a powerful campaign against amphetamines had already begun, and from a surprising source within the drug counterculture. "Let's issue a general declaration to the underground community, contra speedamos ex cathedra," pronounced Allen Ginsberg in 1965.

> Speed is anti-social, paranoid making, it's a drag, bad for your body, bad for your mind, generally speaking, in the long run uncreative and it's a plague in the whole dope industry. All the nice gentle dope fiends are getting screwed up by the real horror monster Franken-stein Speedfreaks who are going around stealing and bad mouthing everybody.[1]

By then a plump guru to the younger generation, Ginsberg explained himself further in this famous underground newspaper interview. Though he had used amphetamine himself for writing, the poet ad-mitted, he had more recently decided that the drug is evil. "Since 1958 it's been a plague around my house. People that I liked or who were good artists have gotten all screwed up on it . . . all the stuff I brought back from India was stolen by speed freaks."[2] This grudge, however, was not mainly personal. Rather, Ginsberg was sounding an alarm that amphetamines posed a deadly threat to the utopia that youthful cultural pioneers were trying to bring to America, and indeed to the world.

This familiar, and now so often stereotyped utopian movement had emerged in the 1960s, as a generation too young to remember the Second World War began demanding explanations for America's per-petual war footing—the countless missiles and endless military ad-ventures to "contain communism" abroad. The pacifist "Flower Chil-dren" or "Hippies" resembled the Beatniks in rejecting traditional American materialism, militarism, competition, and rigid social codes, in valuing authenticity and creativity, and in enjoying the relaxed ca-maraderie of marijuana. Ritualistic and recreational drug taking were central to both countercultures.

But Hippies were unlike the Beatniks in certain ways: they were more hedonistic and less intellectual, seeking mystic enlightenment through an ecstatic fusion with the universe, typically achieved through hallucinogenic or psychedelic drugs (like lysergic acid dieth-ylamide or LSD, psilocybe mushrooms, or peyote cactus). These drugs became the sacraments that Benzedrine Inhalers once had been for Kerouac and his "Angel-Headed Hipster" friends, the Hippies of the 1960s exchanging the Beatniks' prized rush of ideas and improvised poetry for a kaleidoscope of visions and sensations beyond words. Rallying around the call of "peace and love" and offering passive resistance to the Vietnam War, they rejected private property and lived in communal houses in slums, almost ascetically. Bands such as the Jefferson Airplane and the Grateful Dead seemed to herald a total cultural renewal that would spread from psychedelic centers like San Francisco's Haight-Ashbury district, New York's East Village, and the Sunset Strip in Los Angeles, and remake the world.

The idyll was short-lived, and, as Ginsberg seems to have predicted, one of the major forces that devastated urban Hippie culture was a clashing drug subculture that emerged in its midst. The problem was amphetamine—increasingly, methamphetamine—and it became obvious during 1967's legendary "Summer of Love." The doctrine of peace and love, combined with escalation in Vietnam that spelled impending draft for hundreds of thousands of young men, drew flocks of newcomers to San Francisco in search of some combination of enlightenment and escapist pleasure. At the Haight-Ashbury Free Clinic, established by Dr. David E. Smith in the shadow of Alles's old stamping grounds at UCSF Medical Center, more than three hundred people sought treatment that summer for toxic reactions to very high doses of amphetamines. "Speed freaks," as the heavy users were called, injected the drug, and seemed to be spreading like locusts. Herbert Huncke, one-time narcotics instructor to Kerouac and Burroughs, described the feeling of shooting speed:

> I felt it almost instantly, and the rush to my head like a short circuit. My body began to pulsate or grow tiny antennae all quivering in anticipation—and my aliveness took on a new substance and was alerted to the waves of energetic forces sweeping around me. . . . The surroundings were already capable of absorbing force, drive, sprit, and the flow of magic sensed, never seen. I was thoroughly elated.[3]

One of Smith's Haight-Ashbury speed freaks described the "rush" or "flash" of injecting amphetamines as a "full body orgasm." This thrill seemed to appeal to a type of person different from the enlightenment-seeking Hippie. Indeed, the Free Clinic doctors found statistical evidence that speed freaks were not so much converted Hippies as newcomers from outside the San Francisco area.[4]

The speed freaks looked to amphetamines not so much for the buzz and mood elevation that lasts for hours but mainly for the fleeting flash. Seeking to recapture that first taste of chemical nirvana, they would continue injecting, up to ten times a day. At first the doses would be small, equivalent to a few capsules or tens of milligrams, and weeks or even months might pass between binges. But gradually, over perhaps a year, the doses they injected would increase to hundreds or even thousands of milligrams (whole grams, that is). Their "runs," or binges, would continue for several days without rest or food, and then finally end in total exhaustion and a slumber for up to forty-eight hours. In a full-blown speed freak, depression and the craving for more speed would set in immediately after waking up from such a "crash," and another run would begin again within a day or two.[5]

Behavior became increasingly stereotyped and repetitive as a user's amphetamine consumption rose. For instance, doctors from a drug rehabilitation center in Corona, California, described how speed freaks who liked to repair radios and televisions would lose the ability to carry out complex sequences of actions, and would content themselves with tinkering indefinitely. Similarly, they often enjoyed stringing beads or mindless housework like sweeping floors. Inappropriate perseverance, that is, continuing to perform unproductive actions repeatedly, was another consequence, just as Skinner and Brady had noted in their rat behavior work for Merck.

With enough speed, hallucinating paranoia and violent tendencies emerged. One speed freak saw detectives in every tree. Another set up an elaborate system of booby traps and electronic devices to barricade himself into his apartment and thus "outsmart the cops" who never came. A third took his large Doberman on long night walks, hunting his imagined "enemies." A fourth was walking down a New York street feeling like "king of the universe," and then suddenly jumped upon and beat up a man walking near him, after the thought crossed his mind that he might be homosexual. This speed freak could not offer any other explanation of his actions. Whereas most of the cases of amphetamine psychosis that Connell had described in the 1950s had occurred only after years of taking prescription pills to build the habit to such toxic levels, speed freaks got there much quicker, in perhaps a year.[6]

How did this pattern of drug abuse begin? Injecting high doses of amphetamines was not uncommon among heroin users during the 1950s in some American cities, and was often related to heroin shortages. Many heroin users continued to enjoy the two drugs in combination once they tried shooting speed, whereas, for some, speed became their main fix. In the Midwest, speed injectors of the late 1950s preferred amphetamine, but in California methamphetamine was generally favored. Some local observers blamed the Haight-Ashbury outbreak on a core group of San Francisco heroin addicts who had switched to prescription methamphetamine obtained from lax doctors in the early 1960s. Others blamed the motorcycle gangs, which certainly did play a major role in the distribution and dealing of amphetamines.[7]

However it started, street demand for methamphetamine became great enough to fuel an underground cottage industry on the West Coast. Most of the methamphetamine sold on the street in the late 1960s was made in small, illicit factories, even though 80 or 90 percent of amphetamines of all types seized on the street were pills manufactured by U.S. pharmaceutical firms.[8] Making methamphetamine in either solid (salt) or liquid (oily base) form was—and is—not particularly demanding, chemically speaking. One researcher interviewed a fifteen-year-old girl who ran a successful factory, or "speed kitchen," in Haight-Ashbury:

> I moved into this house with a friend of mine in Seattle and this guy was making it in the bathroom, and I'm very interested. I like to learn things, so I just stayed up with him on three different nights and he would go through all the steps and I would write down how to do it. . . . We did this around five times and I learned a lot. I can do it now, and I know most of the chemicals. I have all of it written down and I have to go by it, the temperature and everything.[9]

Naturally, once the national supply of pharmaceutical amphetamines was sharply cut by federal action after 1971, demand for home-made speed grew, driving down drug quality and strengthening the position of the motorcycle gangs. Making a popular drug illegal, without reducing demand, only spurred the development of organized crime to supply consumers—with inferior and often dangerous products. It was the same with alcohol in the days of Prohibition.[10]

At any rate, in 1967 the counterculture in San Francisco began drawing misfits and seekers from elsewhere, and many gravitated to amphetamines. The appearance of the compulsively injecting speed freak spelled the end of the peaceful communalism of the mystic "acid head" wherever the two cultures overlapped. Speed culture differed greatly. Whereas the original Hippies had lived in stable, extended family-like collective households where people worked enough, and with enough harmony, to support themselves indefinitely, the speed freaks were nomadic, according to anthropologists on the spot. Given a place to congregate and a drug supply, a group of users would begin a collective "run," injecting amphetamine every few hours to enjoy as many "flashes" as they could manage. There would be much rapid, garbled talking by several of them simultaneously, as well as plenty of "the fidgets." Soon hostility and paranoia would emerge.[11]

Having lost ten or twenty pounds over just a few days of compulsive talking and injecting, the original users would become exhausted and "crash out," perhaps in the room next door, and new users would take their place as long as the drugs kept flowing. When the drugs ran out or when the police came, often in response to some violent incident, the group would disperse. Because speed freaks react impulsively and violently to any threat or insult—real or imaginary—they frequently set one another off. In 1968–69, the rate of violent crime in Haight-Ashbury predictably rose, including murders and rapes as well as random violence—speed freaks, for example, standing in the middle of the street shooting at anything that moved.[12] The disastrous social chemistry could even be reproduced with animal experiments. David E. Smith and UCSF colleagues found that amphetamine is four times as toxic when mice lived as a group, because they started killing each other when the dosage reached a certain point; "behavioral toxicity" from amphetamine-induced hostility became deadly long before the drug dosage reached biologically lethal levels.[13]

Moreover, as if the direct effects of high amphetamine doses weren't enough, an economic effect aggravated the problems of living around speed freaks. Largely white and middle-class runaways, they lacked the streetwise skills and values of typical heroin users, so they could not competently support themselves either legitimately or criminally. Hence they tended to sponge and steal from anyone foolish enough to tolerate their presence. When they stole from one another, the suspicion and violent reactivity created by the drug itself were naturally exacerbated. Peace no longer ruled the countercultural Eden, and the Hippies soon began fleeing the Haight for rural communes.[14]

Other leaders of the Hippie counterculture and its ideology endorsed Ginsberg's anti-speed edict, mounting a campaign whose rallying cry was "Speed Kills." Buttons spreading the word were common by 1967. A Southern California organization called DoItNow, associated with the recording industry, formed in 1968 to communicate the "Speed Kills" message via popular music. Among their initiatives was a compilation album of songs against needle drugs, called First Vibration (proceeds of which were partly donated to Smith's Haight-Ashbury clinic) (Figure 34), and a series of public service announcements for broadcast on rock radio stations on the theme "put speed down—do it now!" A couple of examples convey the flavor of the campaign:

> This is Frank Zappa from the Mothers of Invention. Hi, wanna die? Start today! Use a little speed—you've got five years. Rot your mind, rot your heart, rot your kidneys . . . cucaracha!

> This is Grace Slick of the Jefferson Airplane. One pill makes you larger, one pill makes you small. And if you shoot up speed you won't be there at all, because you'll be dead, baby. Don't shoot it. Put speed down, do it now.[15]

Involving some of the most credible musicians and philosophical leaders of the psychedelic counterculture, the "Speed Kills" campaign was also noticed and spread by national media, casting amphetamines as "drugs that even scare hippies." The campaign was reinforced by a segment of the medical community concerned with the health of street drug users. Whereas the annual medical conference organized in 1967 by Smith and UCSF drug researchers had as its theme "The Religious Use of Psychedelic Drugs," and featured a sympathetic set of theological and philosophical papers on the place of the new "psychedelic church" in mystical traditions, the tone was drastically different a year later: the 1968 conference dealt with amphetamine abuse, with "Speed Kills" as its official theme. The discussion was totally unsympathetic, focusing on the toxicology of amphetamines, the psychiatry of amphetamine psychosis, and the sociology of the violent world inhabited by compulsive speed users and dealers.[16] A more forceful, self-organized grass-roots effort to reduce drug demand by shaping opinion within a community can hardly be imagined. Unfortunately, no means were in place to assess its impact, so the question of its value remains unresolved. (The "danger" message in the "Speed Kills" campaign, some have suggested, may have attracted as many people to injecting amphetamines as it frightened away.) Still, even if the message could have been better crafted to reduce demand, the "Speed Kills" campaign, in terms of its sheer reach, is a model that deserves study by architects of drug education and harm reduction campaigns to this day.

Though intravenous speed continued claiming new lives, the first wave of Haight-Ashbury speed freaks did not stay long on the drug. The typical pattern of compulsive high-dose amphetamine abuse is very unstable: a heavy speed user either dies in some speed-induced violent situation or from hepatitis or other infectious disease from sharing needles, helped along by starvation. Alternatively, the user stops taking speed, typically by becoming addicted to different drugs —particularly the "downers" he already used to relax and catch some sleep at the end of a run. This is what happened in postwar Japan, when a massive methamphetamine epidemic in the early 1950s was followed by a large heroin epidemic late in the decade.[17]

The same occurred in San Francisco. Whereas two years earlier staff of the Haight-Ashbury Free Clinic had been busy "talking down" Hippies who had gone too high on LSD—sometimes hundreds in a day, when a free rock concert was on—by 1969 heroin overdoses had become their main concern. The neighborhood's atmosphere was now dominated by the "dead cool" of the introverted "smack-head," as contemporary medical observers put it, and heroin addiction remained the biggest drug issue in Haight-Ashbury for years.[18] But the speed injection epidemic did move onward, spreading to cities across the nation and stirring consternation in the halls of Congress, where Smith testified on his experiences at the Free Clinic and foretold that heroin use would soon skyrocket. This prediction essentially promised that a local drug problem in the Hippie subculture would soon, if neglected, feed America's most feared narcotic menace and spawn a national crime wave.[19] Thus, the image of the speed freaks and the havoc they wrought in Haight-Ashbury added to the mainstream political impetus to do something decisive about America's problem with amphetamines.

Amphetamine versus the American Soldier

Another issue that made amphetamine's dark side more prominent in the public eye involved the Vietnam War, that central controversy of the decade. In the late 1960s, America was losing its first war ever. Hundreds of thousands of American soldiers struggled in the jungles to prop up South Vietnam's corrupt regime against a popular communist revolution. The U.S. military threw massive air power at the enemy and its suspected supporters in the countryside to "bomb them back into the stone age" (in the 1965 words of Curtis Lemay, the general in charge of bombing Japan in the Second World War).[20] While this undeclared war wore on and the body count climbed without perceptible progress, the young generation who were called upon to kill and to die revolted in increasing numbers against the culture and government of their parents. Before the war ended, fifty-eight thousand American soldiers had died in Vietnam. The toll on the servicemen who survived was also gruesome. Untold thousands returned so scarred that they could not resume civilian life, and drugs were a huge part of this tragedy. In the late 1960s, congressional investigations revealed that for every soldier killed, ten veterans returned to the U.S. as drug addicts. And the two men per day dying of heroin overdose in Vietnam were just the tip of the iceberg; 10 percent of soldiers in the field had used heroin at least once, and one-quarter of the soldiers regularly abused "hard drugs" (heroin, amphetamines, barbiturates, and psychedelics).[21]

Suspicions fell on the drugs that the military itself fed soldiers. A congressional inquiry disclosed that between 1966 and 1969, the height of the Vietnam conflict, the U.S. Navy was supplying its active duty personnel an average of 210 mg of dextroamphetamine per year per man, and the Air Force used 175 mg and the Army 138 mg. This official speed was equivalent to thirty or forty 5 mg Dexedrine tablets per fighting man per year, enough for an inexperienced user to stay moderately high for a couple of weeks. Indeed, government-issue Dexedrine was distributed "like candy," to quote one veteran, without any limits on the dose or frequency of use. Further, although the military supplied its men no more than the average amphetamine consumption of Americans at the time, it must be kept in mind that soldiers could also buy their own unofficial speed on the street in Vietnam, such as the popular French-made Maxitone Forte—ampoules of

100 mg dextroamphetamine liquid for injection. Naturally, some men took more than others. A large survey by medical researchers found that 7 percent of soldiers in the field were serious amphetamine abusers, and another more detailed study found that after one year in action 5.2 percent of soldiers reported heavy amphetamine use compared to 3.2 percent of the soldiers just arriving in Indochina. Thus, the military was nearly doubling the number of speed abusers among its men in Vietnam.[22]

As one might expect with more than one in twenty soldiers a hard core amphetamine user, problems with the drug emerged in Vietnam itself, well before Congress noticed. On one nighttime river patrol, an elite Green Beret named "Bill" (his last name withheld by his psychiatrists), who had an amphetamine habit of 100 mg per day, was so jumpy after twenty-six sleepless, drugged hours on duty that, when startled by a noise, he machine-gunned an accompanying boat, killing and maiming a number of his colleagues. Officially attributed to enemy action, concealed incidents like this may have been common. For dangerous patrols, men would regularly shoot speed or gobble government-issue Dexedrine to maintain the level of edginess they needed to cope and stay alive, as a commando named Mike Beamon (perhaps a pseudonym) recalled about his excursions behind enemy lines: "When we went on a mission, we took a whole handful of pills, and some of those were Dexedrine. When I hit Dexedrine I'd just turn into a pair of eyeballs and ears." This polydrug approach was shared by a seasoned Special Forces man met by war correspondent Michael Herr, who before night patrols "took his pills by the fistful," Dexedrine from his right pocket and "downs" from his left. The man said that the combination "cooled things out just right," helping him see and move silently in the dark jungle, and making him "one of our best killers" (according to Herr).[23] "When you walk point, man, you get sharp or you get blown away," as another soldier put it. So to stay alert to subtle signs of booby traps or ambushes, men used drugs to achieve the right degree of "paranoia" on patrol: speed or marijuana or a low dose of heroin or all three.[24]

Speed was doubtless involved in numerous incidents of friendly fire in Vietnam, both accidental and intentional, as well as crimes against civilians. Such incidents, of course, do not prove the drug responsible. The underlying situation that created the need for amphetamine or heroin in combat—jungle warfare amid a hostile civilian population—also created extreme tensions that sometimes led to murder. Still, the excess aggression and paranoia generated by amphetamine could only have worsened the situation. And because heavy amphetamine use creates a craving for relaxation and rest, the military's supply of amphetamine to soldiers must also have aggravated the heroin addiction problem, as users moved from one drug to the next, just as they did in Haight-Ashbury.

One would suppose that military authorities had solid grounds for thinking that amphetamine improved performance in combat, given all the Dexedrine they were supplying. However, the medical and psychological evidence for speed's objective performance benefits had grown little since the Second World War. By the end of that war, a great many tests in both simulators and the field had shown that early reports of improvement in work output and performance were based only on subjective impressions. The main reason that the Allied military used amphetamine, despite the failure to demonstrate objective performance gains, was (as I argued in chapter 3) its effect on morale —that is, the way it alters mood to increase aggression and optimism. As the RAF concluded at the end of the war, the drug made men think they were performing brilliantly when, in fact, they were doing an average job or worse, thanks to these mood effects coupled with impaired judgment.[25]

To be sure, a few late-1950s studies in the military and the emerging field of sports medicine had provided evidence that amphetamine objectively retarded the loss of coordination with fatigue.[26] Other studies gauged the effects of the drug on judgment, and some of these confirmed that the drug did cause problems, at least with the judgment of time. In any case, evidence both for and against performance enhancement with amphetamine remained weak, and all studies were open to the criticism that they were far too simple to speak to complex situations in combat. Controversy among scientists in this field continued throughout the 1960s, not that science could have greatly influenced the policy of the U.S. military. As soon as the Korean War flared up in 1950, the military started buying Dexedrine from SKF, still the military's stimulant of choice as of this writing (2006).[27] Whatever the state of scientific opinion, then and now, about amphetamine's contribution to alertness and coordination, the drug's mood-altering effects make soldiers fight harder. Apparently, this is reason enough for the military to continue supplying amphetamine, despite the potential cost to the men who take it and their comrades.[28]

Amphetamine versus Sports

Concern with amphetamine in professional sports began to rise simultaneously with concern about the drug problem on the streets and in the military. The amphetamine scandals began in bicycling, long a testing ground for performance enhancement. This phenomenon is unsurprising given the sport's tradition of extremely grueling events; for example, nonstop six-day races of more than three thousand kilometers were popular in the late nineteenth century, making today's Tour de France seem gentle by comparison. In the early days, combinations of cocaine (for alertness, pain control, and attitude) and strychnine (to combat muscle fatigue) proved popular. In 1939, sports medicine specialists already noted Benzedrine use among professional cyclists, but amphetamine really caught on during the postwar surge in the sport's popularity. In 1948, a British doctor attending cycling teams at the Olympics and World Championship competitions sounded an alarm that the riders were doping themselves "like race horses" with "concoctions of strychnine, caffeine, and Benzedrine." Europe's first postwar mega-star Fausto Coppi, five-time winner of the Giro d'Italia and twice Tour de France champion (Figure 35), made no secret of his use, quipping on camera that he only used the drugs when he absolutely had too—which was "nearly always."[29]

After Coppi, all the serious riders took amphetamines, according to veteran cyclist Rik van Steenbergen. Marcel Bidot, a team manager in the 1960 Tour de France, estimated that three-quarters of the competitors used speed. That year, during the Rome Olympics, the Danish cyclist Knut Jensen died during a time trial from the combination of amphetamine and the heat. Indeed, throughout the 1960s, hardly any professional cycling event was complete without a collapse or death from amphetamine. The spectacular demise of Tom Simpson, 1965 world champion, during the 1967 Tour de France cemented cycling's image as the amphetamine doper's game. The papers had been following Simpson's "comeback" during the race, and journalists recounted in gruesome detail how, after collapsing and insisting on being put back on his bike during a hot, tough climb, he collapsed again and expired, foaming at the mouth. Afterward, stories about his fatal drive to win filled columns around the world for weeks, and methamphetamine turned out to be the main culprit in Simpson's case. France passed a law against drug use in sports later that year.[30] Of course, cycling was a European affair, and Americans paid these scandals little notice.

However, serious worries had already arisen during the 1950s around amphetamine in university and high school sports. In 1957, the American Medical Association launched an inquiry into amphetamine use in college athletics, condemning the alarmingly common practice.[31] Amphetamine was soon banned in college and high school sports as unsportsmanlike and probably dangerous. Professional sports, however, refused to acknowledge its increasingly obvious drug problems in the 1960s. The speed situation in professional football was particularly outrageous, making headlines when well-known players Houston Ridge of San Diego and Ken Gray of St Louis sued their teams for having been forced to take amphetamine and other drugs. The San Diego Chargers' team doctors had kept Ridge in a game with a fractured hip, so high on amphetamine and barbiturates that he had no idea he was injured. And football teams were not just giving speed to injured players. As a doctoral dissertation surveying speed use in thirteen NFL teams discovered (and as evidence in the Ridge lawsuit confirmed), players were taking an average of 60–70 mg of amphetamine in every game, mostly to get them "psyched up." Older players generally took higher doses, which makes sense given that they were plagued more by painful injuries and fears.[32]

A psychiatrist from the University of California, Arnold Mandell, investigated drug use further, at the Chargers' request. Amphetamine, he discovered, was typically used once a week on game days, almost entirely for its psychiatric effects rather than for any technical improvement in performance. Furthermore, players were taking the drug for three distinct purposes, each corresponding to a different dosage, each designed to induce a different psychological state. Quarterbacks, wide receivers, and defensive backs were taking a low 5–10 mg dose, equivalent to a normal prescription for depression or feelings of fatigue. The jobs of these players required alertness and decisiveness under pressure, and the drug was meant to make them think and respond more quickly. For instance, one quarterback reported that amphetamines made "everything slow down while I read the defense."[33]

At the other extreme, defensive ends and defensive tackles, whose jobs require crashing through the offensive side's blockers to attack the ball carrier with maximum velocity, were taking 50–200 mg of amphetamine each game. Except for severe narcolepsy, this huge dose had no medical use. It is the quantity a hardened speed freak would take, with amphetamine psychosis the eventual outcome, but a semi-psychotic rage was just what defensive tackles sought. Speed helped them crush everyone in their way. Still, the impaired judgment and stereotypical behavior brought on by amphetamines could easily make the drugs more of a liability. For instance, Mandell described one game in which a veteran defensive end persistently went "inside on every play, disregarding the linebacker's signals . . . [while the] opposing offense consistently aimed their running attack at the region he could be counted on to leave, and no amount of shouting by the defensive line coach during the game could change the defensive end's behavior."[34]

Between the extremes, offensive backs and linemen were using a "moderate" amphetamine dose (still very high by medical standards) of 15–45 mg. Here the desired psychiatric effect is that of enthusiasm and courage in the face of savage attack. No major loss of judgment would have been tolerable for players in these positions, who had to remain aware both of their quarterback's shifting tactics and those of opponents, and observe stricter rules than the defensive players. As Mandell astutely observed, offensive linemen were using "moderate" amphetamine doses much like the soldiers in Vietnam, altering their moods in similar ways for similar reasons. The calculated way these drugs were employed depending on the player's position indicates— in addition to a callous disregard for their long-term health—a savvy, scientific understanding of the psychotropic effects these drugs were capable of, at least on the part of team management. The amphetamines were, in fact, often prescribed by team doctors.[35]

Football was not the only sport involved. The fights that broke out in ice hockey games so frequently in the 1960s—far more often than previously—may well have arisen from excess reactivity and aggression from amphetamine (plus steroids in many cases). In baseball, several books by players revealed a game awash with amphetamine. "Where's my Dexamyl, Doc," said pitcher Jim Brosman to his team physician before one game, according to his autobiography; "how'm I going to get through the day?"[36] In *Ball Four,* pitcher Jim Bouton's 1970 autobiography, players gobble dextroamphetamine pills, or "greenies," like vitamins, even though everybody knows that their actual impact on performance is not what it seems.

> Some of the guys have to take one just to get their hearts to start beating. I've taken greenies but . . . the trouble with them is that they make you feel so great that you think you're really smoking the ball even when you're not. They give you a false sense of security. The result is that you get gay, throw it down the middle and get clobbered."[37]

Professional athletes knew that the subjective feeling of improved performance often came with impaired judgment, but many of them liked playing on amphetamines just the same. A 1969 exposé in *Sports Illustrated* by journalist Bil Gilbert removed any possible doubt about the problem, and stirred new calls to ban drugs in professional sports— with little immediate effect apart from official denials and attacks on whistle-blowers (including Mandell).[38]

Did amphetamine actually boost athletic performance in any respect? As noted, the military's research into amphetamine effects during and since the Second World War failed to demonstrate any clearcut gain. One influential 1959 study by a Harvard Medical School group compared university swimmers, runners, and track athletes on placebo tablets, on a moderate dosage of amphetamine, and on a small dose of barbiturates (an "active placebo" to control for generic effects when athletes felt the presence of a drug). Most of the weight throwers, runners, and swimmers did better with amphetamine than with the placebos, but these experiments still left room for doubt. To deal with the most serious criticism, that contrived experiments could not measure the difference drugs make in real competitions, the researchers worked with the swimmers more thoroughly. Replicating the excitement and rewards that drive performance in real meets so effectively that many swimmers set new personal records during the study, they found that amphetamine did make a small but significant difference of more than half a second in one-hundred- and two-hundred-yard races. As the Harvard researchers pointed out, a 1 percent gain may not seem dramatic, but because a serious athlete could take months to obtain that kind of improvement by training alone, amphetamine might easily make all the difference between winning and losing. Despite some controversy, this finding stood for more than a decade as the best science concerning amphetamine in sports, and was widely known and cited among athletes.[39]

In the late 1960s, then, player opinion seems to have held that judicious amphetamine use could produce a small gain in quickness, as well as a helpful boost to courage and energy, but considered that these effects had to be balanced against an impairment in judgment also brought on by the drug. The teams and leagues dragged their feet as long as possible; as one critic of inaction put it, "the team was the patient," not the player, as far as the front office was concerned. (Indeed, the NFL instituted drug testing only in the late 1980s, and baseball instituted amphetamine testing only in 2006.)[40] But, by 1969, Americans were already sufficiently concerned about amphetamines that many would agree with Gilbert: it was "high time to make some rules."

Amphetamine versus the Brain

In the late 1960s, while popular sentiment against amphetamines mounted, voices from within American medical research, and to a lesser extent clinical practice, also began to speak a strong message about the harm caused by these drugs. Ultimately, these voices would make a difference in the political arena, for instance, as congressional testimony. Clinical experience with the amphetamine injection epidemic in the U.S. helped remove any lingering doubts that these drugs were dangerous, because the huge doses used by speed freaks made all the consequences of amphetamine overuse more obvious. One widely discussed danger was "addiction," still a pivotal issue politically if not medically. Though new views of "drug dependency" made withdrawal inessential, proof of amphetamine's addictiveness (or "capacity to produce physical dependence," in the new language) was forthcoming: a physically measurable withdrawal or "abstinence syndrome." In a prominent 1967 paper in *JAMA*, California drug rehabilitation doctors highlighted the semi-comatose crash that speed freaks eventually experienced at the end of a run, from which the exhausted user cannot be woken for a day or more. This peculiar sleep reflected the nervous system's rebound downward from excess stimulation, the very opposite of the withdrawal produced in addiction to opiates, alcohol and barbiturates, where agitation marks a rebound upward from the sedation. Actually, in 1963, the same abnormal sleep had already been discovered by Edinburgh physicians studying heavy users of prescription amphetamines, especially Dexamyl "purple hearts." When these users were hospitalized and no longer got their daily handful of pills, they fell into a heavy slumber with an easily measurable reduction in rapid eye movement (REM). Phenmetrazine diet pills showed the same withdrawal syndrome.[41] As we shall soon see, lab researchers also found this distinctive semi-comatose state in monkeys addicted to amphetamine.

In fact, clinical experience with street drug abuse was suggesting that amphetamine's entire extended family of stimulants seemed to have the same set of pleasurable—and less pleasant—cocaine-like effects on the brain. A 1971 letter to a medical journal from a Chicago prison doctor described how a certain prescription drug, advertised as a safer and milder "non-amphetamine" medicine for depression and childhood hyperactivity, was creating a sensation among his patients:

> I was informed by one prisoner who has a 20-year-old heroin habit that he mainlined "West Coast" just once and that he was finding himself "running" (the vernacular for trying to buy it on the street) for it. . . . A second inmate, who is an addict both to heroin and to "West Coast," but mostly to "West Coast," told me today that in the two months that he was out of jail he lost 14 kg (30 pounds) and got little or no sleep. . . . He is nervous and jittery and seeks only more "West Coast" to keep him going. . . . The more proper name for "West Coast" is methylphenidate, or perhaps doctors know it as Ritalin. Yes, it is the most highly addicting and dangerous drug that any of the men can think of, and they have had much clinical experience in the matters of intravenous addiction.[42]

Thus, methylphenidate injection at the right dose is as pleasurable as amphetamine injection. And, when used recreationally, it produces the same kind of depression, craving, and compulsive chasing after the drug supplies run out. Controlled experiments showed that even experienced speed connoisseurs could not tell the difference between comparable doses of methylphenidate, amphetamine, and methamphetamine in a blind "tasting"; that is, subjectively perceived differences are mostly the result of user expectations, and in street drugs impurities, rather than the drug compounds themselves. The widespread abuse of phenmetrazine in diet pills and by injection in the 1960s in Britain and Sweden, complete with cravings, heavy dependency, and psychosis, illustrated much the same thing: the drugs closely related to amphetamine all share the same set of attractive and destructive properties, because they have just the same effect on the mind.[43] To many doctors who treated abusers, the only difference between street speed and the pharmaceuticals was the quality and the dealer's legal status.

Those who helped drug abusers had no specialty of their own at first, but one by-product of the amphetamine injection epidemic in the late 1960s and early 1970s was the formation of a new clinical field in the United States, addiction medicine. It began through the cross-fertilization between an established group of mainly East Coast–based doctors treating alcoholics and a new group of physicians like David E. Smith treating speed freaks and other street drug users mainly on the West Coast. Both shared a common compassion for patients who in many other quarters were scorned for moral weakness. They also shared a theory that there existed a single disease of addiction behind all substance abuse, although one without any essential relation to withdrawal syndromes. (That this concept clashes with the World Health Organization's concept of drug dependency, which never fully displaced the old narcotic addiction concept in America, may help explain why addiction medicine firmly established itself first in the United States.) A number of key meetings brought together American leaders in the treatment of alcohol and drug abuse during the first years of the 1970s, where they hammered out a unified approach to substance abuse treatments and a program for introducing the subject into medical school curricula. As typically occurs when new scientific and medical disciplines establish themselves, new journals proliferated, their titles advertising the new concept of the field, for example, *The Drug Abuse & Alcoholism Newsletter* (1971), *The Addiction and Drug Abuse Report* (1972), *The American Journal of Drug and Alcohol Abuse* (1974), and *Research Advances in Alcohol & Drug Problems* (1974). Supported by emerging research on the brain mechanisms of drug abuse, and by government efforts to respond to a perceived drug epidemic (efforts marked, for instance, by the 1974 foundation of the National

Institute on Drug Abuse), by the late 1970s the new addiction disease concept together with addiction medicine began gaining mainstream medical status. It might never have happened without the speed injection outbreak of the late 1960s, which helped expose underlying similarities among the different drugs.[44]

Meanwhile, beyond clinical medicine, America's alarm over the amphetamine injection epidemic, and drug abuse generally, led to a surge in experimental research into dependency on amphetamines. This research in turn brought two major consequences. First, it led to important discoveries about how the brain works and how amphetamine affects its function. Second, those discoveries reinforced mounting worries about the harmfulness of amphetamines with the certainty of laboratory science.

In the 1960s, psychologists adapted Skinner's methods to study the dependency-producing qualities of any drug as a behavioral rather than physiological issue, by setting up experiments so that animals could dose themselves by pressing a lever. Maurice Seevers conducted some especially dramatic studies late in the decade. (This is the same Seevers who had helped invent the habituation/addiction distinction, and whom SKF had approached in the 1930s to report that amphetamine was not addictive.) Seevers and colleagues at the University of Michigan developed equipment that allowed monkeys to inject themselves, right into the arteries feeding the brain at the back of the neck, yet still move freely so they could build up their own drug problems over weeks. Cocaine proved the most addicting of the stimulant drugs: once hooked, a monkey would compulsively press a lever six thousand times for hours, just to get a single shot. Monkeys on cocaine would inject themselves with the drug almost continuously if allowed, eventually bringing on epilepsy-type convulsions, and then continuing to press the lever as soon as they regained control of their movements. This went on for several days until the animal collapsed. If not dead, the exhausted animals would sleep continuously for a day or two, eat and drink a little, and begin another binge. They gnawed their fingers off, lost interest in food, wasted away, and pulled their fur out in the monkey counterpart of the "crank bugs" that speed freaks imagine infesting their skins. Tested the same way, amphetamine and methamphetamine showed all the same effects. Furthermore, the basic pattern of cyclical binging, together with a semi-comatose crash between binges, was exactly the same for the lever-pressing monkeys as for speed freaks shooting crank. So these experiments proved that the drug itself causes the amphetamine habit; character inadequacies, fashion, and culture do not apply to rats and monkeys.[45]

Given access to enough amphetamine, any rat, monkey, or man would eventually self-destruct. But what, exactly, did speed do to the brain to wreak all this havoc? Measures of lever pressing alone cannot say. By the late 1960s, a new style of brain science emerged—"neuro-psychopharmacology" was one of several awkward names for it—in an effort to answer such questions. The ambition was to look behind the curtains of behavior at the machinery of the mind by linking brain chemistry, the clinical world of biological psychiatry, and animal behavior. For instance, one could look at behavior using Skinner's methods and at the same time surgically or chemically manipulate an animal's brain to see how the manipulations affected lever pressing. This sort of approach showed that animals wired up to stimulate their pleasure centers electrically by pressing a lever acted just the same as animals with coke or speed habits, quickly reaching a state where they did nothing else. When given a chemical that blocks brain signaling by the neurohormone dopamine, animals stop working for rewards, whether the rewards are pleasure center stimulation, food, or drugs. And the same chemical blunts the euphoria felt by a person injecting speed. Thus, researchers concluded, the brain circuits behind normal reward-driven behavior—activity driven by physical pleasure, like mating and eating—were also involved in addiction, and they turned out to function mainly through dopamine. (Thus, part of the amphetamine-enhanceable "energy feeling" that Myerson discussed turned out to be our reward circuits firing with dopamine; if dopamine is involved in natural depression as well as addiction, as some scientists believe today, we would have to credit him with even greater foresight.)[46]

Between the late 1960s and the late 1970s, these pieces of our current understanding of drug dependence were starting to fall into place. Drugs like amphetamine feel pleasurable because they increase dopamine and thus trigger the nerves of our reward circuits directly. But this high dose of pleasure comes at a price: reacting to the excess dopamine, in time the nerves receiving dopamine signals become less sensitive. The drug user then takes more drugs, reducing sensitivity further so that still more drugs are needed, in a vicious spiral. A heavy user ends up with dopamine signaling that is so low without drugs that pleasure is completely impossible, and nothing besides getting more drugs is a strong enough reward to motivate behavior.[47] This line of research helped redefine "addiction" physiologically as well as behaviorally, supporting its revival as a neurochemical disorder—a disease of the nervous system.

Studies with amphetamine did still more for the basic neurosciences, beyond catalyzing this work on reward and drug dependence. Already by the first half of the 1960s, legendary scientists Julius Axelrod and Arvid Carlsson proved that amphetamine does boost adrenaline nerve signaling in the brain (as Myerson's Harvard circle speculated in the 1930s). Furthermore, it did this not just by inhibiting the hormone's breakdown by monoamine oxidase, which was how the newer MAOI antidepressants worked. Amphetamine also raised levels of the hormone at nerve endings by interfering with the recycling, or "reuptake," of released hormone—which was how the tricyclic antidepressants worked. Moreover, it raised levels of signaling by the neurohormone serotonin in the same ways, a finding that kept open both competing hypotheses that natural depression was caused by lack of serotonin, versus lack of adrenaline, in mood-controlling circuits. At very high doses, furthermore, amphetamine raised levels of adrenaline (and serotonin), signaling in yet a third way by causing extra hormone to leak out of nerve cells and thereby depleting stores, thus explaining the deep depression that speed freaks eventually experienced.

By the end of the 1960s, amphetamine was known to cause dopamine release as well, dovetailing with the emerging evidence that reward systems and addiction crucially involved dopamine circuits.[48] Thus, amphetamine became an integral part of knowledge about both phenomena: drugs that did what amphetamine does to dopamine signaling were addictive, whereas drugs that did what amphetamine does to adrenaline and/or serotonin signaling in the brain were antidepressants. (Below I examine how today's leading antidepressants, serotonin reuptake inhibitors like Prozac, are the result of building on and amplifying this second set of amphetamine's many actions.)

Finally, the speed epidemic also gave medical science in the 1960s fresh leads to a better understanding of that most fearsome and common psychotic disorder, schizophrenia. In the 1950s and early 1960s, LSD was thought to produce a "model psychosis" akin to schizophrenia, but increasing experience led psychiatrists to consider amphetamine psychosis, with its paranoid delusions and mainly auditory hallucinations, much more similar to the natural mental illness. If you gave lots of amphetamine to rats in the laboratory, it brought on agitated and repetitive behavior, and antipsychotic drugs like chlorpromazine (which helps people with amphetamine psychosis as well as schizophrenia) reversed this effect. This fit with the finding that amphetamine raises levels of dopamine in the brain, along with adrenaline and serotonin, and that antipsychotics reduce dopamine. Dopamine circuits seemed the culprit. Since around 1970 dopamine excess has remained the leading theory of the cause of schizophrenia, and amphetamine psychosis in animals has served as a key animal model for the disease, proving a productive way to study and discover antipsychotic drugs.[49] One might well ask, however, why any drug known by the later 1960s to produce the ideal schizophrenia and drug addiction for scientists to study in laboratory rats was still widely available by prescription, and immensely popular in family practice.

In Britain, the national penchant for the "purple heart" and "sweetie" raised widespread public concern. In 1964, possession of amphetamines without prescription became a criminal offense, allowing police to raid nightclubs in search of pills, while experts like Connell urged extreme caution in prescribing. Judging from letters in mainstream medical journals, by the mid-1960s British physicians generally began to agree with the WHO view of amphetamine dependency, and to conclude that amphetamines were addictive and too dangerous for routine use in general practice.[50] In 1968, an expert panel of the British Medical Association pronounced that, for the most part, the risks to amphetamine users outweighed the benefits of their use. Around the same time, British family doctors began organizing their own local bans and moratoriums on prescribing the drugs. These doctors felt that, for their communities, amphetamines, on balance, were harmful; except in rare instances such as narcolepsy, they also believed that individual patients would be better off without this whole "group of compounds for which the disadvantages were far greater than the advantages."[51] Although London did experience a short-lived outbreak of methamphetamine injection in 1968, driven by prescriptions to heroin addicts, already in that year there were indications that physician restraint was cutting the supply of amphetamines by as much as 25 percent.[52]

American medicine lagged far behind. Although the American Medical Association's Council on Drugs urged adoption of WHO thinking on drug dependency and abandonment of the opiate-based "addiction" concept in 1963, the professional organization for American doctors proved resistant to applying the logic to amphetamine. For instance, a prominent 1966 AMA statement on "Dependence on Amphetamines" sharply distinguished between drugs producing "physical dependence" and those showing dependence caused "solely by psychic needs," the class in which it placed the amphetamines. This 1966 statement reproduced the old addiction-habituation distinction and, furthermore, did not acknowledge that depression could be a direct consequence of amphetamine withdrawal (though a preexisting depression might be "unmasked"); denied there was any "characteristic abstinence syndrome"; denied that doctors were often responsible for amphetamine dependence (by attributing "most cases" to "illicit channels"); and only suggested moderate caution when prescribing the drugs for long-term and continuous use.[53]

American general practitioners were still happy to defend amphetamine's routine prescription in office practice both vigorously and publicly, in 1970 and after. It was not until 1978 that the AMA issued a revised statement acknowledging that amphetamine withdrawal could cause a "depressive reaction" and that doctors needed to watch out for "signs and symptoms" of "drug dependence." Even this statement did not rule out prescribing amphetamines for weight loss but urged low dosages, short courses of treatment, and "drug holidays" to forestall tolerance and dependency. Finally, in 1980, the AMA issued a call for American doctors to cooperate on the local level to stop prescribing the drugs whenever possible and to get them out of the pharmacies, as the British profession had done a decade and a half earlier.[54] But notwithstanding the AMA's passivity, in mounting political strife over the dangers of drug abuse during the later 1960s, accumulating scientific knowledge would make the defense of amphetamine in medicine an increasingly untenable position.

The People versus Amphetamine

In the mid-1960s, and again in the late 1960s, serious efforts were made to bring the amphetamine problem under greater control through new legislation. Two major laws were enacted by Congress, each failing to solve the speed problem, and then a third, more successful attack on amphetamine was mounted from within government agencies. However, to understand the origins and outcomes of these specific political initiatives, it is necessary to consider the broader picture of drug politics. Throughout the 1960s, the pharmaceutical industry and the problem of drug abuse drew enormous attention in Washington, sometimes separately and sometimes together, in a deep reconsideration of the proper place of drugs in American society. The struggle over amphetamine control in some ways encapsulated the entire political dynamic of the 1960s. It would throw together, in a single melee, the advocates of free enterprise, good government, law and order, nonconforming youth, concerned parents, peace in Vietnam, and American expansionism.

A particularly big change in the politics of drugs occurred in 1962, with legislation expanding the federal government's regulatory authority over pharmaceuticals. Twenty years after the 1938 legislation giving the Food and Drug Administration substantial powers to regulate the drug industry, a set of congressional hearings, in 1958, began to raise serious questions about the adequacy of pharmaceutical regulation. The topic initially was the excessive consumption, and promotion, of the popular new tranquilizers, and it sparked the interest of Tennessee senator C. Estes Kefauver, then famous for an early-1950s Senate inquiry into racketeering and organized crime. Seeing pharmaceuticals as a legal racket needing discipline, Kefauver, in 1959, launched a new investigation from his position as chairman of the Senate Subcommittee on Antitrust and Monopoly. In more than two years of wide-ranging inquiry, Kefauver's committee attacked the huge profits enjoyed by pharmaceutical companies, profits based in retail prices several thousand percent above the actual cost of drug production. At first glance, this indeed looked like profiteering, if not racketeering. As the former FDA counsel W. W. Gooodrich recalled in a 1986 interview:

> The pharmaceutical industry responded to that by bringing in some of their big guns, presidents of companies—Frederick Brown from Schering and what's his name from Parke Davis, and Eli Lilly and those companies all sent their big presidents down here to testify. Their testimony was that drugs were high because it cost a lot of

money to do the clinical research, it cost a lot of money to promote, it cost a lot of money to advertise, and that they were under an obligation to follow the experience with them and they had a short life.

Well, of course, they stepped right into the bear trap when they did that. That just focused attention on these various phases of new drug development and promotion. First of all, was it really all that expensive? Were they really doing all that kind of research? And anyone who had looked at any of the New Drug Applications knew, as I knew, that that was all baloney, and what they were [sending] to us in those early days was essentially a bunch of testimonials.[55]

Kefauver deflated industry claims by looking at the relationship between price and research costs behind individual drugs. One example was chlorpromazine, which Rhone-Poulenc discovered with no help from SKF, but which SKF sold as Thorazine at $3.00 for fifty pills in the U.S. compared to the $0.50 Rhone-Poulenc charged in France for the same quantity under its Largactil brand name. Kefauver also showed through economic analysis that overall profitability and rates of return on investment in pharmaceuticals more than doubled that prevailing in other industries, as they still do. Drug prices obviously exceeded levels required to cover research costs and to return normal profits, several times over.[56]

After dismissing the drug companies' claims that they needed such high prices to finance drug discovery, Kefauver went on to explore the marketing methods and regulatory framework that allowed them to get away with it. This probe allowed the senator to develop a good case that drug firms used tricks of patent law to keep exclusive control of older drugs rightly belonging in the public domain; that most new drugs were not important contributions to medicine, and often were not new discoveries at all; that drug advertising deceived doctors into thinking that patented new drugs worked better than much cheaper older drugs; and that the testing arranged by drug firms to establish the safety and efficacy of their new products was often shoddy and sometimes downright fraudulent. Kefauver also unearthed damning evidence of a level of cooperation (if not collusion) between the drug industry and its federal regulators that threatened the public interest; for instance, the FDA's head of antibiotic regulation had received $300,000 in "honoraria" from the very firms whose products he was charged with monitoring. Kefauver introduced an ambitious bill not only making federal regulation more stringent, and placing special controls on habit-forming drugs, but also including economic policy such as provisions limiting patent rights on drugs in order to stimulate competition, and requiring new drugs to be proven improvements on old drugs if they were to be granted patent protection at all.[57] One can only wonder if the social problems and controversies now surrounding pharmaceuticals could have been averted had Kefauver's bill passed as proposed.

In any event, it did not. The drug industry—whose response was summed up as "dangerous nonsense" by SKF's Francis Boyer—had many friends in Congress. The industry also funded a massive public relations campaign in the pages of medical journals and the popular media to defend its image. In mid-1962, more than a year after its introduction, Kefauver's bill seemed to be going nowhere despite President Kennedy's signal of support as an element of his consumer protection agenda.[58]

Unforeseen by the lobbyists, however, a series of newspaper stories starting that July transformed the situation. A rash of strange birth deformities had cropped up in Europe, leaving infants with stunted, seal-like limbs. Scientists traced the deformities to a new tranquilizer called thalidomide that their mothers had taken while pregnant. It then emerged that the same deformities were occurring in the U.S., although to a much lesser extent. A medical officer new to the FDA, Frances Kelsey, had stubbornly resisted pressure brought by her government superiors and the American firm that owned rights to the German product, holding out for more evidence of drug safety. Nonetheless, the U.S. firm, Merrell, had distributed millions of sample thalidomide pills to thousands of doctors to try on a "research" basis while awaiting approval, and these samples were the cause of the U.S. deformities (suddenly making the old drug industry tradition of so-called research samples appear scandalous). Kennedy acclaimed Kelsey a heroine, and public opinion swung toward Kefauver's view that the drug companies needed disciplining. No congressman was prepared to oppose a bill protecting American babies from deformity, and a version of the bill passed House and Senate in record time. As passed, the 1962 law mainly provided for FDA's more formal involvement in new drug testing, and authority to require proof of a new drug's effectiveness as well as safety before it could be marketed. Old drugs marketed before 1962, including amphetamine and methamphetamine, were exempt. As for the restrictions on patenting and pricing that Kefauver had seen as crucial, and the special restrictions on habit-forming drugs (meaning amphetamines and barbiturates) that Kennedy had endorsed, the bill that actually passed contained none.[59]

Round One: Thrill Pill Crusade

The first concerted effort to control amphetamines with new legislation began before Kefauver's bill, from an extended series of congressional investigations into street crime. Of course, drugs and crime are perennial issues in Washington, as shrewd politicians play to America's craving for ever tougher law enforcement and rampant fear of narcotics. But in the postwar years the "goofball" menace—nonmedical barbiturate use—merged with the narcotics menace in the political imagination, and by the mid-1950s nonmedical amphetamine use (especially from inhalers) was tarred by the same brush. In 1958, a Senate inquiry into juvenile delinquency, headed by Thomas Dodd of Connecticut, began to explore a range of scapegoats for this obsession of the 1950s: broken homes, pornography, psychological harms from bad parenting, but, most of all, demon drugs. "Thrill Pills," the senators called them, rarely distinguishing between the largely opposing effects of barbiturates and amphetamines. A parade of anecdotes about juvenile crime committed under the influence were trotted out before Dodd's committee, supplied mostly by the FDA, possibly in a bid for greater authority. For instance, a fifteen-year-old Illinois girl was found dead in bed from a drug overdose (presumably of barbiturates) given to her at a party by older men, one of whom fell to his death from a window. A girl ran over her mother and dragged the body more than a mile under the car. Young waitresses took thrill pills and drove off with truck drivers, older people furnished them to teenagers in order to "have sex relations" with them, and gangs of teenage boys took them to bolster their courage for committing robberies. In 1961, Dodd introduced legislation to place amphetamines and barbiturates under stricter controls, but it went nowhere thanks to the opposition of pharmacists, doctors, and drug firms.[60]

In 1964, Dodd was coming up for reelection, and he reintroduced his bill to control illegal distribution of prescription amphetamines and barbiturates. Again he was supported by the FDA, whose agents would gain powers under the bill to act more like law enforcement officers (rather than mere health inspectors). This time Dodd's litany of horror anecdotes emphasized highway deaths as the tragic consequence of "thrill pills," as well as the old theme of "juvenile delinquency and promiscuity, and violent and bizarre crimes." In July 1963, the car of an Air Force sergeant and his wife and two children had been struck from behind by a large truck at a highway inspection stop, pushed under another truck and engulfed instantly in flames. In January 1964, a truck crossed to the wrong side of the West Virginia turnpike and collided head on with a postal truck, killing everyone in both vehicles. The amphetamines found on both drivers were blamed (even though one would expect to find amphetamines at many truck accidents, whether or not the drugs had anything to do with the crashes, simply because drivers used amphetamines to stay awake). The trucking industry attracted special attention not only because drivers taking amphetamines were involved in crashes but also because recent FDA investigations had targeted truck stops as major nodes for the wholesale distribution of amphetamines. A cynical view would also suggest that shifting the blame to truck drivers, who lacked lobbying resources, rather than major trucking firms and doctors and pharmacists, who all had powerful lobbies, was an expedient way of packaging legislation to restrict particular prescription drugs.[61]

Apart from turning FDA inspectors into gun-slinging G-men, Dodds's bill required manufacturers of amphetamines and barbiturates to register with the government and keep detailed records of all production and sales. All wholesalers, distributors, and pharmacists would also have to maintain records enabling the FDA to trace the annual flow of 8 billion 10 mg doses of amphetamine made by American drug firms. Pharmaceutical manufacturers at first did not openly oppose the bill, but the pharmacists did, objecting to FDA inspectors checking their records, and also to the fact that doctors who dispensed the drugs directly would be exempted from strict record keeping. The AMA opposed it despite the physician exemption, because the doctors thought it represented "government interference with drugs proven valuable to medicine." President Johnson did not like it either, because by transferring certain aspects of authority over drug control from the Bureau of Narcotics to the attorney general, it indirectly strengthened the hand of his rival then occupying that position, Robert Kennedy.

But the bill passed the Senate anyway in 1964 and moved on to the House of Representatives.[62]

In the House it met fierce resistance, now from the pharmaceutical lobby, too, because of changes introduced shortly before Senate passage. The name of the bill, in 1964 the "Psychotoxic Drug Control Act" ("psychotoxic," poisonous to the mind, was a buzzword adopted by the Kennedy administration to link the problems of narcotics with prescription drug abuse) bothered the drug companies, but most worrisome was the definition of which drugs were to be regulated. Originally, the bill had dealt only with barbiturates and amphetamines—strictly speaking, only amphetamine and methamphetamine —which were older off-patent drugs for which the big drug companies now sold expensive and medically fashionable replacements. But new wording included other drugs that have "a potential for abuse because of its depressant or stimulant effect on the central nervous system or its hallucinatory effect"—or "psychotoxic effects or antisocial behavior" because of their capacity to alter "consciousness, the ability to think, critical judgments, motivations, psychomotor coordination, or sensory perception." This meant that new and profitable medicines might come under the same restrictive rules, including the tranquilizers and some new antidepressants and diet drugs. AMA opposition stiffened as well when, to placate the pharmacists by leveling the playing field, the bill was changed so that doctors dispensing amphetamines and barbiturates would have to keep the same careful records.[63] The bill was stalled and probably doomed.

Then a sensational September 1964 exposé by a CBS news team punctured the drug industry's pretensions to self-regulation by showing how, with only a fake company letterhead, reporters were able to buy more than a million doses of amphetamines and barbiturates from manufacturers for just $600. On national television, CBS-TV news anchorman Walter Cronkite pointedly connected these "seemingly innocent" pharmaceuticals to the creeping evil of narcotics addiction. Newly elected President Johnson decided to make the bill one of the priorities of his "honeymoon" with Congress in 1965, now that Robert Kennedy was a senator and no longer the attorney general. And the physicians' lobby was distracted by another of Johnson's initiatives, government subsidized medical care for the very poor. "The AMA is tied up in its last-ditch fight against Medicare," as the drug trade journal *FDC Reports* put it succinctly in March 1965.[64] Helped by this odd convergence of events, the bill passed.

The most important ingredient for the bill's passage in 1965, however, was probably a rich coating of sugar added for the benefit of the pharmaceutical lobby: tough penalties against the makers of medicines that looked like brand-name products—that is, "counterfeit drugs"—regardless of how safe and effective they might be. We have already seen the commercial problem SKF had with cheaper generic amphetamine mimicking Benzedrine pills even in the 1940s, and numerous small manufacturers and amateurs produced look-alike Dexedrine and Dexamyl from 1950 on, similarly intended for sale by sharp pharmacists or by street dealers. For instance, in October 1964 in New Jersey, the FDA seized more than eight hundred thousand capsules and tablets that looked just like Dexedrines and Dexamyls and that contained the same ingredients, along with the pill-making equipment that produced them.[65] Of course, drug firms other than SKF had similar problems. Any successful drug invited generic knock-offs, but the most popular drugs to counterfeit were the ones with recreational value on the street.

Now under the provisions of the new bill, first known as H.R. 2 and signed into law in July 1965 as the Drug Abuse Control Amendments, the federal government extended assistance to drug companies in their efforts to maintain extraordinary monopolies over their products. Historian Rufus King explains this nicely:

> Nowhere else had criminal sanctions ever been attached directly to mere trade infringements. If, for example, some ambitious manufacturer of film should start putting out his product in a familiar-looking yellow box with a famous word like K-d-k on it, the Eastman Company would have to hire lawyers, commence a civil proceeding, and be content—at most—with an injunction plus whatever damages could be shown to have been caused directly by the infringement of its rights (at the end of which proceedings the infringer might risk wrist-tap punishment if he defied the injunction).
>
> But if the same eager manufacturer decided instead to put out some perfectly pure and efficacious aspirin with a word like B-y-r impressed on the tablets, by the terms of H.R. 2 as it became law he has committed a federal crime for which he can be fined (if he intended

to defraud or mislead) $10,000 and imprisoned three years; the gun-toting drug inspectors will go out and seize all his product wherever they can find it; and even the plant and the equipment he has used for the manufacture of the aspirin may be condemned and forfeited to the United States. Small wonder, then, that the drug lobbyists turned up this time working right along with the proponents of H.R. 2.[66]

The counterfeiting provision applied to all drugs, not just drugs declared dangerous like amphetamines. As for amphetamines and barbiturates, in particular, the law's impact on counterfeit manufacture and nonmedical traffic would supposedly solve the psychotoxic drug problem. But, as passed, the Drug Abuse Control Amendments were soft on the huge grey market in pills emanating from pharmacists and physicians of relaxed scruples—provided, of course, that the pills were genuine brand-name products. Prescriptions for amphetamines and barbiturates drugs could be refilled up to five times, and only then had to be renewed by the doctor, even in phone conversation with a pharmacist (keeping open the possibility of fake calls to the drugstore). Record keeping requirements were not very enforceable, and the bill imposed no restrictions on amphetamine manufacture or commercial distribution. Essentially, the Drug Abuse Control Amendments did nothing to control the major source of abused drugs, pharmaceutical firms. No great wonder, then, that more than four years later, in 1969, another congressional hearing would be devoted to the theme "Crime in America—Why 8 Billion Amphetamines?"[67]

Round Two: Nixon's War on (Unprofitable) Drugs

In 1969, Washington was still filled with sound and fury about drug abuse, when the second major effort to control amphetamines gathered strength. Drugs were now widely identified as the nation's leading social problem, perhaps because they were easier to address than deeper issues like racial and economic inequalities. Apart from worries about the popularity of marijuana and LSD among middle-class youth, consternation about the heroin epidemic blossoming among American soldiers serving in Vietnam, and an estimated one hundred thousand injecting "speed freaks" across the nation inspiring special terror, there was also grave concern that mainstream American culture was suffering a "hidden epidemic" of prescription drug abuse. As we'll remember, New York's Max ("Dr. Feelgood") Jacobson was still at the height of his methamphetamine-prescribing powers. But it was the diet doctors that drew fire first.

Foreshadowing later feminist critiques, the overmedication of women with amphetamines by dubious weight-loss clinics attracted national headlines in 1968–69 and, eventually, congressional attention. In a January 1968 issue of *Life* magazine, a slender journalist named Susanna McBee told how she made the rounds of diet clinics and walked away almost every time with massive jars of prescription amphetamines, sometimes without even a cursory physical examination. Follow-up stories reported how a number of patients had died from the diet pills (most containing thyroid), and this feminist issue also helped spur action to deal with prescription "pill popping" in general. Richard Nixon, finally realizing his dream of presidency at the end of 1968, had promised decisive action on drugs during his campaign. Nixon kept his word in the form of the 1970 Comprehensive Drug Abuse Prevention and Control Act, although, as one astute journalist, James Graham, noted, the result was "an all-out war on drugs which are *not* a source of corporate income."[68]

The bill that became this Act was drafted by Nixon's attorney general, John Mitchell, in close consultation with the major drug companies and, as progressively emerged during Senate and House hearings, came to Congress pre-endorsed and supported by the pharmaceutical lobbyists. The bill gave federal law enforcement authorities new powers and, in particular, gave the Bureau of Narcotics and Dangerous Drugs authority to monitor and control the production of highly abused pharmaceuticals. Five categories or "schedules" of drugs were defined, from harmless drugs in Schedule V to heroin and other drugs with high abuse potential and no medical justification in Schedule I. A new UN agreement on drug control then in the planning stage would contain similar drug categories, and the bill was intended to fit with this international agreement. Drugs in Schedule II would be subject to new, stricter, and more enforceable record-keeping rules allowing easier tracing from production to sale; prescriptions would be non-refillable; and the production of these drugs could be limited by the Bureau of Narcotics to a quota meeting justified medical demand. Reflecting the input of the drug companies, however, all of the more than six thousand different amphetamine products on the U.S. drug market would be listed in Schedule III, where they were subject to no quotas, looser record keeping, and prescriptions refillable five times as before. Tranquilizers like Valium, whose overprescription and abuse had become a major issue akin to the diet pill scandal, were not even listed on lenient Schedule IV.[69]

As the bill came under consideration by lawmakers, "the industry strategy from the beginning was to center congressional outrage on the small minority of persons who injected large doses of amphetamines," Graham observed. This strategy attracted attention to illegal diversion of the drugs in order to avoid the larger problem of lawful abuse. But while the pharmaceutical industry tried to keep certain issues separate like the "speed freak" and "pill-popper hidden epidemic," they did not entirely succeed. The drug fascination of the youth counterculture and prescription pharmaceutical overuse in mainstream American society were, to many, different sides of the same coin. As Senator Thomas Dodd declared in early 1970, America's drug problems were no accidental development; the pharmaceutical industry's "multihundred million dollar advertising budgets, frequently the most costly ingredient in the price of a pill, have pill by pill, led, coaxed and seduced post–World War II generations into the 'freaked out' drug culture" now plaguing the nation. Furthermore, as the head of the Bureau of Narcotics and Dangerous Drugs admitted, up to 90 percent of the amphetamines sold on the street were products of U.S. pharmaceutical firms. This made any effort to deal with street abuse separately from amphetamine overproduction and overprescription practically impossible, as well as hypocritical.[70]

Congressional committees considering the bill in 1969 heard alarming testimony from top medical experts that the amphetamines were truly addictive; that amphetamine and methamphetamine were now proven ineffective treatments for weight loss and depression, and that newer, similar drugs such as Ritalin were no different; and that if these popular uses were banned, the legitimate demand for the drugs would decline from the 8–10 billion doses sold by drug firms to only a few tens of thousands of doses per year. This amount would suffice to treat the few hundred patients suffering narcolepsy, and also the children with an unusual hyperactivity syndrome, nearly as rare as narcolepsy according to some expert witnesses, amounting to perhaps a thousand cases in the entire nation. (Under a new name, Attention Deficit/Hyperactivity Disorder or AD/HD, diagnoses of childhood hyperkinesis would surge a few years later, after amphetamine's other legitimate uses were blocked.) Experts also testified that 8 percent of prescriptions written in the U.S. were for amphetamines and that 9 million Americans were habitual users of amphetamines. (These estimates are exaggerated, the second depending on the definition of "habitual," but my own more conservative estimate of over 10 million active amphetamine users, a million dependent and three hundred thousand or more physically dependent, are dire enough.) Thanks largely to Dodd's influence, along with populist Thomas Eagleton of Missouri, the reforming forces in the Senate overcame stiff opposition and altered the bill so as to classify all amphetamines in Schedule II and tranquilizers like Valium in Schedule III.[71]

However the industry's lobbyists proved stronger in the House, despite a valiant battle by Claude Pepper (ironically, a one-time patient of Max Jacobson), and many of Eagleton's and Dodd's victories in the Senate were reversed. [72] The final version that emerged from the House-Senate conference and passed into law in late 1970 differed only trivially from the Nixon administration's original. Valium and similar tranquilizers were returned to lenient Schedule IV. In a symbolic gesture toward the problem of the methamphetamine-injecting "speed freak" (only one or two hundred thousand in number but high in visibility), injectable liquid methamphetamine was listed on Schedule II—affecting only five of the roughly six thousand amphetamine products on the U.S. pharmaceutical market, even though all the pills could easily be dissolved and injected. As Pepper observed, this gesture was "virtually meaningless," and as Eagleton lamented, "when the chips were down, the power of the drug companies was simply more compelling" than the public's health or safety.[73] Thus failed the second concerted effort to protect the public from the torrent of speed flowing from the pharmaceutical industry. Like the first, it was sabotaged by the drug industry's lobbying power. Under the new law, business as usual, or nearly usual, would continue for all the main amphetamine products and their manufacturers.

Round Three: Rise of the Bureaucrats

The impact of the 1970 Comprehensive Drug Abuse Prevention and Control Act on amphetamine consumption was not great: between

1969 and 1970, reported legal production dropped only 17 percent.[74] Nevertheless, it was a near miss for the drug industry. The Act had established mechanisms for stronger control of prescription drugs, and agitation against amphetamine in Washington did not end with its 1970 passage. That year a scandal broke on the drugging of children for hyperkinetic behavior (now AD/HD) with Ritalin and Dexedrine. In some school districts, the *Washington Post* reported, up to 10 percent of the children were being dosed with the stimulants just to make them more manageable in the classroom. A highly publicized congressional investigation confirmed the reports and revealed that many elementary school students were receiving the drugs with prescriptions from general practitioners, based only on reports of misbehavior from school employees, and that drug company advertising had targeted teachers and principals. The government convened a group of psychiatrists friendly to the practice, and, in 1971, these experts proclaimed that up to 3 percent of elementary school children suffered from hyperkinetic disorder and might need drugs, but still conceded that parents should never be coerced into medicating their kids. That same year, exposés in the *Ladies Home Journal* and elsewhere fanned the flames of concern about overprescription of drugs to women; apparently, a shocking 14 percent of American women were actively using minor tranquilizers, and, lagging not far behind, 3 percent were using amphetamine psychiatric medications and 6 percent diet pills, all essentially amphetamine-based.[75] From the leafy and affluent suburbs to the streets of Haight-Ashbury, public sentiment spoke in favor of stronger controls on amphetamines.

Where the elected lawmakers twice failed, civil servants now rose to the amphetamine challenge. At this point, the FDA had new leadership and was prepared to capitalize on public sentiment to take a less supine, more proactive role in regulating the drug industry. Longtime FDA chief George Larrick, who since the thalidomide affair had borne heavy criticism for his inappropriate intimacy with the industry, stepped down after achieving the sought-after expansion of his agency's law enforcement powers in 1965. The three FDA Commissioners that succeeded him were all medical doctors, reflecting Congress's concern that regulatory decisions reflect a greater understanding of technical issues and a more careful regard for the welfare of patients. The first FDA head to follow Larrick, James Goddard, instituted a far-reaching review of the status of old pharmaceuticals, products introduced before the 1962 laws empowering FDA to judge the efficacy of new drugs. Goddard convinced the U.S. National Academy of Sciences to lend its expertise and authority to the daunting task. Some three thousand old drugs with a total of sixteen thousand claims to effectiveness had to be evaluated. To this end, the Academy established a committee of academic physicians and life scientists to assess the evidence—published studies as well as any other data companies might like to submit—for the effectiveness of all these old drugs, and the Academy favored evidence from recent randomized controlled trials (RCTs).[76]

The RCT is a type of study that involves testing treatments on large numbers of patients, to make statistical analysis meaningful; random distribution of patients among treatment or placebo groups, to eliminate unconscious selective bias; and "double blinding" so that experimenting physicians do not know which patients are taking the drugs and which the placebo. It evolved gradually by several stages from the 1930s, when placebo controls were becoming standard practice, through the 1940s, when new statistical methods and randomization came in.[77] By the 1960s, the RCT was a relatively standardized approach and had become the benchmark of clinical knowledge. Because the RCT was fairly new, many of the older drugs introduced before 1962 lacked any such trials to support their effectiveness. Thus, the National Academy drug evaluation exercise gave the FDA a chance to impose the higher standards of modern medical science retroactively on the drug industry. The reevaluation took time, however, and still had doubtful legal weight. So, for the entire remainder of the 1960s, amphetamines officially remained safe and effective medicines for weight loss and depression.

When the National Academy released most of its verdicts seven years later in 1969, the head of the FDA was then Herbert Ley, who was frustrated with the resistance of the pharmaceutical industry to responsible testing and marketing. "Unless there is a major change in the drug industry emphasis on sales over safety," Ley once said, "the industry as we know it today may well be buried within the next several years in a grave it has helped dig—inch by inch, overpromotion by overpromotion, bad drug by bad drug."[78] The findings of the National Academy gave FDA leverage. For each drug it looked at, the National Academy committee had rated every one of the therapeutic claims as "effective"; "effective, but" with shortcomings; "probably effective"; "possibly effective," or "ineffective." The National Academy study had rated amphetamine-based antidepressants like Dexamyl only "possibly effective," since "controlled studies provide little basis for the use of amphetamines in depressive states." Amphetamines fared particularly badly when tested for severe depressions, although the drugs did seem to help people get through mildly low periods. On the other hand, the National Academy committee had judged amphetamine-containing obesity drugs "effective, but" only for short-term weight loss. Drug companies could still market amphetamines as antidepressants and diet pills, much as before, but had to carry a disclaimer speaking to the National Academy's findings.[79]

In August 1970 Leys's successor, Charles Edwards, took a bold step by revoking the "grandfather" status of amphetamine and methamphetamine. This status had exempted these old products, which had been introduced before the agency gained power in 1938 to require safety testing and in 1962 to require efficacy testing. Arguing that the uses of amphetamines had changed over time, the FDA now declared that all medicines containing the drugs must be considered new products and proved both safe and effective by the agency's current standards. In effect, on its own authority, the FDA demanded that manufacturers wishing to sell amphetamines for weight loss had a year to offer new proof of safety and effectiveness.

Some eighty-five amphetamine makers responded by submitting new drug applications before the 1972 deadline, but most of the studies the drug companies submitted with these applications were not new. (Perhaps the manufacturers expected to overturn the FDA's creative new exercise of authority in court.) Backed by older, more impressionistic non-RCT studies, amphetamine and methamphetamine fared poorly. To support Benzedrine Sulfate, SKF submitted only studies from the 1940s showing the drug to be effective in weight loss, and none of these was double-blind. Furthermore, even the most favorable studies showed that weight loss slowed after the first few weeks; later, patients either gained back the weight or had to take ever more amphetamine to stay thin. And, of course, by the 1970s, it was known that if patients did take increasing quantities of amphetamine as they developed tolerance, they would spiral into dependency and eventually psychosis. So, given these serious safety concerns as well as the limited evidence for effectiveness in weight loss, the FDA denied approval. After almost thirty-five years on the pharmaceutical market, and twenty-five years as a diet medicine, Benzedrine—the original amphetamine—was finished.[80]

While the bureaucratic wheels of FDA reapproval were in motion, public outcry and congressional hearings on the dangers of amphetamines continued. There were fresh scandals such as the delivery of huge shipments of U.S.-made pharmaceutical speed direct from the manufacturer to addresses such as the 11th hole at the golf course in Tijuana, Mexico.[81] In mid-1971, the Bureau of Narcotics and Dangerous Drugs engaged in its own creative exercise in independent authority to attack the diversion problem at its source. Under the 1970 Comprehensive Act the agency had gained administrative power to reschedule drugs, and now they used it to shift all amphetamines to Schedule II, including methylphenidate (Ritalin) and the diet drug phenmetrazine (Preludin), both of which had proved themselves attractive to high-dose injection abusers from Seattle to Sweden. Drugs in Schedule II required a fresh prescription each time they were filled, and doctors and pharmacists had to keep strict records or face prosecution. Soon after the change was announced, prescription sales of amphetamines and related drugs shot upward, as users stocked up for the coming drought, and then plummeted 60 percent below their original level once the rules came into effect.[82] Protestations of medical need notwithstanding, many patients and doctors obviously knew their "medical" use of amphetamines would not stand scrutiny.

The move to Schedule II also allowed the Bureau of Narcotics and Dangerous Drugs to set production quotas limiting the manufacture of amphetamines to quantities required by medicine. Consultation with FDA would establish total production levels sufficient to meet medical needs in the United States in a given year, and manufacturers would apply for their share of that total based largely on their past production and compliance record. The FDA, busily reducing legitimate amphetamine demand by applying science to de-legitimize prescription uses, now worked with Narcotics to shut off the speed supply at the source. The initial 1971 quotas allowed the manufacture about 14,000 kg of amphetamine and methamphetamine base, 40 percent less than the 25,000 kg (around 4 billion 10 mg doses of amphetamine salts) that government figures suggest were legally prescribed in 1969. Another 40 percent cut in the amount of amphetamine produced in the U.S. was slated for 1972, but given the sharp downward trend that followed the Schedule II listing, Narcotics, with FDA agreement, instead set production levels for 1972 at one-fifth the 1971 levels, and one-tenth the 1969 levels: enough for about 400 million 10 mg doses of amphetamine salts.[83] It was a dual-agency pincers movement against both supply and medical demand.

At first, major manufacturers including SKF, still the industry's top amphetamine producer, threatened to delay action indefinitely by using their rights to review and appeal, but they eventually relented in the face of bad publicity. (And, as *Fortune* observed, SKF's $20 million in amphetamine sales by now accounted for only 6 percent of the firm's total revenue, the firm having acquired, over time, a range of still patented and more profitable products at earlier stages in their life cycle.) There may also have been pressure from the Nixon administration, which was under fire for pushing its harsh cannabis and opiate controls on other countries in the 1971 United Nations Convention on Psychotropics, while resisting provisions inconvenient to U.S. drug firms.[84]

In any case, the critics had been vindicated: the United States managed perfectly well on the 400-million-pill amphetamine quota allowed for 1972. Therefore, not only must the 8–10 billion amphetamines produced by drug manufacturers in the late 1960s have vastly exceeded medical consumption, but the 4 billion prescribed by American doctors in 1969 must have been ten times higher than they were prepared to justify medically only two years later. Further, the prescription and production of amphetamines stayed down through the 1970s. The only remaining legitimate uses were narcolepsy and that still uncommon disorder of hyperactivity in children, AD/HD. It must have seemed, for a time, that apart from minor quantities produced by illicit speed kitchens, America's amphetamine problem was basically solved. There can be no more powerful indication of this sea change than Dexedrine and Dexamyl finally dropping off the drug industry's list of best sellers in 1974 and 1975, after a solid run of more than two decades.[85] It was an astonishing victory of democracy and good government over corporate and professional interest groups, a telling example of how the cultural revolt of the 1960s helped purify and restore the integrity of the American political system. We might well reflect on why such governmental fortitude in the face of corporate interests has become so rare since the 1970s, and contemplate how the acquiescence in corruption that this rarity suggests may affect the nation's well-being.

Gordon Alles never lived to see the downfall of his invention in both medical doctrine and popular opinion. Perhaps inspired by the psychic effects he discovered in methylenedioxyamphetamine (MDA, the original ecstasy) in 1930, Alles devoted almost the whole of his career to mind-altering drugs. In the 1930s and early 1940s, while still working closely with SKF, he produced hallucinogens related to amphetamine and mescaline, including MDA, for the firm to test in low doses as diet drugs and antidepressants. Alles also worked with SKF at isolating medically useful drugs from cannabis.[86] Starting in the late 1950s, having become an honorary pharmacology professor at the medical school of the University of California, Los Angeles, he worked on developing hallucinogenic amphetamines such as MDA and even more powerful derivatives, partly funded by the U.S. Army's chemical warfare program.[87] He investigated hallucinogenic and stimulant chemicals in the Khat plant, starting with a 1955 expedition to Ethiopia to study how it was used in traditional medicine. In January 1963, upon returning from a Tahiti trip to investigate the traditional Kava root as a source of new tranquilizers, Alles died. The cause of death of this biochemist who had begun his career by studying insulin was, ironically, diabetes, a disease Alles never knew he had.[88] Insulin could have saved his life, of course, but no matter how marvelous a drug may be in itself, it is only beneficial when accompanied by the right diagnosis and prescription.

8

Fast Forward

Still on Speed, 1971 to Today

AMPHETAMINE AND METHAMPHETAMINE passed through the complete life cycle between the mid-1930s, when they were first heralded as miracle drugs, and the mid-1970s, by which time both drugs were widely viewed as public enemies and their medical use diminished to a trickle. With declining medical consumption, street consumption declined sharply too, as recreational users had to rely mainly on illicit manufacturers for amphetamine supplies. Illicit speed remained available, but by the late 1970s cocaine far outstripped amphetamines as America's favorite stimulant.[1]

Amphetamine's rise and fall was dramatic but hardly unique. From cocaine to chloral hydrate to the barbiturates, many psychotropic pharmaceuticals had followed the same career path driven by the same major forces—drug industry marketing, trends in medical science, and the practical demands of doctor-patient relationships particularly in general practice.[2] Many non-psychotropic drugs had followed a trajectory from glory to infamy as well, although, when medically obsolete, they tended to retire more peacefully, without police intervention. Once dead, these drugs stayed dead or much diminished as mainstream medicines (an afterlife as a recreational drug is not unusual, particularly with a naturally sourced drug like cocaine). What is so unusual about amphetamine is that, within two decades, the drug had returned from the dead in multiple new forms, and in force. For not only are amphetamines back as a widespread and devastating drug of abuse—particularly methamphetamine (known as "meth," "ice," "crank," etc.), the old scourge of Haight-Ashbury—but, as we shall see, so, too, have the drugs made a major and troubling resurgence in medicine.

Illicit Use: The Speed Freak's Back in Town

The speed freak or "meth-head" or, less colloquially, high-dose amphetamine abuser has made a frightening comeback in recent years. Certainly amphetamine injection never went away, but it declined in the mid-1970s after production quotas imposed by narcotics authorities finally turned off pharmaceutical industry taps. Eventually, however, the illegal drug industry, arguably as adaptable as the pharmaceutical industry, found ways around government restrictions on the starting chemicals used by speed kitchens. By the 1980s, the main type of speed sold on the street in the United States shifted from amphetamine to methamphetamine, and was being made from ephedrine (or its synthetic substitute, pseudoephedrine). Ephedrine is easily extracted from over-the-counter cold medicines, and making it into methamphetamine is easier than amphetamine synthesis—so easy that, given the starting materials, anyone can do it at home. All an amateur chemist needs is the ephedrine, lighter fuel, and a few other common odds and ends like phosphorous from match heads. When knowledge of the process began to spread, illicit production surged.[3]

U.S. government statistics suggest that the high-dose methamphetamine resurgence began in centers in California, Colorado, Oregon, Oklahoma, and Texas, and has continued growing in these Western areas while spreading eastward since the mid-1980s. Based on emergency room admissions mentioning amphetamines, serious meth abuse doubled nationally from 1983 to 1988, doubled again between 1988 and 1992, and then increased fivefold further from 1992 to 2002. Though the problem has not diminished, the form in which meth is taken has changed since the trend began; since 1992, when around 12 percent of users smoked the drug, smoking became the dominant method of taking it in 2002, with over 50 percent of users preferring this method. Snorting powdered speed up the nose has dropped off radically, whereas injection has remained fairly stable as the second most popular method, at around 30 percent. The preferred method varies, however, with the local drug culture: in 2000, users mostly smoked meth in Southern California, snorted it in Minnesota, and injected it in Texas.

The number of people involved is astonishing. In 2004, almost 1.5 million Americans used methamphetamine and 3 million used amphetamines of some kind nonmedically, twice the number of a decade earlier. And although national survey data indicate that for the past few years the overall number of nonmedical speed users has stabilized, the number of heavy users with addiction problems has doubled since 2002. So the national amphetamine problem is still growing more severe. Recent national surveys show that about 600,000 Americans use amphetamines nonmedically at least weekly and that 250,000 to 350,000 are addicted, twice the number addicted to heroin. Put another way, there are perhaps 3 million misusers and abusers of amphetamines in the country now (almost as many nonmedical users as in 1969), 1 percent of the total population, and a tenth of them are currently being destroyed by the drugs.[4]

Several reasons are usually cited for the speed freak's return. There is the attraction of price: cocaine is both expensive and highly addictive in the same way, so that those who are hooked can economize by switching to much cheaper amphetamines. Apart from being cheaper to buy, dose for dose, speed lasts up to eight hours—three or four times longer than cocaine. Furthermore, purified "crystal" meth (a form of methamphetamine like clear, rock salt), easy to prepare from crude home-cooked meth, has caught on. Because this form of the drug is more concentrated and the dose usually higher when injected, it is more addictive. Another factor is the introduction of new chemical forms of amphetamine that can be smoked: methamphetamine in base form and also methylmethamphetamine, weaker than methamphetamine or amphetamine gram for gram but actually legal when first introduced in the 1980s. Inhaling "ice" or "glass," as the smokable form of amphetamines are often called, gives much the same immediate rush that used to be available only from injection, and being able to smoke the drug is a key feature for users switching from smoking freebase cocaine or for the needle-shy. (As illicit brand names cannot be protected by trademarks and lawsuits, the high-status label "ice" is now often used, confusingly, of any crystalline-looking amphetamine product.) Sheer availability is another major reason for the speed freak's return, as methods of simple underground chemistry travel quickly via the Internet. Recently, large-scale supply from illicit Mexican factories has stepped in to compete with American home-brew, making matters even worse with crystal meth that is 80 percent pure instead of just 40 percent, and bringing with it guns and all the other problems that come with organized crime.[5]

What about the demand for meth behind the statistics, the users and the types of use? Speed is a macho drug especially when injected or smoked in high doses; the typical nonmedical amphetamine user today is male and in his twenties or thirties. Speed goes well with hard drinking, allowing the user to party longer, with hard erections and rough sex, and with fighting. Though meth freaks come in all flavors—Caucasian and Islander, gay and straight, white collar and blue —the drug is particularly popular with rural working-class white men of a type that previously would not have used illegal drugs (except perhaps marijuana). Because of this last demographic, many see it as a redneck drug or a disease of the heartland. Communities are badly damaged when heavy users stop doing what others rely on them for, whether it is holding down a job or taking care of children and the elderly at home. Many even stop eating and bathing. When parents make the drug themselves, their children may be poisoned by the toxic chemicals left in the fridge or burned when the solvents used in making the drug catch fire. People on meth don't just drop out of their communities, they sometimes turn against them, like the meth-using social circle of Terry Nichols and Timothy McVeigh, the right-wing extremists who blew up the federal government offices in Oklahoma City.[6] Probably the paranoid psychosis and violent reactivity brought on by heavy speed use has a lot to do with antisocial behavior among users, just as David Smith noted when speed destroyed the Haight-Ashbury dream of universal harmony around 1968. Social alienation could well be a cause, as well as a result, of the meth epidemic. People in the American heartland have a greater reason than ever to seek euphoria in the drug when their livelihoods have been lost to Asian factories and their town centers gutted by monster chain stores in peripheral malls.

For some meth is just a party drug, but for others there is another, old explanation that still has a lot to offer: illicit use of amphetamines (and cocaine) may represent self-medication by people needing help to "adjust" but without easy access to psychiatry. The following recent interview with a meth addict reported by journalist Dirk Johnson captures beautifully what some users feel when they first encounter meth: "Wow! This is amazing. I felt smarter, stronger, better looking, more articulate. I felt like I was simply a much better person. For the first time, I felt like the person I was meant to be." Now consider what patients say about the antidepressant Prozac, as reported by psychiatrist Peter Kramer. One named John felt "strong . . . resilient . . . confident" on the drug, and that with it he became "who I am." Another, Tess, loved the way it made her more outgoing and "confident," but when she went off Prozac she became "not myself."[7] Thus, some people are using methamphetamine in the same way others use Prozac, for help with living up to expectations that we be upbeat, smart, articulate, productive, and good looking—exactly the same medical needs that pharmaceutical amphetamines like Dexamyl once satisfied.

One could argue that today methamphetamine does for the poor and medically underserved what amphetamine once did for everyone, but that the new antidepressants now do for the rich. Moreover, the use of illicit amphetamines partly for their antidepressant action can explain why speed abuse appears to be higher among people with a record of mood disorders.[8] Unfortunately, for people who are actually depressed, amphetamines are not very effective. The drug's mood-elevating action quickly fades as tolerance develops, requiring increased doses and pushing users down the path to addiction, brain damage, and all the other toxic effects of high doses.

Ecstasy, from Chemical Weapon to Love Drug

Another, utterly different manifestation of amphetamine has also returned to the collective consciousness: ecstasy. With a reputation as the ultimate party drug, ecstasy is an amphetamine that combines the euphoria sought by speed freaks with the insight and universal communion sought by acid heads. Actually, "ecstasy" is a small family of amphetamines: here I use the term to refer both to MDMA (methylenedioxymethamphetamine) and MDA (methylenedioxyamphetamine). Their story must be told together, because the fate of the two compounds has been intertwined; furthermore, they are as similar to each other chemically as amphetamine and methamphetamine, and it takes a pharmacologist to describe the subtle distinctions in action. (The most experienced ecstasy user probably could not tell the difference in a blind tasting.[9] In any case, ecstasy bought on the street only contains MDMA or MDA if the buyer is lucky; "ecstasy" pills are often a cocktail containing neither drug.)

Ecstasy's journey from promising new pharmaceutical to notorious drug of abuse was particularly long and winding. Remember that Alles himself discovered MDA in 1930, the year after he discovered amphetamine. He noticed then that MDA was pleasant, and that it seemed to make him super-sensitive to sound, alter his sense of time, and cause mild visual hallucinations. Though intrigued, Alles never found a use for the drug, at least not until he tried to turn it into a chemical weapon for the Army. In the 1950s his old business partner, SKF, ran MDA in clinical trials as a possible antidepressant under the name "SKF-5" or "amphedoxamine." Although results were promising for both mild (neurotic) and major (psychotic) depression, as well as for obsessive-compulsive behavior, the drug did not work consistently enough to commercialize. Sensibly, in such medical trials, doses were kept lower than the 100–200 mg needed for dramatic changes in perception; patients receiving 120 mg/day complained of these side-effects, thus setting an upper limit. MDA was also patented as a diet drug, a tranquilizer, and even a cough suppressant, and presumably tested for all these uses with results too disappointing to publish.[10]

Not strong stimulants like amphetamine, nor hallucinogens as powerful as mescaline, MDA and MDMA were neither fish nor fowl. Indeed, pharmacologists found evidence in these drugs that the "alerting" effects of amphetamines must have a separate biological basis from their perception-altering effects, since MDA has little of the first but lots of the second. And the perception-altering effects are noteworthy. In 1969 Alexander Shulgin, the legendary drug chemist then researching compounds like DOM for Dow Chemicals, concisely described the difference in subjective effects between the strongly hallucinogenic mescaline-like drugs and LSD, on the one hand, and the MDA-type semi-psychedelic amphetamines, on the other.

> There is little if any of the profound insight or religious significance that is so characteristic of the indolic pyschotomimetics [such as LSD] or of the methoxylated amphetamines [mescaline-like drugs such as TMA]. This is the loss of the property most generally accepted as "psychedelic." In its place there is the generation of a form of dream-world; for some subjects this is structured in the framework of past events, while for others it appears to be merely a dream-like entertainment.[11]

MDA found its way in the late 1960s from the laboratory to the Haight-Ashbury streets, as the "Love and Harmony Groove Pill," "Love," and the "hug drug." According to credible rumors at the time, the drug was stolen from a Bay Area military installation, suggesting that by the 1960s the Army had moved beyond the pure research stage with its nonlethal chemical weapons program. In any event, despite Shulgin's lukewarm tasting notes, MDA gained a number of converts to its energetic yet relaxing and mood-lifting effects, along with the less intensely hallucinogenic, "dream-like" trip. And apart from "entertainment," it also offered a distinctive increase in sensitivity to the feelings of others, leading (a few years later) to the coining of the term "empathogen" for this class of drugs. In 1970, a California underground newspaper raved about the new "love drug" and recommended MDA highly as a legal alternative to LSD and speed. Without a commercial backer or a mainstream medical use, MDA was quickly outlawed in the United States, but the ban was specific to that chemical and did not include closely related derivatives. Thus, medical researchers and drug pioneers like Shulgin were able to continue exploring these psychedelic amphetamines legitimately by working with minor chemical variants of MDA, such as its still legal sister MDMA.[12]

MDA was still being made and taken in the American drug culture through the late 1970s, judging from occasional arrests and emergency room crises, but it would take two decades before the methylenedioxyamphetamine family seriously caught on as recreational drugs. Meanwhile, during the 1970s until 1985, MDA and especially MDMA, legal until that latter year, were both explored as promising new medicines for psychiatric healing. Shulgin—no longer working for Dow—seems to have been a key figure in interesting psychiatrists in this class of drugs, which were labeled "feeling enhancers" by Shulgin's therapist collaborator, Claudio Naranjo, as opposed to the more frankly hallucinogenic "fantasy enhancers" like LSD.

The "feeling enhancers" promoted exceptional self-honesty, openness, and a sense of heightened authenticity, believed Naranjo, as well as a non-possessive, empathic kind of love. Thus, for psychiatrists working with MDA and MDMA (which Naranjo came to consider the subtly superior compound), it made sense that these drugs are helpful in psychotherapy not only by bringing repressed feelings and thoughts to the surface—like LSD and barbiturates—but also by generating a sense of well-being, supporting the patient's conscious efforts to accept and process what was long repressed. The drugs boost confidence and lower defenses enough for a more honest approach to self and others, according to this view, making them especially suitable for relationship therapy. Studies employing moderately strong doses (up to 200 mg) of MDA and MDMA in conjunction with 1970s-style psychoanalytically informed therapy reported good results for depression, anxiety, guilt, emotional withdrawal, and low self-esteem. Known as "Adam" especially on the West Coast, MDMA acquired the reputation of restoring the soul to a childlike, original state of innocence. Informal estimates place therapeutic usage of MDA and MDMA during the later 1970s and early 1980s in the high hundreds of psychiatrists and thousands of patients.[13]

Although the psychotherapists using "Adam" did not trumpet its potential as a penicillin for the soul, the scenario they feared did eventually emerge. As with LSD before it, word of the mind-altering wonder drug spread too widely, via circles near the therapists and their patients—including LSD's champion Timothy Leary, whose first use of the drug with his girlfriend, Barbara, around 1980 led immediately to their marriage and left him very impressed. MDMA finally attracted the harsh attentions of U.S. drug enforcement agencies in 1984, when a large-scale "pyramid"-style scheme to sell the still legal drug emerged in Texas; people were recruited not only to sell the product to their acquaintances but also to recruit new dealers, whose profits the recruiter would share. One company was manufacturing around 3 million tablets a year under the label "Sassyfras." You could even buy MDMA by ringing a toll-free number with a credit card handy. Frustrating those advocating the drug's potential for psychiatry, in 1985 the government placed MDMA in the most stringently controlled category (Schedule I), along with MDA, LSD, and heroin, thus squelching clinical research.[14] Nevertheless, throughout the 1980s, recreational use of the drug, by now known in this context as "ecstasy," continued to grow among upper-middle-class university students, "yuppies," and spiritual seekers.

By the late 1980s, another context of use had evolved. MDMA was now associated with a particular "young and arty" crowd (according to the *New York Times*) that frequented nightclubs and parties in what was becoming known as the "rave" scene. Like the LSD scene of the 1960s, this new ecstasy subculture enjoyed a particular sonic atmosphere with its drug sacrament, a style of music known as "acid house." Originating in Britain (or, as some stories have it, among Britons on perpetual holiday in the Spanish island of Ibiza), acid house has been aptly described by Bruce Eisner as a "propulsive,

trance-inducing . . . throbbing sonic collage" of snippets from previously recorded music, set against a heavy synthetic drumbeat. Buoyed
by ecstasy, the dance party throbs on forever, a hypnotic rapture of
bodies swaying in synchronized drumbeats and strobe lights all pre-
sided over by the "electronic shaman" or DJ. So it seemed, at any rate,
to a journalist who attended the 1991–92 New Years Eve rave in San
Francisco's Fashion Center. Still, the phenomenon was selective, not
huge; from 1979, when a small blip of new users showed up in national drug use surveys, first-time users of ecstasy gradually climbed
from almost nothing to about 200,000 Americans per year in 1987, a
level of new recruits that remained stable through the early 1990s.
Compared to LSD, which was still initiating 600,000 to 800,000 new
users every year since 1969, ecstasy remained a minor drug.[15]

Then suddenly in 1995 ecstasy use took off in the United States,
with 400,000 trying it for the first time, a count rising steadily to 1.8
million new users in 2000, after which new recruits began to decline.
Some commentators have attributed the late-1990s leap not only to the
drug's reputation and inherently attractive properties but also to the
entry of large-scale organized crime in manufacturing and distributing MDMA to this now substantial market (the drug is made from
ephedrine much like methamphetamine but with a few extra steps).
Whatever the reason, around 3 million Americans used the drug in
2002, but most were not using it constantly like speed freaks, nor were
they turning into paranoid, violent, sickly and emaciated shadows of
their former selves.[16]

The typical pattern of use for ecstasy is occasional or episodic, as
LSD and other hallucinogen use has always been, not compulsive like
high-dose amphetamines. Few users take it more than once a week,
and the great majority only a few times a year, so it cannot be highly
addictive. Recent survey data show changes in the ecstasy user profile, with the educated avant-garde taking the drug less, and poorer
non-white groups taking it more, and more often with other drugs.
Still, even if recent figures showing a decline in active (past year)
ecstasy users to 2 million do not herald the drug's disappearance, the
"hug drug" presents much less to worry about than methamphetamine—which is more common, more addictive, and more toxic in the
quantities typically used than MDMA.[17] Finally, research on the use of
MDMA in psychotherapy is again under way. It may yet find a place
in respectable medicine, although any treatment requiring the close

personal attention of a psychiatrist will inevitably be too expensive and exclusive to transform society.

Thus far we have counted 5 million Americans misusing and abusing amphetamines in the past year, about 3 million on methamphetamine and similar stimulants, and 2 million on ecstasy. These numbers reflect nonmedical amphetamine use nearly equivalent to the height of the first epidemic in 1970, when the number of people using amphetamines nonmedically in the United States was about 4 million, which would be 6 million when adjusted for today's population.[18] But even if methamphetamine and ecstasy use were somehow eliminated tomorrow, we could not stop worrying about a resurgence of amphetamine addiction and psychosis. The medical consumption of amphetamines has also made a comeback, in some ways at least as worrisome.

Brain Fuel: Attention Deficit and Medical Amphetamine Use

Before the tough controls of the 1970s, amphetamine's main medical uses were, of course, for weight loss, depression, and a range of vaguely related psychiatric problems involving a lack of energy and efficiency. Today, the most popular medical use of speed is not so very different from this last, poorly defined category of dysfunction. The trend began with children. In the late 1930s, as we have seen, psychiatrists already knew that certain children with disruptive behavior reacted "paradoxically" to amphetamine in that they calmed down and could focus better on schoolwork, but Benzedrine was not marketed for that purpose. In the 1950s, hyperactive misbehavior received increasing attention from child psychologists, who refined its definition and called it "Emotional Disturbance" if they were inclined to Freudian theory and blamed childhood trauma, or "Minimal Brain Damage" if they were biologically inclined (because the behavioral pattern resembled what occurs after certain viral infections in the brain). The problem was also known by more neutral names like "Hyperkinetic Disorder of Childhood." As we have further seen, even in the late 1960s medical experts testified to Congress that the condition was so rare that a few thousand prescriptions for amphetamine would meet the needs of these patients nationally. Even allowing for exaggeration because of the charged amphetamine politics of the time, mainstream medical opinion in that decade placed the number of children suffering from the disorder in the United States in the tens of thousands. This market niche was just large enough to attract drug makers in the 1960s with would-be antidepressants like Deaner (deanol) and Ritalin (methylphenidate).

In the 1970s, however, something remarkable happened: suddenly the disorder became a lot more common than it had been in the 1960s. Prescriptions for stimulants to treat it began an inexorable climb, just as prescription amphetamines were being cut off for almost all other legitimate medical purposes. Already in 1970, as many as 150,000 children in the United States were given medication for hyperactivity, triggering a wave of scandal around drugging children for the convenience of schools. Notwithstanding controls on the drugs prescribed for it, by 1980 that number had roughly tripled to perhaps 500,000. In that year the official psychiatric definition of the childhood disorder changed, along with its name. With the new label of Attention Deficit Disorder (ADD), as it then was called, failure of attention became central so that a child could be diagnosed with the condition without hyperactive behavior.

Diagnosis rates increased still more during the 1980s, so that by 1990 the number of children receiving medication for it climbed to nearly 1 million. Then, in the 1990s, diagnosis of the condition rocketed upward, increasing about fivefold by the early 2000s, so that now between 4 and 5 million Americans are receiving medication each year for Attention Deficit. Some experts hold that not only do 10 percent of today's children have the condition, 5 percent of adults do as well, implying that close to 20 million people nationally are candidates for medication.[19] Thus, many millions more may soon be taking drugs for Attention Deficit. It appears that America suffered an increase in this psychiatric disorder of 100,000 percent in just one generation, from tens of thousands in the 1960s to tens of millions today.

What can explain this massive outbreak? This question has attracted much discussion in recent psychiatric literature (along with the question of whether Attention Deficit Disorder is a "real disease").[20] It is possible, of course, that something goes wrong with human brains these days much more commonly than before—especially with the brains of Americans, who seem to suffer more attention deficit than people in other nations. Perhaps video games or junk food or modern advertising methods are causing neural damage. It is also possible that a large fraction of the population have always had this same condition, only doctors now understand and recognize it much better.

There are, however, a number of factors to consider that make both these answers too simple, if not altogether wrong. Although it has always been true that a very large proportion of patient visits to doctors are for complaints which the doctor cannot attribute to any distinct disease or physical problem (see chapter 5), evidence suggests that today patients more aggressively demand a medical diagnosis for a given level of discomfort.[21] Thus, one factor that could explain the increase in Attention Deficit is that today a given level of mental distraction is more likely than before to count as a medical problem. But apart from this creeping inflation of symptom severity (which probably applies to all forms of distress), a second factor in rising diagnosis rates is that the definition of the condition we now call Attention Deficit/Hyperactivity Disorder has expanded throughout all its changes in name since the 1960s. As noted, around 1980, hyperactive behavior became optional, so that people could be diagnosed just on the basis of problems in attention, concentration, and impulsiveness. Then, in the 1990s, the idea was abandoned that Attention Deficit was something that could only affect children. The broader the definition, the more people it has applied to, even if the prevalence and experience of the symptoms have remained unchanged over time.

A third factor is that parents may have learned to appreciate the benefits of having their children diagnosed with the neurological disorder, since it relieves them of blame for their child's behavior and may give access to special school programs. The diagnosis can also confer benefits for adults, especially in contexts where disability is compensated by competitive advantages, such as special consideration for a student at a university or extra protection from dismissal for the working adult. One commentator has even gone so far as to call Attention Deficit Disorder "affirmative action for white people," referring to the middle-class, predominantly white majority who receive the diagnosis.[22] This third explanation fits with much lower diagnosis and medication rates outside the United States.

So does a fourth factor: the presence of highly active support and lobby groups for Attention Deficit sufferers that spread the word about how common and terrible the condition is, push for special benefits for sufferers, and try to make the drugs more widely available.

These groups are funded by the makers of medications for the disorder, evidently as an aspect of their marketing efforts—particularly in the U.S., where drug prices are high. And though evidence suggests that doctors are less enthusiastic for the diagnosis than parents and patients are, as a fifth factor we might include incentives from within the medical system for doctors to make the Attention Deficit diagnosis for complaints of distraction, bad behavior, and poor performance. Child psychiatrists may depend on the diagnosis for business, whereas, in the case of pediatricians, prescribing drugs wastes less physician time. Prescriptions also cost health insurers less than psychotherapeutic approaches to childhood misbehavior. Certainly, some combination of all these distorting factors is needed to explain why, in certain parts of the country, up to 20 percent of the school population is not only diagnosed with Attention Deficit but are taking medications, four times the national average (according to a recent government study). Serious overdiagnosis must be occurring at least locally.[23]

In addition to all these factors raising diagnosis rates of Attention Deficit are the effects and attractions of the medications themselves. About half the prescriptions for Attention Deficit in the United States are for amphetamine, especially popular under the Adderall brand name (also DextroStat, Vyvanse, etc.). In all of these the active drug is not just *an* amphetamine, it is *the original amphetamine,* chemically the same as Benzedrine and/or Dexedrine. Almost all the rest of the pills prescribed for the disorder are methylphenidate, best known by the brand names Ritalin and Concerta (more rarely prescribed in most other countries, where amphetamine is regarded as equivalent). By most definitions, methylphenidate is also an amphetamine, and both drugs affect the concentration of all people in the same way, not only those diagnosed with Attention Deficit.[24]

Psychological experiments with amphetamines going back to the war era suggest that gains in test performance may stem from improved mood and confidence rather than objective increase in intellectual function but, in any case, the use of the drugs in schools and universities confers what many *perceive* as an advantage. Thus, even if there were no risk of abuse of Attention Deficit drugs, we should be concerned about the subtle but widespread social harm generated by allowing selected people drugs offering perceived performance enhancement, very like the situation created when professional sports turn a blind eye to steroids and amphetamines. When a few players take drugs to gain an edge, whether real or imagined, all the other players feel forced to do drugs so they can keep up. As pediatrician Lawrence Diller put it, when doctors diagnose Attention Deficit and prescribe medication, are they not "promoting an anti-humanistic, competitive environment that demands performance at any cost?"[25] One might ask something similar about modern antidepressants, when one of the key features leading to their discovery is the power to make rats press levers on command even when the work becomes extremely unrewarding, much as they do on amphetamine. But let us leave the issue of how the social environment creates a "need" for such drugs until later, when we have fully taken the measure of that demand today.

The consumption of Attention Deficit medications has now grown to staggering levels in the United States—and much more in the United States than elsewhere. Since at the right dose the drugs are essentially the same—15 mg of methylphenidate is roughly equivalent to 5 mg of dextroamphetamine—we can use the government's production quotas on these controlled substances to track America's Attention Deficit drug habit in terms of standardized amphetamine doses. Expressing production levels for Attention Deficit drugs in standard doses, defined arbitrarily as 10 mg amphetamine and 30 mg methylphenidate base per dose (quite large doses for Attention Deficit, in fact, enough for a full day and more than enough to produce a high when taken all at once), America's annual consumption of pharmaceutical speed has risen almost tenfold since 1995, and in 2005 exceeded 2.5 billion such defined doses.

In 1969, at the height of the amphetamine epidemic, U.S. drug firms manufactured roughly 25,000 kg of amphetamine and methamphetamine base for actual prescription use, or 2.5 billion standard doses defined as 10 mg base, plus much smaller quantities of methylphenidate (e.g., Ritalin) and phenmetrazine (e.g., Preludin). (This quantity is enough for about 4 billion 10 mg tablets of amphetamine salts, and was only half the amphetamine actually manufactured in 1969 but a fair estimate of the amount of amphetamine distributed through medical channels.)[26] So, in absolute volume, with Attention Deficit medications the nation has now returned to roughly the same level of medical speed consumption that prevailed at the height of the amphetamine epidemic in 1969–70 (Figure 36). It also seems that this same quantity of drugs is being consumed by a smaller number of patients, 5 million now compared to 7 million medical amphetamine users in 1970 (assuming all the Attention Deficit drugs manufactured today are only being consumed by prescription—which they are not, as we shall see).

It might be true that, as medication advocates argue, people taking drugs for their Attention Deficit Disorder not only concentrate better with the low doses prescribed but that for this action—unlike the mood elevation, appetite suppression, and the other speed effects the medications produce—a small dose remains effective without ever building up tolerance. Regardless, there is abundant evidence that people do take the medications for elevated mood and for pleasure, methylphenidate and amphetamine alike, and when used this way tolerance will occur and lead to increasing doses, addiction, and ultimately psychosis. Reports of medication abuse have increased in step with Attention Deficit drug prescriptions for adolescents and adults. One 2003 survey found that 2.6 percent of eighth-grade students in the United States and 4 percent of high school seniors used Ritalin recreationally and without prescription, an abuse level more than ten times greater than in 1988. Other surveys place the current percentage of high school students abusing the drugs still higher.[27] Abuse of the medications at some universities has become even more popular than marijuana, according to student informants. And the shift from misusing unprescribed Ritalin as an occasional study aid to straightforward abuse can happen easily, as one Harvard student discovered when she became "an absolute speed-freak—up all night and strung out all day," and ultimately doing much worse in her courses. The reference to "speed freaks" is apt: this is an old, familiar slippery slope, as writer Elizabeth Wurzel also found when, recovering from cocaine addiction, she lapsed into compulsive Ritalin snorting only a week after her psychiatrist added the drug to her antidepressant regimen. The middle classes now are discovering the same thrills and pitfalls that junkies fond of "West Coast" have known since the early 1970s: Ritalin is "simply an amphetamine" (as Wurzel put it), very pleasurable and very addictive once you start taking it for the mood lift.[28]

In 2005, 600,000 Americans consumed psychiatric stimulants other than methamphetamine nonmedically at least monthly, according to government surveys, and given that methamphetamine is the main illegally manufactured drug of the type, these frequent abusers must be taking legally manufactured Attention Deficit medications like Adderall and Ritalin.[29] Indeed, as a detailed recent study of medication abuse based on these national survey data found, of the nation's 3.2 million past-year nonmedical amphetamine users, more than 750,000 had never misused any stimulants but Attention Deficit pharmaceuticals *in their entire lives.* Those who only used pharmaceutical-type amphetamine in the past year (that is, Attention Deficit medication misusers), together account for a third of the approximately 300,000 Americans estimated to be suffering serious amphetamine abuse or dependence in this study.[30] With so many billions of prescription amphetamine and methyphenidate pills flowing through the nation's population each year for Attention Deficit, it should come as no surprise that hundreds of thousands are abusing them. It should also come as no surprise if today, just as in the 1960s, tens of thousands of Americans are falling prey to medical amphetamine addiction. Research into the precise number should be a high-priority concern.

How heavy is America's amphetamine consumption now compared to the past? In 1969–70, at the peak of the first amphetamine epidemic, we estimated that more than 10 million Americans, or 5 percent of the total population, were using amphetamines, medically and nonmedically.[31] In our discussion of amphetamine's resurgence, we have so far estimated the number of Americans now using Attention Deficit stimulants by prescription at 5 million each year and probably rising, and the number using meth and other amphetamines nonmedically at about 3 million and steady. There are also about 2 million using ecstasy, mostly occasionally. This brings the number of Americans actively using all three types of amphetamines, medically and nonmedically, each year to around 10 million just as in 1969–70. This is more than 3 percent of the total population and quite an alarming figure. As noted above, with Attention Deficit drugs, *medical* amphetamine consumption has now reached a level equal to that prevailing during the peak of the first speed epidemic in 1969–70, in terms of drug volume. In terms of prevalence of use, however, the current outbreak of amphetamine use has not yet reached the magnitude of the first speed epidemic: the 10 million American medical and nonmedical amphetamine users in 1970 would be equivalent to 15 million speed users today, since the American population has grown from about 200 million to 300 million. With 10 million speed users now, we are only two-thirds of the way there. However, if we expand our definition of "speed" just slightly, the tally continues to rise.

Diet Drugs: Speed by Any Other Name

In the late 1960s, 4 or 5 million Americans were using amphetamines each year by prescription for weight loss (half to two-thirds of all prescription amphetamine consumers, 2 to 3 percent of the total population). More than three-quarters of these diet pill users were women.[32] Other than the particular drugs involved, this situation has changed little since. Recent evidence suggests that over 3 percent of the American population takes diet pills each year, and they switch readily between prescription and nonprescription medications depending on whether the trendiest diet drug at any given time is available by prescription only.[33] Diet pill users are still mainly women; indeed, according to surveys in the 1990s, 33–40 percent of adult women in the United States were trying to lose weight at some time, and about 14 percent of these were taking diet drugs. This makes the overall proportion of American women actively taking pills to lose weight around 5 percent, amounting to perhaps 6 million women at any given moment (or 2 percent of the total population, which suggests that 3 percent of the whole population using diet pills each year may be a low estimate). About half the women trying to lose weight had no significant weight problem, by medical standards, at the time of these studies. In contrast, despite increasing male self-consciousness about appearance, even in the 1990s only half as many men were trying to lose weight as women, the vast majority of them officially overweight or obese.[34]

It appears, then, that since the late 1960s, approximately 3 percent of the American population has continued using diet pills. Ever since amphetamines became the leading diet drugs, and especially after they became tightly controlled substances in 1971, the pharmaceutical industry, the weight-loss doctors, and, increasingly, the natural food industry have all vied to fill the dieters' demand for an amphetamine replacement. A continuing stream of "non-amphetamine" diet drugs would be advanced, purportedly free of the side effects of amphetamine but nevertheless acting on the brain to reduce appetite much like amphetamine. Eventually, one after another, they would be discredited by harmful side effects. But there was always yet another drug ready to take its place, each one a chemical relative of amphetamine, with similar pharmacological characteristics. As we shall see, the result has been that the most popular diet drugs have remained close relatives of amphetamine—speed, at their core—into the twenty-first century.

The first crop of new "non-amphetamine" diet drugs actually began to flow from the pharmaceutical industry's research labs in the late 1950s, all of them close amphetamine derivatives (Figure 37). Diethylpropion was introduced by Merrell in 1959 as Tenuate, a product represented as free from all stimulating effects on the brain and on blood pressure, and not interfering with sleep. Phentermine was introduced into the U.S. that same year under the brand name Ionamin, by the small Strasenburgh firm. Never as pleasant nor quite as effective as amphetamine, both compounds remain on the market today (diethylpropion is still known by the old brand names Tenuate and Tepanil among others, and phentermine is now widely know under the brand name Adipex).

A more popular appetite-suppressing drug was phenmetrazine, introduced into the U.S. in 1956 as Preludin by the Swiss firm Geigy. Preludin advertisements promised "potent appetite-suppressant action" with minimal risk of "discomfort from side reactions." Though emphatically "not an amphetamine," Preludin also offered the benefit of "mild elevation of mood conducive to an optimistic and cooperative attitude" toward the other aspects of weight loss programs. By 1962, the drug manual of the American Medical Association was already warning that addiction and amphetamine psychosis could occur with the product, which was widely abused in 1960s British counterculture (as "Sweeties"). Sweden made this "non-amphetamine" diet drug a controlled substance in 1959, but the United States waited until 1971, when phenmetrazine was listed together with amphetamine and Ritalin as Schedule II narcotics.[35]

By the later 1960s, many more new drugs crowded the weight-loss market, all of them chemical derivatives of amphetamine, although they could be advertised as "non-amphetamine" since they contained neither amphetamine nor methamphetamine (still the leading prescription diet drugs). For example, there was phendimetrazine, chlorphentermine, and benzphetamine (see Figure 38), none of which ever gained a large following. After the wave of phenmetrazine abuse and addiction, the next weight-loss drug disaster appeared in Europe in 1968. In Switzerland, Austria, and Germany, a surprising number of young people—mainly in their twenties and thirties, and 80 percent of them women—began coming to cardiology clinics gasping for breath, suffering from a particular heart condition. Called pulmonary hypertension, the problem was excessive blood pressure in the vessels flowing from the heart to the lung, which caused the overworked heart to fail, and the condition is quite rare in those under sixty. As the young patients began to die, medical researchers racked their brains trying to explain this bizarre outbreak. Surveying victims about everything from their cleaning products to their eating habits, cardiologists discovered that all used a popular new diet pill—some for just a month —six to twelve months before their shortness of breath, swollen ankles, and other symptoms of heart disease appeared. The suspect drug, aminorex, had a chemical structure less like amphetamine than most diet drugs, and also had less toxicity in animal tests as well as little stimulating effect; it was therefore rated safe enough to sell without prescription. Amid objections that the case against the drug was inconclusive, aminorex was removed from the market in late 1968, and by the end of 1969 the pulmonary hypertension outbreak was receding. Most of the English-speaking world missed this particular pharmaceutically induced epidemic, because the applications to market aminorex in the U.S. and U.K. were still pending when the story broke in Europe. Clinical trials supporting the application to sell the drug in the United States, based in a Veterans Administration clinic, had only followed the patients for four weeks—just long enough to show significant weight loss but short enough not to see signs of heart disease.[36]

Although lucky to have escaped aminorex, the American public would bear the full brunt of the next diet drug catastrophe. In the late 1970s, the top diet pill in the United States was Dexatrim (the uncanny resemblance of the product's name to Dexedrine presumably no accident). Like all its major competitors in the nonprescription diet drug market, at the time this pill was based on phenylpropanolamine, or PPA. Close in structure to ephedrine as well as amphetamine, PPA had been in use since the late 1930s, mainly as a decongestant. Although PPA's action on the central nervous system had never been carefully studied, it definitely affected the brain the same way as amphetamine; the euphoric effects were weaker compared to its power to raise blood pressure, but it caused jitters and irritability and, at high enough doses, hallucinations as well.

In 1981, an estimated 4 million Americans consumed 10 billion PPA-containing diet pills, and consumption rose still further through the later 1980s. But, as so often happens, as the drug's use increased, so, too, did medical awareness of its toxic effects. There were reports of paranoid psychosis from PPA, just like amphetamine, and dangerously high blood pressure, and also strokes—such as the one suffered by a thirty-five-year-old businesswoman and mother of four, who reported to a Chicago hospital with a headache and nausea after taking Dexatrim, and had to have emergency brain surgery to save her from paralysis or death. Others were less fortunate.[37] Dieters might actually have been better off with amphetamine, which does not raise blood pressure very much at appetite-suppressing doses. Despite accumulating reports of adverse events and successful lawsuits against diet pill makers, PPA remained available in nonprescription diet pills, and cold remedies, throughout the 1980s. Indeed, PPA was only removed from over-the-counter sale at the end of 2000, a delay that provoked controversy about the FDA's apparent interest in protecting manufacturers rather than consumers.[38]

In the 1990s, the hottest diet pill was phentermine, this time in combination with a newer drug, fenfluramine, and it was available only by prescription. Like phentermine (FDA-approved in 1959), fenfluramine was actually not at all new but FDA-approved for U.S. sales in 1973. The combination was what was new. Fenfluramine, like phentermine, is related to amphetamine (Figure 37), but fenfluramine works slightly differently, affecting serotonin in brain circuits more than adrenaline, a balance opposite that of phentermine and amphetamine. And unlike phentermine and most diet drugs in the extended amphetamine family, fenfluramine does not cause a pleasant buzz and so carries less risk of abuse or addiction. On the contrary, the drug could cause depression, which helps to explain why it never became popular in the period dominated by PPA diet pills.

In the mid-1990s, however, the drug was reintroduced as dexflenfuramine (best known under the trade name Redux), the right-hand isomer in pure form. As with amphetamine, the right-handed isomer is responsible for most of the action on the central nervous system, allowing a lower dose for the same effect. Furthermore, when fenfluramine was combined with phentermine, both drugs worked together against appetite, while the mood-lifting effect of the phentermine balanced the depressing effect of fenfluramine. The rationale was that, in combination, neither phentermine addiction nor fenfluramine depression would develop, and the lower doses would allow safer long-term usage so that people could maintain their weight loss.

Through weight-loss doctors and clinics, the "Fen-Phen" dexfen-fluramine-phentermine combination caught on like wildfire, driving the number of Americans using prescription diet pills to more than 10 million in 1996, up from 4 million the year before (the difference probably balanced by reduced consumption of nonprescription diet pills). It took only a year more for the lethal effects to become obvious. Not only did an outbreak of pulmonary hypertension occur, much like that created by aminorex, but also an outbreak of another kind of heart disease. The diet drugs were inducing cancer-like overgrowth of cells in the heart valves of some people, so that they died or needed heart transplants and valve replacements. Dexfenfluramine was found to be responsible, and the drug was removed from the U.S. market in late 1997.[39] That same year another amphetamine relative came on the market for weight control, a drug called sibutramine that suppresses appetite like amphetamine but supposedly lacks euphoric effects (although its elevating effect on mood has been mentioned as a potential positive feature). Meanwhile, pharmaceutical firms continue to seek the next miracle diet medicine in the amphetamine family, one that ideally would affect the appetite like amphetamine but not the heart and blood vessels, nor, to any great extent, the pleasure centers in the brain. Pharmaceutical optimism springs eternal.[40]

The diet pill that enjoyed the greatest boost since the "Fen-Phen" catastrophe was one of the oldest—even older than amphetamine. Older does not always mean "safer," however. Ephedrine, extracted from ephedra plants (Ma Huang) and touted as an "all natural" product, rose to prominence in the nonprescription charts during the early 1990s. Although these ephedrine-based pills were mainly found in the food supplement and vitamin sections of drugstores, or else in a natural food store, some of these "food supplements" were commercial blockbusters rivaling major prescription drugs (for instance, Metabolife 365, with sales in 1999 around $900 million). Ephedrine aids weight loss exactly like amphetamine, mostly by suppressing appetite but also by boosting physical activity and metabolism slightly. Ephedrine also has similar side effects—judgment loss, stroke, agitation, even psychosis—only worse than amphetamine, in that little more than the dose needed for weight loss brings on these undesirable effects. Yet, because of a quirk in U.S. drug law, many of the ephedra diet pills carried no warning labels: the FDA is authorized to regulate the safety and efficacy only of products that claim medically therapeutic effects, and these "herbal food supplements" typically made no such claim. So, after industry lobbyists foiled an effort to put warning labels on ephedrine-containing pills, the FDA could only sit back as the reports of adverse events accumulated.

Previously sane and secular bank managers suddenly began raving of biblical revelation; healthy clothing designers suffered lethal strokes at health clubs; and so forth. By 1999 the ephedrine "events list" had grown to include more than a thousand cases, among them thirty-five deaths from heart attack, stroke, and other blood-pressure-related effects of the drug. Finally, in 2004, the FDA removed the diet products from sale.[41] Metabolife and the other brands had ephedra-free formulations waiting in the wings, but, without ephedrine, the natural supplement makers must again be losing a large share of the diet pill market to the pharmaceutical industry.

The series of drugs that have occupied amphetamine's dominant position in the diet pill market is a succession of chemical derivatives of amphetamine. Each, in turn, was trumpeted as much less toxic and less liable to abuse, yet each one—after being used for weight loss by millions—was in fact revealed to be addictive and prone to abuse in much the same way as amphetamine, to be more toxic than amphetamine, or both. Since all resemble amphetamine chemically, affect appetite like amphetamine, affect the brain in other ways very much like amphetamine, feel similar subjectively, and cause the same dangerous "side effects," at least to some extent, it is reasonable to describe all these past "non-amphetamine" diet pill blockbusters as "speed" of a sort. And, although the evidence from millions of users of the current best-selling weight loss drugs is not yet in, the lessons of this repetitive history argue caution and pessimism. It may be that no drug will ever be better than amphetamine for suppressing appetite in terms of balancing safety and effectiveness. That, however, is not saying much.

In any case, at least until the 2004 removal of ephedra from its dominant place in the diet pill market, it would be fair to count the 10 million Americans taking weight-loss drugs in any given year as speed users. Adding these to the 10 million users of illicit amphetamines and Attention Deficit drugs classed as amphetamines, which we have already counted, we reach a tally of 20 million Americans actively using speed in the mid-2000s. This figure, representing over 6.5 percent of the total population, indicates a national level of speed use, medical and nonmedical combined, higher than American amphetamine consumption at the height of the first epidemic in 1969–70, which, at that time, was 5 percent of the total population, or roughly 10 million users (which would be about 15 million adjusted for today's higher population). Thus, based on these numbers, America's current speed habit is significantly worse than ever before.

Depression after Amphetamine

We have finished counting the Americans currently consuming speed, taking the term broadly (including stimulants like methylphenidate and diet drugs like phentermine and ephedrine), with a tally of around 20 million Americans using amphetamine-like drugs in a given year. But we could continue counting still further if we seek the answer to another related question, not about this particular drug family but about our culture. Sociologically rather than pharmacologically speaking, what is the demand for speed today? Or to put the question another way, how many Americans now use drugs for the same reasons that they once took amphetamine, when it was an ordinary pharmaceutical? To answer this question, we must count not just those who today are taking amphetamine-like drugs recreationally, for weight loss, and for Attention Deficit. We must also count the drugs that took amphetamine's place in its original, major market: minor depression and emotional distress in general practice. For as we shall see, even though not closely related to amphetamine, these drugs are prescribed and consumed in ways very much like that psychiatric amphetamine blockbuster of the 1950s, Dexamyl. They meet the same perceived medical need.

To understand how today's antidepressants have regained this market for the drug industry, let us take a brief historical detour into the history of depression since the 1970s. The end of amphetamine as an antidepressant for commonplace depression, brought on by restrictions imposed by the FDA and federal narcotics authorities in 1971, left a gaping hole in the prescription drug business. The MAOI and tricyclic drugs never captured more than a fraction of the psychiatric market that amphetamine antidepressants once enjoyed—no matter how much better they fared in clinical testing on severe depression, and no matter how enthusiastically the psychiatric specialists recommended them over amphetamine. In 1970, about 2 percent of the U.S.

adult population reported taking one of the newer antidepressants in the previous year compared to more than 5 percent taking amphetamines by prescription, and these newer drugs did not gain much ground even when amphetamines were restricted.[42] Thus, family doctors needed a new pill that could replace Dexamyl for everyday emotional distress, one their patients would accept. The drug industry never neglects such a large unmet demand. But what was the right strategy to develop a replacement for amphetamine as a general practice antidepressant? The right answer, for a drug company, depended on picking the best theory of depression—best both in terms of discovering new drugs and impressing prescribing doctors.

Depression had become a hot scientific topic in the 1970s, thanks to advances in research fields from neurobiology to experimental psychology to molecular genetics. Psychiatrists, psychologists, and laboratory biologists of many different stripes studied the condition intensively. According to all schools, from psychoanalysts to existentialists to behaviorists to neurochemists, enormous breakthroughs in understanding depression's causes had been made—although few could agree on exactly what those breakthroughs were: alienation, learned helplessness, low self-esteem, or low serotonin.[43] But somehow a way of tying together all these pieces into a more unified view of depression, serviceable enough to reduce friction among the various experts, began to take shape in the mid-1970s. Whether caused by early trauma or disappointments later in life or bad genes for weak pleasure circuits or drugs like reserpine, depression appears when the nerve circuits for drive and reward are depleted of their signaling hormones, causing reduced drive and helpless agitation. Helplessness leads to renewed incapacity to manage stress and improve the situation, setting up a vicious cycle of failure and reaction to it.[44]

This new consensus theory had the advantage of explaining how depression could be treated either by changing people's behavior to more rewarding patterns (as the behaviorist and cognitive-behaviorist therapy schools proposed), by changing people's attitudes so that they less readily accepted punishment (as Freudian psychotherapists tended to think), or by using medication that stimulated the brain's reward centers. One could break the cycle of reduced activity, reduced pleasure and reward, and reinforced loss of drive by intervening at any point with all these therapeutic techniques, much as Myerson argued in the 1920s and 1930s. In 1980, the American Psychiatric

Association produced revised psychiatric disease categories, collectively known as *"DSM-III"* (*Diagnostic and Statistical Manual,* 3rd ed.) in a style that avoided theoretical terms like "neurosis" in favor of easily observable signs on which different groups of psychiatrists could agree. *DSM-III* defined depression, now labeled "Major Depressive Disorder" or milder "Dysthymia," chiefly in terms of anhedonia: "loss of interest or pleasure in all or almost all activities and pastimes." Although the *DSM-III* is often portrayed as the overthrow of Freudian dominance by biologically oriented psychiatrists, the handling of depression shows how the new consensus granted a valid place to every major type of psychiatric practitioner, reducing the need for factional conflict and improving the profession's scientific standing. (To be sure, psychoanalysts regretted the abandonment of "neurosis," which much of Freudian thought had been devoted to explaining.)[45]

The pharmaceutical industry noted these developments in the depression field and, indeed, was responsible for some of the 1970s ferment in the brain sciences. As mentioned earlier, one of the ways that amphetamine was thought to elevate mood was by blocking the mechanisms responsible for the recycling or "reuptake" of serotonin, as well as adrenaline, after the neurohormones are released in particular brain circuits. Tricyclic antidepressants work mainly in this way, affecting both adrenaline and serotonin circuits to differing degrees depending on the particular drug's chemical structure. So many drug companies looked for new chemicals that would block reuptake of just one or the other neurotransmitter, more selectively. For various reasons, including accidents and the politics of science, serotonin emerged as the favored neurotransmitter. As psychiatrist and historian David Healy has argued, once the drug industry settled on serotonin-affecting drugs and amplified the research supporting serotonin-based theories of depression in order to market them, alternative theories of depression were overshadowed.[46]

Swedish neurochemists created the first drug that blocked the reuptake of serotonin much more efficiently than it blocked adrenaline, selectively amplifying the serotonin circuits. Called zimelidine, the Swedish firm Astra patented it as an antidepressant in 1971. Although proper clinical studies showing it to be an effective antidepressant were not published until 1980, other pharmaceutical firms followed closely in Astra's footsteps and during the 1970s invented many such "selective serotonin reuptake inhibitor" (SSRI) drugs. The French firm

Duphar marketed one called fluvoxamine (best known under the brand name Luvox) in Europe in 1983, a year after Astra launched zimelidine. Then, in 1988, the American firm Lilly marketed its own SSRI in the U.S., fluoxetine or Prozac, fifteen years after that drug was first invented.[47]

These new antidepressants took a surprisingly long time to get from discovery to marketing. One suspects that, in the 1970s and early 1980s, drug company managers were not trying very hard to bring new antidepressant drugs to the market. Perhaps the industry had become pessimistic and decided, after the failure of MAOIs and tricyclics to take off like the amphetamines, that the general practice antidepressant market had dried up forever, and that there was only a limited market in major depressive illness at stake. Indeed, Healy suggests that certain drug company managers at the time believed that no more than a hundred people per million (0.01 percent of the population) would be prescribed an improved antidepressant.[48]

But if drug companies were skeptical about market prospects for SSRI antidepressants, they must have quickly changed their minds shortly after Prozac was released in the United States. It took little more than a year for a portrait of the pill to feature on the cover of *Newsweek* magazine, where it was hailed as a huge breakthrough in the treatment of depression. Actually, the carefully controlled studies comparing Prozac and other SSRIs to tricyclics found them only equally effective as these older drugs in the treatment of major depression: with certain patients they worked better, with many other patients not so well. Nevertheless, Prozac caught on with family doctors like the tricyclics and MAOIs never had, partly because it had fewer of the side effects and dangers that made doctors hesitant to prescribe the older antidepressants.[49]

Another reason Prozac and the other SSRI antidepressants caught on is the way they made the patients feel and perform socially. As psychiatrist Peter Kramer described their effects in his influential book, *Listening to Prozac*, these drugs lowered inhibitions and increased outgoing, confident behavior in many people. Since our culture values these traits, even normal (non-depressed) individuals using the drugs may feel a benefit reinforced by society. The reward for outgoing confidence is especially great in certain high-paying, competitive occupations, making antidepressants like Prozac performance-enhancing "steroids for the business Olympics."[50] Kramer goes on perceptively to equate the use of Prozac, particularly by people with mild or no depression, to the use of amphetamines on the street: in both cases, the drugs are taken "for overcoming inhibitions and inspiring zest," for boosting confidence, and for accelerating thought and speech.[51] The main difference is that Prozac is taken by the well-to-do with prescriptions, whereas amphetamines are now taken mainly by poorer people, outside the law, or else by prescription for Attention Deficit.

Basically, according to this view, Prozac and similar SSRI drugs have proven so much more popular than the tricyclics not because of their effectiveness for treating serious depression (which is undeniable but not remarkable), nor just because they have fewer unpleasant side effects. They caught on because they boost drive and capacity for pleasure, whether or not the user is depressed, just like amphetamine. And they also offer pleasant amphetamine-like side effects that many people find socially desirable, like confidence and talkativeness. Some of Kramer's patients even gave weight loss—another common side effect—as a reason why they liked Prozac so much. Like amphetamines, SSRIs can make people feel and look "better than well."[52]

If Kramer is right and Prozac boosts what Myerson called "zest for living" much like amphetamine, whether or not the user is clinically depressed, this subjective "zest" effect can explain why SSRIs have inherited amphetamine's old psychiatric market. In any case, patients responded enthusiastically to the drugs, and physicians saw no reason to resist. In the 1990s, heavy drug company marketing carried the message to family doctors that they should never leave depression untreated: now that SSRIs offered a safe option, there was no harm in trying drug therapy with patients suffering possibly depressive emotional distress. Government-endorsed depression awareness-raising campaigns, motivated by the high economic costs attributed to depression, backed up the marketing.[53]

Sales of the new antidepressants boomed throughout the decade, finally beginning to plateau in the early 2000s at stratospheric levels. In 2003, the SSRI antidepressants were being dispensed in the United States at a rate of 100 million prescriptions per year, which translates minimally (assuming every user accounts for twelve one-month prescriptions) to more than 8 million Americans and, more realistically, between 15 and 20 million. Seventeen million is a reasonable estimate of the number of Americans using Prozac and other SSRI antidepressants each year, a figure which assumes that each user on average accounts for six monthly prescriptions.[54] But even taking the minimum figure of 8 million, a larger proportion of the American population is now using the drugs than ever took amphetamines by prescription for psychiatric purposes. And if 17 million is a close estimate of how many now use the drugs each year, the SSRI antidepressants are actually being taken by the same proportion of Americans (about 5 percent of the total population) that used amphetamines *for any purpose* at the height of the amphetamine epidemic in 1969–70. Like the amphetamines but unlike any antidepressants that succeeded them, the SSRI drugs not only impress psychiatrists but also fulfill the wishes of distressed patients as well as the patient-management needs of the family doctors who still prescribe a great many of them. They must also suit the health insurers that have to foot the bill.[55] Otherwise, they would never be as popular.

Thus, with Prozac, the buzz finally came back, that elated feeling of extra energy that patients once expected when they saw their family doctor about trouble coping and which tricyclic antidepressants failed to deliver. Moreover, given authoritative pronouncements that there are millions more who still need the drugs, not just for depression but also for new uses such as "Social Anxiety Disorder" and "Premenstrual Dysphoric Disorder," consumption of SSRIs is set to grow even further, beyond the 10 percent of the American population currently said to be suffering depression or related mood disorders.[56]

Although depression actually may have grown more common since the 1970s, such enormous numbers, reflecting at least a tenfold increase in medically recognized depression (and, by some reckonings, a thousandfold increase), can only reflect a loosening of the definition of "depression" to include the sort of "situational emotional distress" for which Dexamyl once proved such a popular treatment.[57] It is worth remembering that solid RCTs in the early 1960s found placebos to be just as effective as both Dexamyl and the tricyclic antidepressants for mild depression and "situational emotional distress." Recent studies with moderately to seriously depressed patients have found that tricyclics and SSRIs work about equally well, and although both antidepressant drug types help these patients somewhat better than placebos, placebos work so well that about 75 percent of the response to the drugs is actually a placebo response. In other words, placebos and modern antidepressant drugs both work, and the real drugs work, at most, one-third better than placebos as a treatment for moderate depression. Moreover, in experiments where unsuitable drugs are used as "active placebos" instead of inert sugar pills, the placebos work still better and narrow the apparent superiority of antidepressants still further—simply because patients can detect some sort of drug effect. These studies, furthermore, were with patients showing true depression of moderate or worse severity; with milder depressions, specific drug effects are even less, and the superiority of SSRIs over placebos is undetectable.[58]

All this suggests that the great majority of SSRI antidepressants dispensed today for milder depressions serve as placebos, much like Dexamyl. And they seem to be working, much as Dexamyl did. Even patients who are significantly depressed will respond to the side effects of the SSRIs while they wait for the delayed antidepressant effects, whereas the others, emotionally distressed but not depressed by strict medical standards (probably the majority), will enjoy the benefits of the side effects while their distress passes on its own. Everybody wins—provided we do not count the costs of drugging people who only need a sugar pill or emotional support, and a little time.

Speed, America's Persistent Drug Habit

We have now counted 5 million using Attention Deficit medications, 3 million using methamphetamine and related stimulants nonmedically, and 2 million using ecstasy, making a total of 10 million more using amphetamines, rather strictly defined. We have also counted 10 million or more Americans taking diet pills each year, virtually all of these still (or, until quite recently) very speed-like, even if they are not strictly amphetamines (see Figure 37). Further, as I have argued, at least 8 million and probably over 17 million more Americans are taking today's SSRI antidepressants. Even though SSRI antidepressants are not closely related to amphetamine and are safer, they are largely dispensed and appreciated, like Dexamyl, for their amphetamine-like side effects and placebo action, rather than for their genuine antidepressant action. Although these are conservative estimates, they would still add up to 37 million Americans, assuming no overlap, for instance, between diet pill and antidepressant users. (Evidence from 1970 suggests that the overlap then, at least, was not great.)[59] Even if not quite 12 percent of the total U.S. population, the actual combined prevalence of use of these drugs is enormous.

Today's users take their amphetamines and pharmaceutical amphetamine derivatives in order to lose weight, cheer up, work harder, think faster, or just for fun, in essentially the same way that Americans took amphetamine in 1969. Others take SSRI antidepressants to cheer up, work harder, and even lose weight. Consumption of all these medications and illicit amphetamines together represents the demand that amphetamine alone once met, at the height of the first speed epidemic. Since up to 12 percent of the total U.S. population today are using drugs (whether or not these are pharmacologically related to amphetamine) that serve the same purposes that amphetamine originally served, as compared with about 5 percent (10 million) of the total population using amphetamines, medically and nonmedically, in these same ways each year at the end of the 1960s, it is fair to conclude that the American population's appetite for drugs that do the various things that speed does has ballooned. Indeed, the percentage of Americans using such drugs has doubled in one generation.

Why this massive, expanded national demand for speed's effects? Consider the major types of medical use that first made amphetamine a successful pharmaceutical during the 1940s. Doctors prescribed it to fight mild ("reactive") depression and emotional distress, particularly when patients showed anhedonia and lack of "zest"; doctors prescribed it for weight loss; and people also used it with and without a prescription as a pick-me-up and energizing aid for studying or working. Using pharmaceuticals to counteract disappointments and emotional distress means turning to medicine in order to become outgoing, upbeat, and assertive when we would otherwise be sadder and more reflective. Using pharmaceuticals to lose weight means turning to medicine to alter our eating habits just because our body doesn't live up to standards of beauty (at least for the vast number of diet pill users who are not in fact medically obese) or because we have an insufficiently active lifestyle or possibly both. Using pharmaceuticals to stay focused, alert, and productive means turning to medicine in order to perform work at a grueling pace instead of resting more frequently and taking longer to do the job or else finding more inspiring and inherently rewarding work. The diverse group of drugs that have each partly replaced amphetamines today—SSRI antidepressants,

Attention Deficit medications, crystal meth, and diet pills that work much like amphetamine—are all popular for exactly the same three reasons.[60] These drugs are simply the current "technologies of the self" that do what amphetamine once accomplished for everyone.

The amphetamines and related drugs no doubt tap into universal human mechanisms of pleasure and excitement. Nevertheless, our interest in them depends as much on our particular society and culture as on our biology. Our culture rewards outgoing, upbeat behavior and discourages introspection. It respects vigorous, focused work in pursuit of career advancement, material rewards, and personal betterment, while it discourages modest ambitions and so-called laziness. And our culture prizes a youthful physique and slimness, but does not provide most people with quality foods or the time to cook them or the opportunity to exercise. When Americans cannot live up to society's values and norms, they may seek help in medicine. Medicine, aided and urged by the pharmaceutical industry, welcomes the opportunity to manage such mismatches between individuals and social norms as treatable medical problems. In the process, sickness has been generated, in the sense that certain behavioral patterns become recognized as illness—usually in concert with shifting social conditions that make those behaviors seem more problematic.

The sociologist Ivan Illich once described this as the general pattern attending the expansion of medicine's domain: the medicalization of social problems. The concept certainly applies to the rise of amphetamine. Viewed through the lens of medicalization, this then is how we would reconstruct what happened when amphetamine was welcomed as a miracle drug. In 1940s and 1950s America, low interest in pleasurable pursuits and advancement became recognized as depressive illness in the form of anhedonia, bringing vindication to Myerson's prescient theories from the 1920s. Unusually high food intake and largeness became recognized as the psychiatrically inflected disorders of overweight and obesity. Helping to validate the new pathology, amphetamine provided a corrective remedy for both these new forms of illness, these postwar disorders of consumption. Soon millions seeking help for failing to meet society's standards around good cheer, ambition, accomplishment, and physique received absolution with a diagnosis and, with the wave of a prescription pen, an amphetamine benediction. What might have been a moral issue of substandard conduct, or instead might have brought standards of conduct into question, became commonplace mental health problems, managed medically with amphetamines.

No doubt, the later twentieth century has seen a gradual shift in power within the medical system, drug companies gaining and physicians losing. Still, considering the system as a whole, medicine's role in upholding the normality of what Rose has called (echoing Illich) "the enterprising subject" has not wavered since the 1940s, when amphetamine was first widely prescribed. Sadness and discouragement are still drugged, now mainly with SSRI antidepressants. Wandering focus and poor work discipline are drugged with amphetamine and other Attention Deficit medications. (It is worthwhile, in this context, to consider Jean Baudrillard's characterization of asthenia and apathy —depression—as passive rebellion against the competitive consumerist social order, the unconscious and private equivalent of the collective factory "slowdown.")[61] And largeness is still drugged, both by prescription and self-medication, with amphetamine-like diet pills.

Is this mass recourse to drugs necessarily a bad thing? Doubtless some individuals, on balance, benefit from the medicalization of their failure to meet norms. But, as Illich argued, the net effect of medicine's participation is harmful, because the process "creates not only biologically formulated legitimacy for man-the-consumer but also new pressures for escalation" of the pressures to conform.[62] Indeed, as Illich's theory predicts, the cultural-medical process that made anhedonia into depression, plumpness into pre-obesity, and amphetamine into a remedy for both has escalated. Judging by today's expanded drug consumption for the conditions that drove amphetamine use in the 1960s, we are now considerably sicker with the ailments that amphetamines remedy—twice as sick, if we combine medical and nonmedical speed use as equivalent "technologies of the self." But if amphetamines and their substitutes are medicines for a social disease, it might now be time to question whether the ailment may lie not chiefly in the physiology of the one out of every eight or ten Americans now taking drugs with amphetamine-like effects. Perhaps we should consider that the problem lies instead in a sick social system fundamentally at odds with natural human capacities and fulfillments.

It is hardly a novel view that the system that supposedly meets our needs and makes us richer in fact makes us sicker. Those who raised questions in the late 1960s about how we expect pills to fix problems of living often suggested as much. The view that medicines are really technological fixes for social ills may even apply to most best-selling drugs, not just psychotropics, insofar as they keep us alive and if possible contributing economically, despite our bad habits and unwholesome environments. This does not mean we are necessarily passive victims of our drugging. That amphetamine demand never went away even after the drug was all but condemned medically, and that with or without prescriptions Americans have found ways to consume as much as ever, proves that drug users make active choices about altering their minds and bodies. The insight remains profound nevertheless: individual shortcomings and disorders exist only by contrast with society's standards of normality and health. Thus, drugs often say more about society than biology, whether viewed as correctional instruments or as self-fashioning tools that help us become more what we want to be. Distinguishing the two is harder than it first appears: the self we struggle to become may be one designed to meet the expectations of others. When those expectations require us—come what may—to work hard, play hard, be outgoing, control our appetites, and feel optimistic, the success that drugs can bring is, at best, a doubtful liberation.

Conclusion

The Lessons of History

ALTHOUGH MAJOR CHANGES in social structures and values may be needed if America's craving for speed is ever to diminish, this is no reason to neglect the search for simpler, smaller-scale changes that might help mitigate the harms, both direct and indirect, of today's heavy consumption of amphetamine-like drugs. And history does suggest, moreover, that harmful consequences will accrue beyond the immediate and obvious effects of crystal meth. Apart from an increase in cases of amphetamine psychosis by the thousands and the other harms of amphetamine-type addiction by the tens of thousands, as well as hepatitis and AIDS from amphetamine injection, America can expect redoubled problems with other drugs. "What happens when a major speed scene develops," testified David E. Smith of the Haight-Ashbury Clinic before Congress in 1971, is that "a downer or depressant scene follows" inevitably.[1] His predictions were borne out on the national level, in America's late-1970s heroin epidemic.

Heroin is not so easy to get as in the 1970s, and pharmaceutical barbiturates are no longer widely available, but we may already be seeing the same rebound effect in the recent massive wave of prescription pain-killer abuse in the United States. In the decade from 1993 to 2003, the number of first-time abusers of these drugs—most of them related to heroin, like Vicodin and Oxycontin—tripled to 2.5 million per year. This means that a huge wave of people has been turning to these mind-numbing opiates, tracking the rising tide of meth and Attention Deficit medications. And because these opiates are addictive, first-time users often become long-term abusers: in 2004, 11 million Americans used prescription pain relievers and 5 million used tranquilizers nonmedically, more than double the number a decade earlier. The relation of current opiate and sedative abuse to prior stimulant use is a question that demands further research, given that 10 million

Americans are now using amphetamines both for Attention Deficit Disorder and recreationally.[2]

Whether or not the rise in speed use (both medical and recreational) is behind the rise in opiate abuse, the direct consequences of heavy methamphetamine use are bad enough to warrant strong and immediate action. The first lesson from the original speed epidemic that we might apply involves the way drug abusers are treated by society. While the U.S. has clung to a punitive "zero tolerance" approach that wages "war" on (illicit) drugs and drug abusers alike, much of the developed world has taken another path called "harm reduction." Harm reduction seeks to take pragmatic action to limit the damage drugs cause society, by treating drug abusers as people that need medical help whether or not they are currently trying to quit. Apart from providing medical services in ways that do not scare away drug users (such as informing law enforcement or compelling detox), a key harm reduction strategy in the context of amphetamines would be needle exchange. People who shoot speed may inject very frequently while on a run, which helps explain why amphetamine injectors are at much higher risk of AIDS than people who only inject heroin.[3] Providing clean needles helps prevent users from getting AIDS, or hepatitis, which means not only do they not get sick but they don't make others sick, costing everyone a lot of money and trouble.

Harm reduction works, both to lower infection rates and save society money. In Australia, for example, despite heroin and amphetamine drug abuse rates as bad as those in the U.S. and the early appearance of AIDS in the country, twenty years of effective needle distribution has led to a situation in which only about 5 percent of all new infections with the AIDS virus are caused by drug injection. Only about 2 percent of injecting drug users are infected with the AIDS virus in Australia. The rate of AIDS virus infection among injecting drug users in the United States is *twenty times higher,* thanks to hostility toward needle exchange. Moreover, America's national rate of new AIDS virus infections (incidence) is about thirteen times higher than Australia's. One-fifth of the forty-two thousand new AIDS virus infections in the United States each year occur among injecting drug users, and in addition most infections transmitted through heterosexual contact—about a third of all new infections with the AIDS virus—originate from injecting drug use. So, essentially, around half the new AIDS virus infections in the United States, twenty thousand per year, would not be happening if needle exchange were conducted on the same scale as in Australia. Harm reduction has worked elsewhere, too, and is now containing the wildfire spread of AIDS in the former Soviet Union.[4] Even if it were morally defensible to treat drug abusers as sub-humans unworthy of medical help, it would still be foolish to refuse them clean needles, because, from the virus's perspective, we are all the same pool of potential victims.

Harm reduction needs to be coupled to initiatives that reduce demand for illicit amphetamines, like rehabilitation and aftercare for those who quit, and education and health promotion campaigns that reduce the number that become drug abusers. While helping people get off and stay off amphetamines will help limit damage, demand reduction needs to be accompanied by supply reduction in order to reduce both new use and consumption levels among users. This is the domain of vigorous, traditional law enforcement and federal regulation. To cut small-scale illicit methamphetamine supplies, there needs to be strong, federally imposed national restrictions on sales of cold medications containing ephedrine and pseudoephedrine or, better yet, complete removal of products with these ingredients from over-the-counter sale. Congestion never killed anyone, and, in any case, sinus sprays without ephedrine will still be available. Of course, stopping small-scale local production is not enough, since organized crime has stepped in to import manufactured methamphetamine from countries where raw materials are easily obtained. Thus, well-resourced law enforcement efforts to deal with the large-scale methamphetamine trade are also needed, for example, continued efforts to find and imprison wholesale dealers in meth. Strong penalties are needed for unauthorized possession of large quantities of pure ephedrine and pseudephedrine, since even though these are medically valuable drugs in themselves, their only use in this form is the illicit manufacture of amphetamines. All these measures are not likely to create any great controversy, given the traditional emphasis in the U.S. on supply reduction approaches to illicit drugs; indeed, changes along these lines are well under way.

However, supply control measures cannot end with law enforcement against illicit speed. In the 1960s, the pharmaceutical industry manufactured and distributed massive quantities of amphetamines, and these pills not only fueled medical addiction but also supplied most recreational use. Now that the consumption of prescription

amphetamine and methylphenidate for Attention Deficit has reached
2.5 billion defined doses annually, and with six hundred thousand
Americans evidently misusing these medications in any given month,
widespread diversion may already be returning. Even granting that
Attention Deficit is a genuine neurological disorder, rather than just
above-average distractibility, and that the medications effectively treat
it in those correctly diagnosed, with billions of pills per year flowing
through medical channels the risk to public health posed by these
medications is huge. In the mid-1960s, the British medical profession
decided that the risks of prescribing drugs like amphetamine and
methylphenidate far outweighed the benefits, and that the drugs were
simply too dangerous for routine prescription. Patients might demand
the pills, and they might even work for some, but patients on the
whole were still better off without them. Society certainly was: by 1968
medical amphetamine use in the U.K. had leveled off at half the U.S.
levels and had begun to decline, possibly saving Britain from the same
sort of high-dose amphetamine injection outbreak in the late 1960s
and 1970s that afflicted the U.S.[5] History suggests that American doctors today should ask themselves whether they really ought to be supplying large numbers of basically healthy children—and now adults
—with the same addictive drugs that give medical research its best experimental simulation of schizophrenia. Perhaps the FDA and Drug
Enforcement Administration will have to make that decision for them
if the American medical profession fails to control itself, just as they
did in 1971.

     This brings us to a final set of policy lessons we might draw from
this history, lessons as relevant to all drugs as they are to amphetamine. No matter how pleasant a medicine or how socially desirable its
effects, patients only get a chance to try it when drug companies convince prescribing doctors—mainly family doctors for the really big
sellers—that a new drug is safe and effective. Amphetamine became
the first mass-market antidepressant in the 1940s through the construction of a convincing scientific case for the drug, thanks to astute
management of the medical research literature on depression and
clever marketing. This set the stage for the pharmaceutical speed epidemic that followed in the 1950s and 1960s. Drug marketing in current
times is far more sophisticated, pervasive, and lavish, and proven effective in influencing prescribing habits.[6] Despite great advances in
the methods used to test drugs in the laboratory and clinic since the

1930s, published scientific studies today still reflect a measurable (and often large) bias in favor of drug company sponsors.[7]

All these factors together mean that the drug industry, in its normal course of business, still generates a constant threat to society: thanks to company marketing, the wrong drugs may be prescribed to the wrong people, or excessive drugs to suitable people. Occasionally new drugs with runaway popularity are created that turn out to be deadly or addictive, or both, in ways that initial testing does not detect. None of these old problems surrounding the drug industry has disappeared. Therefore, in order to make medical science the main driver of prescribing decisions, strong restrictions are needed on pharmaceutical marketing and promotion, as well as stronger limits on the methods used by drug firms to manage medical research for marketing purposes.[8] The independence of regulatory authorities like the FDA, since the 1980s increasingly solicitous of the desires of the drug industry it regulates, badly needs restoration so that the public health can be protected. Only by keeping the pharmaceutical industry on a tight leash will more patients receive drug treatments that benefit them, and fewer get drugs that cause them more harm than good. Even doctors have an imperfect ability to see through the fog of company-generated information about drugs, so clearly the medically untrained public are still less able to judge how to use pharmaceuticals appropriately. An obvious conclusion is that the United States should return to the standard followed everywhere else in the world (except New Zealand) by banning direct-to-consumer prescription drug advertising.

Over-prescription, excessive marketing, and the American tolerance of outrageous drug prices (whether from affluence or helplessness or both), which drives the entire problem by making it all pay off, help explain why the United States has the costliest and least efficient medical system in the developed world. Moreover, the American medical system provides health, as measured by life expectancy of an infant born now, near the bottom of the list of developed countries, at 77.8 years, about the same as Denmark's and worse than Korea's (78.5 years), according to the latest OECD figures. And our medical system's mediocre performance is purchased at outrageous cost. Combining both public and private expenditures, most developed nations spend 7–10 percent of their wealth (gross domestic product [GDP]) compared to 15 percent spent by the U.S. in 2005, a figure still spiraling up and out of control. Denmark, although not an especially healthy nation, spends 9 percent of its wealth, or, in real dollars, less than half as much money per person as the U.S. spends; for similar results, Korea only spends about one-third as much of its wealth, or, in real dollars, one-fifth as much money per person. Even Mexico achieves health results close to those in the United States, a life expectancy at birth only 3 percent (2.3 years) lower, while spending 6 percent per capita of its much smaller GDP, or, in real dollars, one-ninth as much money on health per person. In 2005, ten of thirty OCED nations outperformed the United States in health by at least this same margin, at much lower cost—including Canada.[9]

Perhaps the time has come for the United States to learn a lesson from the rest of the world and adopt the sort of national health insurance systems (privately supplemented to varying degrees) that, in virtually all the other developed nations, deliver equally good or better health at a fraction of the cost. Of course, pharmaceuticals are not the only cause of the spectacular inefficiency of American medicine, but they are certainly part of the problem. A major function of government health insurance systems is to negotiate best value in pharmaceuticals, subsidizing only medically appropriate drug use. A "free market" in pharmaceuticals, in any case, has been pure fiction for at least a century, since FDA and AMA regulation had to step in to protect the public from the total market failure in drugs prevailing in 1905. We cannot expect a miracle cure for our medico-economic ailments to come from the pharmaceutical industry. The longer Americans fail to change their ways and address the glaring issue of their dysfunctional medical system, the more that future historians will marvel at the nation's inappropriate perseverance.

Notes

Notes to the Introduction

1. On Paul Ehrlich and his quest for Salvarsan and other antibiotics, see Timothy Lenoir, "A Magic Bullet: Research for Profit and the Growth of Knowledge in Germany around 1900," *Minerva* 26 (1988): 66–88; on the sulfonamides, see John Lesch, *The First Miracle Drugs: How the Sulfa Drugs Transformed Medicine* (Oxford: Oxford University Press, 2007); on insulin, see Michael Bliss, *The Discovery of Insulin* (Chicago: University of Chicago Press, 1982).

2. On antipsychotics, see Judith Swazey, *Chlorpromazine in Psychiatry: A Study of Therapeutic Innovation* (Cambridge, Mass.: MIT Press, 1974); on tranquilizers, see Mickey C. Smith, *Small Comfort: A History of the Minor Tranquilizers* (New York: Praeger, 1985). The worthwhile sources on the history of penicillin are too numerous to mention, but one might profitably begin with John C. Sheehan, *The Enchanted Ring: The Untold Story of Penicillin* (Cambridge, Mass.: MIT Press, 1982); Milton Wainwright, *Miracle Cure: The Story of Penicillin and the Golden Age of Antibiotics* (Oxford: Blackwell, 1990); and Robert Bud, *Penicillin: Triumph and Tragedy* (Oxford: Oxford University Press, 2007).

3. Toine Pieters and collaborators have attributed recognition of this pattern of a new medication's high reputation and popularity, followed by a period of disrepute and unpopularity, followed finally by rational and moderate reassessment to the early-twentieth-century psychiatrist Max Siege. The first stage of enthusiasm is what begs explanation. See Stephen Snelders, Charles Kaplan, and Toine Pieters, "On Cannabis, Chloral Hydrate, and Career Cycles of Psychotrophic Drugs in Medicine," *Bulletin of the History of Medicine* 80 (2006): 95–114.

4. Campbell Gibson, "Population of the 100 Largest Cities and Other Urban Places in the United States: 1790 To 1990," U.S. Census Bureau, 1998, available at http://www.census.gov/population/www/documentation/twps0027.html (accessed February 12, 2007).

5. In 1975, medical writers Lester Grinspoon and Peter Hedblom published an influential book titled *The Speed Culture: Amphetamine Use and Abuse in America* (Cambridge, Mass.: Harvard University Press, 1975). In it they reviewed the harmful effects of amphetamines, condemned the use of these

drugs as medicines (thus joining a chorus of opinion at the time), and explained the popularity of amphetamines in terms of patient demands for a technological fix for increasingly stressful lives—in combination with a ruthless drug industry eager to profit from this need. This book discusses the same series of events that these authors sketched out, and also brings the amphetamine story up to date. Although I do not disagree essentially with the views of Hedblom and Grinspoon, this book draws on a larger body of evidence and adds to their project in three main ways. First, it offers a detailed historical account of the processes by which the drug industry interacted with the medical research and clinical communities to make amphetamine into a successful pharmaceutical in the first place. Second, it more closely examines the cultural side of these same processes that made amphetamine a successful pharmaceutical, the ways in which previously unmedicated problems of living came to be understood as amphetamine-treatable medical conditions (that is, medicalized), especially in the United States between the 1930s and the present day. Third, it capitalizes on hindsight, and on the much more sophisticated understanding of drug abuse available today, to relate the amphetamine epidemic of the previous generation to the one now rampant.

Notes to Chapter I

1. For animal experiments, see, for example, Gordon A. Alles, "Experiment 2," November 27, 1928; "Experiment 6," December 1, 1928; for the first human test, see Alles, "B-Phenyl-isopropyl amine Action on Circulation—Man—Subcutaneous Administration," June 3, 1929; both in Gordon Alles Papers, California Institute of Technology Archives (hereafter, GAP), box 5, folder "SKF vs. Alles: Alles Lab Records."

2. Throughout the book I refer to the main hormonal secretion of the adrenal medulla, as well as the main adrenergic neurotransmitter, as "adrenaline," even though the former is now known to be a mixture of adrenaline and noradrenaline (or, in American parlance, epinephrine and norepinephrine), and the latter is known to be noradrenaline. In calling it by this archaic name I conform to common medical usage of the early twentieth century, and indeed most colloquial usage today.

3. Tom Mahoney, *Merchants of Life: An Account of the American Pharmaceutical Industry* (New York: Harpers, 1959): 73–74; J. J. Abel, "On Epinephrine and Its Compounds," *American Journal of Pharmacy* 75 (1903): 301–25. John Parascandola, "John J. Abel and the Early Development of Pharmacology at the Johns Hopkins University," *Bulletin of the History of Medicine* 56 (1982): 512–27; Walter Sneader, *Drug Discovery: The Evolution of Modern Medicines* (London: Wiley, 1986), 96–99; Miles Weatherall, *In Search of a Cure: A History of Pharmaceutical Discovery* (Oxford and New York: Oxford University Press,

1990); Tetsumori Yamashima, "Jokichi Takamine (1854–1922), the Samurai Chemist, and His Work on Adrenalin," *Journal of Medical Biography* 11 (2003): 95–102; Anon., "Timeline: The Hundred-Year History of Sankyo," Sankyo, http://www.sankyo.co.jp/english/history/history1900.html (accessed February 2, 2004); Horace Davenport, "Epinephrin(e)," *Physiologist* 25 (1982): 76–82; Jonathan Simon, "Adrenalin, Epinephrin, or Suprarenin? Identifying the True Hypertensive Principle," paper presented at the conference "Drugs Trajectories: Historical Studies of Biology, Medicine, and Industry," Max Planck Institute for History of Science, Berlin, June 7–8, 2002.

    4. Paul Starr, *The Social Transformation of American Medicine* (New York: Basic Books, 1982), chap. 3; Kenneth Ludmerer, *Learning to Heal: The Development of American Medical Education* (New York: Basic Books, 1985).

    5. James Harvey Young, *The Toadstool Millionaires: A Social History of Patent Medicines in America before Federal Regulation* (Princeton, N.J.: Princeton University Press, 1961), chap. 9, and passim.

    6. Young, *The Toadstool Millionaires*, esp. chap. 10; Joseph F. Spillane, *Cocaine: From Medical Marvel to Modern Menace in the United States, 1884–1920* (Baltimore, Md.: Johns Hopkins University Press, 2000).

    7. Young, *The Toadstool Millionaires*, chap. 10; Harry Marks, *The Progress of Experiment: Science and Therapeutic Reform in the United States, 1900–1990* (Cambridge: Cambridge University Press, 1997), chap. 1; Peter Temin, *Taking Your Medicine: Drug Regulation in the United States* (Cambridge, Mass.: Harvard University Press, 1980).

    8. James Harvey Young, *The Medical Messiahs: A Social History of Health Quackery in Twentieth Century America* (Princeton, N.J.: Princeton University Press, 1967), chap. 2; John Francis Marion, *The Fine Old House* (Philadelphia: SmithKline Corp., 1980), 76. On strychnine tonics, see Ray Sturgess, "The Magic Bottle," *Pharmaceutical Journal* 263 (1999): 1015–17, available at http://www.pharmj.com/Editorial/19991218/articles/magicbottle.html (accessed May 1, 2006). On neurasthenia, see Barbara Sicherman, "The Uses of a Diagnosis: Doctors, Patients, and Neurasthenia," *Journal of the History of Medicine and Allied Sciences* 32 (1977): 33–54; Francis G. Gosling, *Before Freud: Neurasthenia and the American Medical Community, 1870–1910* (Urbana: University of Illinois Press, 1987); Evelyn Kim, "A Brief History of Chronic Fatigue Syndrome," *JAMA* 272 (1994): 1070–71; Robert L. Martensen, "Was Neurasthenia a 'Legitimate Morbid Entity'?" *JAMA* 271 (1994): 1243; John Stea and William Fried, "Remedies for a Society's Debilities: Medicines for Neurasthenia in Victorian America," *New York State Journal of Medicine* 93 (1993): 120–27; David G. Schuster, "Neurasthenia and a Modernizing America," *JAMA* 290 (2003): 2327–28.

    9. Marks, *The Progress of Experiment*, chap. 1; Young, *The Medical Messiahs*; Young, *The Toadstool Millionaires*; John Parascandola, *The Development of Ameri-*

can Pharmacology: John J. Abel and the Shaping of a Discipline (Baltimore, Md.: Johns Hopkins University Press, 1992); Jonathan Liebenau, *Medical Science and Medical Industry: The Formation of the American Pharmaceutical Industry* (Basingstoke, U.K.: Macmillan, 1987); George Simmons, "The Commercial Domination of Therapeutics and the Movement for Reform," *JAMA* 48 (1907): 1645, discussed in Marks, *The Progress of Experiment*, 23–28.

10. For simplicity here I adopt anatomical terminology for the nervous system consistent with common usage today and in the interwar era. Then, as now, various alternative classifications of the nervous system were used, such as those where central is distinguished from autonomic rather than peripheral, and sensory-motor nerves count or do not count as parts of the central nervous system. The terminology adopted here fits with influential texts of the time, for example, Henry Gray, *Anatomy of the Human Body*, 20th ed., revised by Warren Lewis (Philadelphia: Lee & Febiger, 1918), available at http://www.bartleby.com/107 (accessed November 1, 2005), chap. 9, esp. sec. 7; this source, however, uses the term "cranial-sacral sympathetics" instead of "parasympathetics." On chemical transmission, see Walter B. Cannon, *Bodily Changes in Pain, Hunger, Fear and Rage: An Account of Recent Researches into the Function of Emotional Excitement* (New York: Appleton, 1915); Louis Goodman and Alfred Gilman, *The Pharmacological Basis of Therapeutics* (New York: Macmillan, 1941), chap. 23; and J. D. Robinson, *Mechanisms of Synaptic Transmission: Bridging the Gaps (1890–1990)* (Oxford: Oxford University Press, 2001). Elliot S. Valenstein, *The War of the Soups and Sparks: The Discovery of Neurotransmitters and the Dispute over How Nerves Communicate* (New York: Columbia University Press, 2005), provides an excellent account of the lingering resistance to chemical transmission, although in my view this author overvalues the strictly electrical camp's influence in later years, particularly outside academic neurophysiology.

11. See George Barger and Henry Dale, "Chemical Structure and Sympathomimetic Action of Amines," *Journal of Physiology* 41 (1910): 19–59, and sources cited therein. On Dale and chemical nerve transmission, see E. M. Tansey, "What's in a Name? Henry Dale and Adrenaline, 1906," *Medical History* 39 (1995): 459–76; idem, "Sir Henry Dale and Autopharmacology: The Role of Acetylcholine in Neurotransmission," *Clio Medica* 33 (1995): 181–93; Robinson, *Mechanisms of Synaptic Transmission*, chap. 3; Zenon Bacq, *Chemical Transmission of Nerve Impulses: A Historical Sketch* (Oxford: Pergamon, 1975). On sympathomimetic drugs, also see Sneader, *Drug Discovery*, 99–100. Some chemists also responded to adrenaline's commercial development by pursuing natural substitutes; see Albert Crawford, "The Use of Suprarenal Glands in the Physiological Testing of Drug Plants," *U.S. Department of Agriculture Bureau of Plant Industry Bulletin* 112 (1907): 7–29.

12. On the American drug industry between the wars, see Jonathan Liebenau, "Ethical Business: The Formation of the Pharmaceutical Industry in Britain, Germany, and the United States before 1914," *Business History* 30 (1988): 116–29; idem, *Medical Science and Medical Industry*. On academic-industry collaborations generally, see John P. Swann, *Academic Scientists and the Pharmaceutical Industry* (Baltimore, Md.: Johns Hopkins University Press, 1988); and Nicolas Rasmussen, "The Moral Economy of the Drug Company–Medical Scientist Collaboration in Interwar America," *Social Studies of Science* 34 (2004): 161–86. On insulin, see Michael Bliss, *The Discovery of Insulin* (Chicago: University of Chicago Press, 1982); and Swann, *Academic Scientists,* chap. 5, and passim. For a discussion of endocrinology and especially sex hormones as a "gold rush," see Nelly Oudshoorn, *Beyond the Natural Body: An Archaeology of the Sex Hormones* (London: Routledge, 1994), 88 (quoted is biologist Robert Frank, 1929). Abel quote is from John J. Abel, "A National Institute for Drug Research," *Journal of Industrial and Engineering Chemistry* 10 (1918): 969–70. I am grateful to Harry Marks for this citation.

13. Williams Haynes, *American Chemical Industry: Decade of New Products,* vol. 5 (New York: Van Nostrand, 1954), chap. 18; Alan Parkes, "The Rise of Reproductive Endocrinology," *Journal of Endocrinology* 34 (1966): 20–33; Jean-Paul Gaudilliere, "Better Prepared Than Synthesized: Adolf Butenandt, Schering AG and the Transformation of Sex Steroids into Drugs (1930–1946)," *Studies in History and Philosophy of Biological and Biomedical Sciences* 36 (2005): 612–44. On the sex hormones, also see George Corner, "The Early History of the Oestrogenic Hormones," *Journal of Endocrinology* 31 (1965): 3–17; Roy Greep, "The Saga and the Science of the Gonadotropins," *Journal of Endocrinology* 39 (1967): 2–9; Merriley Borell, "Organotherapy and the Emergence of Reproductive Endocrinology," *Journal of the History of Biology* 18 (1985): 1–30.

14. Gordon Alles, "Experiments on the Chemical Behavior of Insulin," master's diss., Department of Chemistry, California Institute of Technology, 1924; idem, "The Comparative Physiological Action of Some Derivatives of Guanidine," doctoral diss., Department of Chemistry, California Institute of Technology, 1926. Alles appears to have collaborated with Abel on insulin around 1924; see Anon., undated [1963] obituary draft, GAP, box 5, folder "SKF vs. Alles Documents"; Alles, "Draft Description of Piness-Alles Patent Situation," January 20, 1948, GAP, box 15, folder "Originals January 1948."

15. See K. K. Chen and C. F. Schmidt, "The Action of Ephedrine, an Alkaloid from Ma Huang," *Proceedings of the Society for Experimental Biology and Medicine* 21 (1923): 351–54; idem, "The Action and Clinical Use of Ephedrine," *JAMA* 87 (1926): 836–42; K. K. Chen, Chang-Ken Wu, and Erle Henriksen, "Relationship between the Pharmacological Action and the Chemical Constitution and Configuration of the Optical Isomers of Ephedrine and Related

Compounds," *Journal of Pharmacology and Experimental Therapeutics* 36 (1929): 363–400. Goodman and Gilman, *Pharmacological Basis of Therapeutics,* 423–35. See also Sneader, *Drug Discovery,* 100.

16. Alles to Piness, October 22, 1927, GAP, box 14, folder "Originals–1927." Alles to Lamson, January 8, 1928; Alles to Piness, February 28, 1928; Hyman Miller to Alles, February 29, 1928; and Alles to Piness, March 6, 1928, all in GAP, box 14, folder "Originals–1928." On the Harvard-Lilly collaborations, see Swann, *Academic Scientists,* chap. 5; Alles to Piness, February 24, 1928, GAP, box 14, folder "Originals–1928."

17. For animal experiments, see, for example, Alles, "Exp. #2," November 27, 1928; Alles, "Experiment 6," December 1, 1928; both in GAP, box 5, folder "SKF vs. Alles: Alles Lab Records." See also Alles [and Leake?], "Amphetamine and Related Substances," undated [mid-1950s] MS, GAP, box 5, folder "SKF vs Alles Documents," 11–14.

18. Robert Baker, "The History of Medical Ethics," in *Companion Encyclopedia of the History of Medicine,* ed. W. F. Bynum and Roy Porter, Vol. 2, 852–87 (New York: Routledge, 1993); Lawrence K. Altman, *Who Goes First? The Story of Self-Experimentation in Medicine* (Berkeley: University of California Press, 1998); Susan Lederer, *Subjected to Science: Human Experimentation in America before the Second World War* (Baltimore, Md.: Johns Hopkins University Press, 1995).

19. Alles, "B-Phenyl-isopropyl amine Action on Circulation—Man—Subcutaneous Administration," June 3, 1929; Alles, "B-Phenyl-isopropyl amine Action on Circulation—Man—Action on Respiration—Man," June 5, 1929; Alles, "Miss Waddele," June 14, 1929; all in GAP, box 5, folder "SKF vs. Alles: Alles Lab Records."

20. Alles, "Mrs. Bender," June 12, 1929; Alles, "Mr. Rubenstein," June 10, 1929; Alles, "B-Phenyl-isopropyl amine Action on Circulation—Man—Local Application," November 14, 1929; all in GAP, box 5, folder "SKF vs. Alles: Alles Lab Records." George Piness, Hyman Miller, and Gordon Alles, "Clinical Observations on Phenylethanolamine Sulfate," *JAMA* 94 (1930): 790–91. Also cf. Alles [and Leake?], "Amphetamine and Related Substances," 12–14.

21. Sean Dennis Cashman, *America in the Twenties and Thirties: The Olympian Age of Franklin Delano Roosevelt* (New York: New York University Press, 1989); David Kennedy, *Freedom from Fear: The American People in Depression and War, 1929–1945* (New York: Oxford University Press, 1999), chaps. 1,2, and passim. Alles, "Draft Description of Piness-Alles Patent Situation."

22. Alles, lab records, January–February 1930, GAP, box 5, folder "SKF vs. Alles: Alles Lab Records." Gordon A. Alles, "Salts of 1-Phenyl-2-Aminopropane," U.S. Patent 1,879,003, September 27, 1932.

23. Alles, "90 kg," "b-3,4-methylene-dioxyphenyl-isopropylamine hydrochloride," July 16, 1930, GAP, box 5, folder "SKF vs. Alles: Alles Lab Records."

24. Bruce Eisner, *Ecstasy: The MDMA Story*, 2nd ed. (Berkeley: Ronin, 1993), chap. 1.

25. Leake to Langley Porter, October 14, 1931, GAP, box 2, folder "SKF vs. Alles: Documents Received from Alles Office."

26. This arrangement seems informally to have begun in the winter of 1931–32; see Alles [and Leake?], "Amphetamine and Related Substances," 14–16. On Alles's place in the UCSF lab, see also, for example, Leake, "Contributions from the Pharmacological Laboratory of the University of California Medical School, 1932–1934," UCSF Special Collections.

27. Gordon A. Alles, "dl-Beta-Phenylisopropylamines," *Journal of the American Chemical Society* 54 (1932): 271–74; idem, "The Comparative Physiological Actions of dl-Beta-Phenylisopropylamines, I: Pressor Effect and Toxicity," *Journal of Pharmacology and Experimental Therapeutics* 47 (1933): 339–54; Gordon A. Alles and Myron Prinzmetal, "The Comparative Physiological Actions of dl-Beta-Phenylisopropylamines, II: Bronchial Effect," *Journal of Pharmacology and Experimental Therapeutics* 48 (1933): 161–74.

28. Alles [and Leake?], "Amphetamine and Related Substances," 16–17; Alles to Boyer, December 26, 1934, GAP, box 1, folder "Sale of Invention and Patent 1,879,003 on Benzedrine Salts as Medicinal Agents"; J. B. Doyle and L. E. Daniels, "Symptomatic Treatment of Narcolepsy," *JAMA* 96 (1931): 1370–72; Myron Prinzmetal and Wilfred Bloomberg, "The Use of Benzedrine for the Treatment of Narcolepsy," *JAMA* 105 (1935): 2051–54; M. Nathanson, "The Central Action of Beta-Aminopropylbenzene (Benzedrine)," *JAMA* 108 (1937): 528–31.

29. Gordon A. Alles, "Salts of 1-Phenyl-2-Aminopropane," U.S. Patent 1,879,003, September 27, 1932; L. Edeleano, "On a Few Derivatives of the Phenylmeth-Acrylic Acid and of the Phenyl-Iso-Butyric Acid," *Berichte der Deutschen-Chemischen Gesellschaft* 20 (1887): 616; Deposition of Maxy Pope Alles, November 21, 1967, in *SKF vs. Alles* records.

30. F. P. Nabenhauer, "Therapeutic Substituted Benzyl Carbinamines," U.S. Patent 1,921,424, August 8, 1933; Anon., "Nabenauer and Alles Amine Work," 1937, GAP, box 2, folder "SKF vs. Alles: Documents Requested by SKF on Discovery"; Council on Pharmacy and Chemistry, "Benzedrine," *JAMA* 101 (1933): 1315. On the presence of SKF observers at the Oregon meeting, such as Albert G. Young, see Alles to W. F. Thompson, December 12, 1942, GAP, box 2, folder "SKF vs. Alles: Documents Received from Alles Office."

31. On SKF in the 1930s, see Mahoney, *Merchants of Life*, 33–35; Marion, *This Fine Old House*, 114–30.

32. Alles to Leake, April 27, 1934, GAP, box 16, folder "Correspondence Not Listed in Card File." Francis Boyer to Alles, June 5, 1934; Alles to Boyer, June 26, 1934; Boyer to Alles, July 6, 1934; Alles to Boyer, August 1, 1934; all in GAP, box 1, folder "Sale of Invention and Patent 1,879,003 on Benzedrine Salts

as Medicinal Agents." Alles to Boyer, September 8, 1934; Boyer to Alles, September 17, 1934; Alles to Boyer, September 25, 1934; Boyer to Alles, October 22, 1934; Alles to Boyer, November 12, 1934; Boyer to Alles, December 6, 1934; Alles to Boyer, December 17, 1934 and attached contract; all in GAP, box 1, folder "Sale of Invention and Patent 1,879,003 on Benzedrine Salts as Medicinal Agents." See also Theodore Wallace memo, November 8, 1935, GAP, box 15, unlabeled folder.

Notes to Chapter 2

1. Harry Marks, *The Progress of Experiment: Science and Therapeutic Reform in the United States, 1900–1990* (Cambridge: Cambridge University Press, 1997), chap. 3; Peter Temin, *Taking Your Medicine: Drug Regulation in the United States* (Cambridge, Mass.: Harvard University Press, 1980); John Swann, "FDA and the Practice of Pharmacy: Prescription Drug Regulation before the Durham-Humphrey Amendment of 1951," *Pharmacy in History* 36 (1994): 55–70; Harry Marks, "Revisiting 'The Origins of Compulsory Drug Prescriptions,'" *American Journal of Public Health* 85 (1995): 109–15.

2. Wallace research memos of February 27, 1936; May 29, 1936; July 16, 1936; February 8, 1937; and August 3, 1937; all in GAP, box 15, unlabeled folder. W. E. Ehrich and E. B. Krumbhaar, "The Effects of Large Doses of Benzedrine Sulfate on the Albino Rat: Functional and Tissue Changes," *Annals of Internal Medicine* 10 (1937): 1874–88.

3. On Dyer's study, see Wallace memos of March 14, 1935; May 9, 1935; December 6, 1935; February 10, 1936; September 17, 1936; January 1, 1937; GAP, box 15, unlabeled folder; Thompson research memo, January 25, 1937; and Anon., June 8, 1938, in GAP, box 2, folder: "SKF vs. Alles: Documents Received from Alles Office." W. W. Dyer, "The Pressor Effects of Amphetamine ('Benzedrine') on Normal, Hypotensive, and Hypertensive Patients," *American Journal of Medical Science* 197 (1939): 103–8. On regulation, see Charles O. Jackson, *Food and Drug Legislation in the New Deal* (Princeton, N.J.: Princeton University Press, 1970); on ethics, see A. C. Ivy, "The History and Ethics of the Use of Human Subjects in Medical Experiments," *Science* 108 (1948): 1–5; Henry Beecher, "Ethics and Clinical Research," *New England Journal of Medicine* 274 (1966): 1354–60; Robert Baker, "The History of Medical Ethics," in *Companion Encyclopedia of the History of Medicine,* ed. W. F. Bynum and Roy Porter, Vol. 2, 852–87 (New York: Routledge, 1993).

4. On the interactions of drug firms and clinical researchers in the 1930s, see Nicolas Rasmussen, "The Drug Industry and Clinical Research in Interwar America: Three Types of Physician Collaborator," *Bulletin of the History of Medicine* 79 (2005): 50–80. Rein Vos, *Drugs Looking for Diseases: Innovative Drug Research and the Development of the Beta Blockers and the Calcium Antagonists* (Dor-

drecht: Kluwer, 1991). "Sixty-odd men" in Wallace memo, July 16, 1936, GAP, box 15, unlabeled folder. The multiple sclerosis researcher was the eminent neurologist Richard Brickner, Wallace memo of March 13, 1936, while colitis was being studied by the similarly eminent Grier Miller, according to Wallace memo September 17, 1936; both in GAP, box 15, unlabeled folder.

5. Wallace memo, "Possibilities on Benzedrine Sulphate," March 13, 1936, and Wallace memo, February 11, 1936, both in GAP, box 15, unlabeled folder. On "hunches," see Walton, minutes of "Research Meeting of Wednesday November 20th, 1935," November 21, 1935, GAP, box 15, unlabeled folder.

6. Wallace memos of January 7, 1936; May 29, 1936 (where a physician named Toland is said to have found no effect on dysmennorhea); December 8, 1936 (where Drs. Howard and Vaux in Phildelphia are named as dysmenorrhea trialists); and June 25, 1937: GAP, box 15, unlabeled folder. Anon., "SKF Research Program #25," December 14, 1938, GAP, box 2, folder "SKF vs. Alles: Documents Received from Alles Office." J. M. Hundley, Jr., J. C. Krantz, and J. T. Hibbets, "Dysmenorrhea—Including Clinical and Pharmacological Studies on Benzedrine Sulfate," *Medical Clinics of North America* 23 (1939): 273–93, quote at 275; see page 284 for trial results. On allergy and asthsma (Drs. Glaeser and Friedman are named as trying the drug on this condition, as well as Prinzmetal), see Webb to Alles, July 14, 1936, GAP, box 2, folder: "SKF vs. Alles: Documents Received from Alles Office"; also Wallace memos of January 7, 1936; March 13, 1936; "Possibilities on Benzedrine Sulphate," July 16, 1936; all in GAP, box 15, unlabeled folder.

7. William Sargant and J. M. Blackburn, "The Effect of Benzedrine on Intelligence Scores," *Lancet* 2 (1936): 1385–87; the Maudsley group's discovery evidently began with the idea that by increasing blood pressure the drug might increase blood flow in the brain. See George Carl and William Turner, "The Effects of Benzedrine Sulfate (Amphetamine Sulfate) on Performance in a Comprehensive Psychometric Examination,"*Journal of Psychology* 8 (1939): 165–216. A doctor employed by SKF to "work very closely with the men at the Institute to direct, insofar as possible, the general trend of the study" monitored the SKF-funded Penn psychology project; Wallace memo of June 25, 1937, GAP, box 15, unlabeled folder.

8. M. Molitch and J.P. Sullivan, "The Effect of Benzedrine Sulfate on Children Taking the New Stanford Achievement Test," *American Journal of Orthopsychiatry* 7 (1937): 519–22; M. Molitch and A. K. Eccles, "The Effect of Benzedrine Sulfate on the Intelligence Scores of Children," *American Journal of Psychology* 94 (1937): 587–90. On the placebo effect as understood in midcentury America, see Henry Beecher, "The Powerful Placebo," *JAMA* 159 (1955): 1602–6. Wallace memo, February 11, 1936, GAP, box 15, unlabeled folder. On differing opinion over when and why placebo controls and double blinding became standard in medical research, see Abraham Lilienfeld, "Ceteris Paribus: The

Evolution of the Clinical Trial," *Bulletin of the History of Medicine* 56 (1982): 1–18; Marks, *The Progress of Experiment*; Ted Kaptchuk, "Intentional Ignorance: A History of Blind Assessment and Placebo Controls," *Bulletin of the History of Medicine* 72 (1998): 389–433; Iain Chalmers, "Comparing Like with Like: Some Historical Milestones in the Evolution of Methods to Create Unbiased Comparison Groups in Therapeutic Experiments," *International Journal of Epidemiology* 30 (2001): 1170–78.

9. Charles Bradley, "The Behavior of Children Receiving Benzedrine," *American Journal of Psychiatry* 94 (1937): 577–85; Katherine Cutts and Herbert Jasper, "Effect of Benzedrine Sulfate and Phenobarbital on Behavior Problem Children with Abnormal Electroencephalograms," *Archives of Neurology and Psychiatry* 41 (1939): 1138–45; Charles Bradley and Emily Green, "Psychometric Performance of Children Receiving Amphetamine Sulfate," *American Journal of Psychiatry* 97 (1940): 388–94. For further details about Bradley and research at the Bradley Home, see Ilina Singh, "Bad Boys, Good Mothers, and the 'Miracle' of Ritalin," *Science in Context* 15 (2002): 577–603; and Elizabeth Bromley, "Stimulating a Normal Adjustment: Misbehavior, Amphetamines, and the Electroencephalogram at the Badley Home for Children," *Journal of the History of the Behavioral Sciences* 42 (2006): 379–98. Bradley's work is listed among studies other than those sponsored by SKF in Wallace, "Research Memo," August 3, 1937, GAP, box 15, unlabeled folder. M. Molitch and S. Poliakoff, "The Effect of Benzedrine Sulfate on Enuresis," *Archives of Pediatrics* 54 (1937): 499–501. Thus, authors on the history of Attention Deficit who have supposed that SKF funded his work appear to be mistaken; see Peter Conrad and Deborah Potter, "From Hyperactive Children to ADHD Adults: Observations on the Expansion of Medical Categories," *Social Problems* 47 (2000): 559–82.

10. Anon., "Efficiency of Brain Held Due to Its 'Fuel'; Cells Found Speeded Up by Synthetic Drug," *New York Times,* April 10, 1937, 36; Anon., "Pep-Pill Poisoning," *Time* 29 (May 10, 1937): 45; Editorial, "Benzedrine Sulfate 'Pep Pills,' " *JAMA* 108 (1937): 1973–74; Ivor Davies, "Discussion on Benzedrine: Uses and Abuses," *Proceedings of the Royal Society of Medicine* 38 (1938): 385–88; William Minkowsky, "The Effect of Benzedrine Sulphate on Learning," *Journal of Comparative Psychology* 28 (1940): 349–61. Wallace memo, May 18, 1937, GAP, box 15, unlabeled folder.

11. Richard Webb to Alles, March 23, 1936, GAP, box 2, folder "SKF vs. Alles: Documents Received from Alles Office." See H. Houston Merritt, "Minutes of the 431st Meeting of the Boston Society of Psychiatry and Neurology, of March 19, 1936," *Journal of Nervous and Mental Diseases* 85 (1937): 202–6.

12. Wallace memo, December 6, 1935, GAP, box 15, unlabeled folder. SKF's interest in Myerson evidently reflected his influence more than the inherent value of his work; "uncertain of worth of his clinical work, but he is a

'name,' " wrote an SKF manager a few years later; R.S. Fox memo re: "Meeting on Alles Patent Cases 7/28/42," July 30, 1942, GAP, box 15, unlabeled folder. Details of his Smith, Kline & French personal grant are unknown, but typically it would be around $1,000 per year.

13. Myerson's Rockefeller research grant averaged more than $13,000 annually from 1935 until after the Second World War. Myerson to Alan Gregg, June 18, 1935; Myerson, "Boston State Hospital—Psychiatry Annual Report March 1936–March 1937," April 1938; and Myerson, "Boston State Hospital—Psychiatry Annual Report December 1, 1937–November 30 1938," December 1939; all in RAC, RG 1.1, Ser. 200A, box 73, folder 875. Also, e-mail from Susan Irving, Rockefeller Archive Center, to author, April 23, 2004. Abraham Myerson, *The Nervous Housewife* (Boston: Little, Brown, 1920), chaps. 2–3 and passim. On Myerson's background, see Lunbeck, *The Psychiatric Persuasion: Knowledge, Gender, and Power in Modern America* (Princeton, N.J.: Princeton University Press, 1994), 32–33 and passim. On eugenics, see Daniel Kevles, *In the Name of Eugenics* (Berkeley: University of California Press, 1985); Diane B. Paul, *Controlling Human Heredity: 1865 to the Present* (Atlantic Highlands, N.J.: Humanities, 1995); Garland Allen, "The Biological Basis of Crime: An Historical and Methodological Study," *Historical Studies in the Physical and Biological Sciences* 31 (2001): 183–222.

14. Abraham Myerson, "Anhedonia," *American Journal of Psychiatry* 79 (1922): 87–103; and idem, *When Life Loses Its Zest* (Boston: Little, Brown, 1925). On the prehistory of concepts cognate to anhedonia, see German Berrios and J. M. Olivares, "The Anhedonias: A Conceptual History," *History of Psychiatry* 6 (1995): 453–70.

15. Myerson, "Anhedonia," 91; idem, *When Life Loses Its Zest*. On neurasthenia, see Barbara Sicherman, "The Uses of a Diagnosis: Doctors, Patients, and Neurasthenia," *Journal of the History of Medicine and Allied Sciences* 32 (1977): 33–54; Francis G. Gosling, *Before Freud: Neurasthenia and the American Medical Community, 1870–1910* (Urbana: University of Illinois Press, 1987); Evelyn Kim, "A Brief History of Chronic Fatigue Syndrome," *JAMA* 272 (1994): 1070–71; Robert L. Martensen, "Was Neurasthenia a 'Legitimate Morbid Entity'?" *JAMA* 271 (1994): 1243; John Stea and William Fried, "Remedies for a Society's Debilities: Medicines for Neurasthenia in Victorian America," *New York State Journal of Medicine* 93 (1993): 120–27; David G. Schuster, "Neurasthenia and a Modernizing America," *JAMA* 290 (2003): 2327–28.

16. Myerson, "Anhedonia," quotes at 91, 101); idem, *When Life Loses Its Zest*.

17. Abraham Myerson, "Effect of Benzedrine Sulfate on Mood and Fatigue in Normal and Neurotic Persons," *Archives of Neurology and Psychology* 36 (1936): 816–22, quote at 118; Anon., "Trial and Error," *Time*, September 14, 1936, 33.

18. For more on the eclectic character of early-twentieth-century American psychiatry, see Lunbeck, *The Psychiatric Persuasion,* and Jack D. Pressman, *Last Resort: Psychosurgery and the Limits of Medicine* (Cambridge: Cambridge University Press, 1998); see also John Burnham, "Jack Pressman and the Future of the History of Psychiatry," *Bulletin of the History of Medicine* 74 (2000): 778–85. On Adolf Meyer, a key founder of the American approach, see Ruth Leys, "Types of One: Adolf Meyer's Life Chart and the Representation of Individuality," *Representations* 34 (1991): 1–28. For a nice example of the ecumenical attitude toward Freud in general medicine, see Henry Christian, *The Principles and Practice of Medicine, Originally Written by the Late Sir William Osler and Revised by the Late Thomas McCrae,* 13th ed. (Boston: Appleton, 1938), 1380. See also Gerald Grob, *Mental Illness and American Society, 1875–1940* (Princeton, N.J.: Princeton University Press, 1983), although this author does not acknowledge the union of neurology and psychiatry in the interwar period; and, similarly, Mitchell Wilson, "DSM-III and the Transformation Of American Psychiatry: A History," *American Journal of Psychiatry* 150 (1993): 399–410. For the view that the conflict between the Freudians and biological psychiatrists which marked the 1960s was already under way in the 1940s, see, for instance, Edward Shorter, *A History of Psychiatry: From the Era of the Asylum to the Age of Prozac* (New York: Wiley, 1997), chaps. 6–7; also see Judith Swazey, *Chlorpromazine in Psychiatry: A Study of Therapeutic Innovation,* (Cambridge, Mass.: MIT Press, 1974). Even Joel Braslow, to whom a great historiographic debt is owed for enriching the picture of early-twentieth-century biological psychiatry, depicts drugs before chlorpromazine as mere chemical restraints; see his *Mental Ills and Bodily Cures: Psychiatric Treatment in the First Half of the Twentieth Century* (Berkeley: University of California Press, 1997), chap. 2.

19. On lobotomy, see Pressman, *Last Resort;* and on electroconvulsion, see Jonathan Sadowsky, "Beyond the Metaphor of the Pendulum: Electroconvulsive Therapy, Psychoanalysis, and the Styles of American Psychiatry," *Journal of the History of Medicine and Allied Sciences* 61 (2006): 1–25. On the impact of physical therapies in early-twentieth-century psychiatry, see Joel Braslow, "The Influence of a Biological Therapy on Physicians' Narratives and Interrogations: The Case of General Paralysis of the Insane and Malaria Fever Therapy, 1910–1950," *Bulletin of the History of Medicine* 70 (1996): 577–608; and idem, *Mental Ills and Bodily Cures.* On the still active controversy concerning qualitative distinctions between depressive neuroses and psychoses, see P. Boyce and D. Hadzi-Pavlovic, "Issues in Classification: I. Some Historical Aspects," in *Melancholia: A Disorder of Movement and Mood,* ed. G. Parker and D. Hadzi-Pavlovic, 9–19 (Cambridge: Cambridge University Press, 1996).

20. Wallace memo, "Possibilities on Benzedrine Sulphate," March 13, 1936; Wallace memo, July 16, 1936; both in GAP, box 15, unlabeled folder (A). Nathanson, "The Central Action of Beta-Aminopropylbenzene."

21. D. L. Wilbur, A. R. Maclean, and E. V. Allen, "Clinical Observations on the Effect of Benzedrine Sulfate," *Proceedings of the Staff Meetings of the Mayo Clinic* 12 (1937): 97–104; idem, "Clinical Observations on the Effect of Benzedrine Sulfate," *JAMA* 109 (1937): 549–54.

22. S. A. Peoples and E. Guttman, "Hypertension Produced with Benzedrine," Lancet 1 (1936): 1107–9; E. Guttman, "The Effect of Benzedrine on Depressive States," *Journal of Mental Science* 82 (1936): 618–25.

23. Wallace memo, January 11, 1937, GAP, box 15, unlabeled folder (A).

24. More precisely, Cannon attributed fight-or-flight to adrenergic activity, which he in turn attributed to a neurohormone he called "sympathin" since he could not prove it was actually adrenaline. See J. D. Robinson, *Mechanisms of Synaptic Transmission: Bridging the Gaps (1890–1990)* (Oxford: Oxford University Press, 2001), chap. 3; and Walter B. Cannon, *Bodily Changes in Pain, Hunger, Fear, and Rage: An Account of Recent Researches into the Function of Emotional Excitement* (New York: Appleton, 1915); idem, *The Wisdom of the Body* (New York: Norton, 1939).

25. Myerson, "Boston State Hospital—Psychiatry Annual Report December 1, 1937–November 30 1938," 1–2. See also Abraham Myerson, Julius Loman, and William Damashek, "Physiologic Effect of Benzedrine and Its Relationship to Other Drugs of the Autonomic Nervous System," *American Journal of Medical Science* 192 (1936): 560–74; Abraham Myerson, "Human Autonomic Pharmacology XII. Theories and Results of Autonomic Drug Administration," *JAMA* 110 (1938): 101–3; and idem, "The Rationale for Amphetamine (Benzedrine) Sulphate Therapy," *American Journal of Medical Science* 199 (1940): 729–37. The debate between electrical and chemical nerve transmission is recounted in Robinson, *Mechanisms of Synaptic Transmission*, chap. 3, and Elliot S. Valenstein, *The War of the Soups and Sparks: The Discovery of Neurotransmitters and the Dispute over How Nerves Communicate* (New York: Columbia University Press, 2005).

26. Wilfred Bloomberg, "Effects of Benzedrine in Altering Mental and Emotional Processes," *Proceedings of the Association for Research on Mental and Nervous Diseases* 19 (1939): 172–79, quote at 177. Of course, Myerson and his circle of neurologists went much further than neurophysiologists of the day in embracing a thoroughly chemical, rather than electrical, view of the nervous system. The pharmacology Bible of the day acknowledged the currency of these theories obliquely by pronouncing it premature to speculate on the relationship between the amphetamine's sympathomimetic action and its action in the central nervous system; see Louis Goodman and Alfred Gilman, *The Pharmacological Basis of Therapeutics* (New York: Macmillan, 1941), 437.

27. E. W. Anderson, "Further Observations on Benzedrine," *British Medical Journal* 2 (1938): 60–65; E. Guttman and W. Sargant, "Observations on Benzedrine," *British Medical Journal* 1 (1937): 1013–15; E. Davidoff and E. C.

Reifenstein, "The Stimulating Action of Benzedrine Sulfate," *JAMA* 108 (1937): 1770–76; C. L. Carlisle and C. H. Hecker, "Use of Benzedrine Sulphate in Catatonic Stupors: Case Reports," *Medical Bulletin of the Veteran's Administration* 13 (1937): 224–27; P. G. Schube et al., "The Effect of Benzedrine Sulphate on Certain Abnormal Mental States," *American Journal of Psychology* 94 (1937): 27–32.

28. Wallace memo, March 19, 1936, GAP, box 15, unlabeled folder. Council on Pharmacy and Chemistry, "Present Status of Benzedrine Sulfate," *JAMA* 109 (1937): 2064–69; Thompson, "Supplementary Research memo," October 20, 1937, GAP, box 15, unlabeled folder (A). For example, "Benzedrine Sulfate Tablets," advertisement, *California and Western Medicine* 49 (November 1939): 29a. Sales figures from "Smith, Kline & French's Answers to Defendant's Interrogatories, First Set," filed February 26, 1968, Exhibit 32, in *SKF vs. Alles* records.

29. On present-day "Disease Mongering," see Ray Moynihan, Iona Heath, and David Henry, "Selling Sickness: The Pharmaceutical Industry and Disease Mongering," *British Medical Journal* 324 (2002): 886–89 (2002); and Ray Moynihan and Alan Cassels, *Selling Sickness: How the World's Biggest Pharmaceutical Companies Are Turning Us All into Patients* (St. Leonards, Australia: Allen & Unwin, 2005). See, too, the special issue of *PLoS Medicine* 3 (April 2006).

30. "The Patient with Mild Depression," Benzedrine Sulfate advertisement, *New England Journal of Medicine* 223 (July 18, 1940): unpaginated. On hypochondria, see Myerson, *Nervous Housewife*, chap. 2.

31. On today's crisis of confidence in authorship and autonomy of commercially sponsored research, see A. Gelijins and S. Thier, "Medical Innovation and Institutional Interdependence," *JAMA* 287 (2002): 72–77; H. Stelfox et al., "Conflict of Interest in the Debate over Calcium-Channel Antagonists," *New England Journal of Medicine* 338 (1998): 101–6; M. Friedberg et al., "Evaluation of Conflict of Interest in Economic Analysis of New Drugs Used in Oncology," *JAMA* 282 (1999): 1453–57; Sheldon Krimsky, "Journal Policies on Conflict of Interest: If This Is the Therapy, What's the Disease?" *Psychotherapy and Psychosomatics* 70 (2001): 115–17; Lisa Cosgrove et al., "Financial Ties between DSM-IV Panel Members and the Pharmaceutical Industry," *Psychotherapy and Psychosomatics* 75 (2006): 154–60. On bias in published clinical trials, see Lise L. Kjaergard and Bodil Als-Nielsen, "Association between Competing Interests and Authors' Conclusions: Epidemiological Study of Randomised Clinical Trials Published in the *BMJ*," *British Medical Journal* 325 (2002): 249–52; Joel Lexchin et al., "Pharmaceutical Industry Sponsorship and Research Outcome and Quality: Systematic Review," *British Medical Journal* 326 (2003): 1167–70; Mohit Bhandari et al., "Association between Industry Funding and Statistically Significant Pro-Industry Findings in Medical and Surgical Randomized Trials," *Canadian Medical Association Journal* 170 (2004): 477–80. This is a rapidly developing field and the above citations are by no means exhaustive at

time of writing. For a nontechnical survey of the many issues, see Richard Smith, "Medical Journals are an Extension of the Marketing Arm of Pharmaceutical Companies," *PLoS Medicine* 2 (2005): 364–66; Jay Cohen, "The Medical Profession and the Culture of Corruption: Part 1," and idem, "The Medical Profession and the Culture of Corruption: Part 2," *Medication Sense E-newsletter,* January–April/May–August, available at http://www.medicationsense .com (accessed July 1, 2006). For an ethical analysis, see L. McHenry, "Ethical Issues in Psychopharmacology," *Journal of Medical Ethics* 32 (2006): 405–10.

32. For opposing views about the independence of medical researchers in the 1930s, see Rasmussen, "Drug Industry"; Marks, *The Progress of Experiment,* chaps. 1–2 and passim.

33. Wallace memos, February 7, 1935, and May 9, 1935 (respectively), GAP, box 15, unlabeled folder. Louis Sulman, "Certain Conditions in Which a Volatile Vasoconstrictor Has Proved of Particular Value—A Preliminary Report," *Medical Times* 63 (1935): 374–75.

34. Wallace memos, September 17, 1936 (quote), and January 11, 1937; both in GAP, box 15, unlabeled folder. Thompson memo to Research staff, January 25, 1937, GAP, box 2, folder "SKF vs. Alles: Documents Received from Alles Office." Dyer, "The Pressor Effects of Amphetamine."

35. Wallace memos of February 7, 1935, May 9, 1935, and July 11, 1935; all in GAP, box 15, unlabeled folder. For more on Scarano's relationship with SKF, see Rasmussen, "Drug Industry." For an exceptional example of disclosure, see Wilfred Bloomberg, "Treatment of Chronic Alcoholism with Amphetamine Sulfate," *New England Journal of Medicine* 220 (1939): 130–35, 130. Bloomberg had an academic appointment at Harvard Medical School, like Myerson, who also published in this same journal, in the same year, without disclosing his SKF funding.

36. Ella Roberts of Philadelphia Women's Hospital did a study for SKF under a contract explictly giving the firm the right to discontinue the trial on the basis of preliminary data, or to disapprove publication; C. M. N. Killen to Medical Committee, "Grant for Proposed Study of Dexam by Dr. Ella Roberts at the Woman's Hospital in Philadelphia," February 25, 1948, GAP, box 15, folder "Originals March 1948." Robert Bookhammer of Philadelphia General Hospital undertook a study under similar explicit conditions; see R. S. Fox memo to Theodore Wallace et al., "Dr Bookhammer's Study" and attached "Program," August 6, 1943, GAP, box 2, folder "SKF vs. Alles: Documents Received from Alles Office." As far as I can determine, Bookhammer's study appears, indeed, never to have been published.

37. On the apparently unpublished Diehl "cold abortion" trial, see Wallace memos, June 20, 1935, and August 3, 1937 (quote), GAP, box 15, unlabeled folder; also Rasmussen, "Drug Industry." For his studies of cold medicines both effective and ineffective, see Harold Diehl, "Medicinal Treatment of the

Common Cold," *JAMA* 101 (1933): 2042–49; idem, "Treatment of the Common Cold," *Journal of Industrial Hygiene* 17 (1935): 48–65; idem, "Studies of the Treatment of Colds," *Lancet (Minneapolis)* 56 (1936): 533–35; Harold Diehl, A. B. Barker, and D. W. Cowan, "Cold Vaccines: An Evaluation Based on a Controlled Study," *JAMA* 111 (1938): 1168–73.

38. Wallace memo, April 8, 1936; Wallace memo, November 25, 1936; Thompson memo, April 19, 1937; Wallace memo, September 20, 1937; all in GAP, box 15, unlabeled folder. Professional qualifications taken from the 1938 American Medical Association Directory, the 1941 Directory of the American College of Physicians and Surgeons, and the 1953 Directory of Medical Specialists. Kaptchuk, "Intentional Ignorance," and Marks (personal communication) rate the status of Diehl and his trial methodology highly. For further analysis of funding relationships, see Rasmussen, "Drug Industry."

39. Wallace memo, August 27, 1936, GAP, box 15, unlabeled folder.

40. Wallace memo, April 8, 1936, GAP, box 15, unlabeled folder.

41. Esther Everett Cape, *Medical Research: A Midcentury Survey*, vol. 1 (New York: American Foundation, 1955): 585.

42. Wallace memo, May 9, 1935, GAP, box 15, unlabeled folder. On the clinic and other SKF funding for Weiss, see Boyer to Weiss, October 14, 1938, and Weiss to Dean Sidney Burwell, April 4, 1939; Wallace to Weiss, January 15, 1940; Weiss to Wallace, January 16, 1940; all in Soma Weiss papers, Harvard Medical School Archives, Countway Library, box 4, folder "Smith, Kleine [*sic*], and French (1928–43)." Weiss asked SKF whether they would like an acknowledgment of their generous funding to him, but the resulting publications bear no acknowledgment, suggesting a mutual preference; Weiss to Boyer, August 14, 1940; Weiss papers, box 4, folder "Smith, Kleine [*sic*], and French (1928–43)." See Eugene Stead and Paul Kunkel, "Mechanism of the Arterial Hypertension Induced by Paredrinol (alpha-n-Dimethyl-p-Hydroxy-phenethylamine)," *Journal of Clinical Investigation* 18 (1939): 439–46; Paul Kunkel, Eugene Stead, and Soma Weiss, "Effect of Paredrinol (alpha-n-Di-methyl-p-Hydroxyphenethylamine) on Sodium Nitrite Collapse and on Clinical Shock," *Journal of Clinical Investigation* 18 (1939): 679–85; Eugene Stead and R. V. Ebert, "The Action of Paredrinol after Induction of Hemorrhage and Circulatory Collapse," *American Journal of Medical Science* 201 (1941): 396–99. The prominent review article was Soma Weiss, "Chemical Structure: Biological Action: Therapeutic Effect," *New England Journal of Medicine* 220 (1939): 906–11.

43. On the Inhaler "danger" problem, Wallace memos of May 31, 1935; December 6, 1935; December 19, 1935; September 17, 1936; January 11, 1937; August 3, 1937; September 20, 1937; all in GAP, box 15, unlabeled folder. N. A. Simpson and E. Simon, "Experimental Determination of Amount of Benzedrine in Therapeutic Dose from Benzedrine Inhaler," *American Journal of Pharmacy* 109 (1937): 343–47; A. W. Proetz, "Further Experiments in the Action of

Drugs on the Nasal Mucosa," *Archives of Otolaryngology* 30 (1939): 509–15. See advertisements quoting Proetz, e.g., "A Less Irritating Vasoconstrictor," *California and Western Medicine* 63 (September 1945): 57; and "No Appreciable Ciliary Inhibition," *California and Western Medicine* 63 (November 1945): 39. In contrast, see Eldon Boyd and W. F. Connell, "Vasoconstrictor Properties of Benzedrine and Its Use in the Relief of the Common Cold," *American Journal of Medical Science* 194 (1937): 768–72 (1937); Eldon Boyd, "The Effect of Benzedrine on Ciliary Movement," *American Journal of Medical Science,* 196 (1939): 44–46; and Sydney Waud, "The Effects of Toxic Doses of Benzyl Methyl Carbinamine (Benzedrine) in Man," *JAMA* 110 (1938): 206–7. On collaborations between drug companies and biomedical researchers in the period generally, see Nicolas Rasmussen, "The Moral Economy of the Drug Company–Medical Scientist Collaboration in Interwar America," *Social Studies of Science* 34 (2004): 161–86; and idem, "Drug Industry."

44. Council on Pharmacy, "Benzedrine Sulfate—A Warning," *JAMA* 110 (1938): 901; Edward Reifenstein and Eugene Davidoff, "The Treatment of Alcoholic Psychoses with Benzedrine Sulfate," *JAMA* 110 (1938): 1811–12. H. Wayne Morgan, *Drugs in America: A Social History, 1800–1980* (Syracuse: Syracuse University Press, 1981), chap. 7. Thompson, research minutes, "Discussion on Reports in Both Medical and Lay Press of Dangers of Benzedrine Sulfate (Addiction and Habit-formation)" April 8, 1938, GAP, box 15, unlabeled folder. The Syracuse psychiatrists were part of the SKF research collaboration network, meaning that SKF would at least have been sent prepublication drafts.

45. Wallace memo, September 17, 1936; GAP, box 15, unlabeled folder.

46. Jackson, *Food and Drug Legislation,* and Temin, *Taking Your Medicine;* Swann, "FDA and the Practice of Pharmacy"; John Swann, "The 1941 Sulfathiazole Disaster and the Birth of Good Manufacturing Practices," *Pharmacy in History* 41 (1999): 16–25. On the nascent consumer movement and the drug industry, see Arthur Kallett and F. J. Schlink, *100,000,000 Guinea Pigs: Dangers in Everyday Foods, Drugs and Cosmetics* (New York: Vanguard, 1933); and Nancy Tomes, "Merchants of Health: Medicine and Consumer Culture in the United States, 1900–1940," *Journal of American History* 88 (2001): 519–47.

47. David F. Musto, *The American Disease: Origins of Narcotic Control* (New York: Oxford University Press, 1999); Morgan, *Drugs in America;* Jill Jonnes, *Hep-Cats, Narcs, and Pipe Dreams: A History of America's Romance with Illegal Drugs* (New York: Scribner's, 1996); David T. Courtwright, *Dark Paradise: A History of Opiate Addiction in America* (Cambridge, Mass.: Harvard University Press, 2001).

48. Thompson, "Discussion on Reports in Both Medical and Lay Press of Dangers of Benzedrine Sulfate." Leake, "Drug Addiction," *California Monthly* 40 (1938): 14–15, 41–43, quote at 15. For the response to "addiction" caused by today's antidepressants, see McHenry, "Ethical Issues in Psychopharmacology."

49. Anon., memo: "SKF Research Program (#18)," June 8, 1938, GAP, box 2, folder "SKF vs. Alles: Documents Received From Alles Office"; Anon., memo: "SKF Research Program (#24)," December 6, 1938, GAP, box 2, folder "SKF vs. Alles: Documents Received from Alles Office"; A. L. Tatum and M. H. Seevers, "Theories of Drug Adddiction," *Physiological Reviews* 11 (1931): 107–21; Lawrence Kolb, "Drug Addiction as a Public Health Problem," *Scientific Monthly*, May 1939, 391–400.

50. Myerson, "The Rationale for Amphetamine Sulphate Therapy"; Goodman and Gilman, *The Pharmacological Basis of Therapeutics*, 445; Lester Grinspoon and Peter Hedblom, *The Speed Culture: Amphetamine Use and Abuse in America* (Cambridge, Mass.: Harvard University Press, 1975), 22; Chauncey Leake, *The Amphetamines: Their Actions and Uses* (Springfield, Ill.: C. Thomas, 1958), chap. 7.

51. Sidney Friedenberg, "Addiction to Amphetamine Sulfate," *JAMA* 114 (1940): 956–57. Anon., "SKF Research Program (#24)." On the use of new drugs to reduce opiate withdrawal, see Caroline Jean Acker, *Creating the American: Addiction Research in the Classic Era of Narcotic Control* (Baltimore, Md.: Johns Hopkins University Press, 2002), chap. 3.

52. Lowell Smith, "Collapse with Death Following the Use of Benzedrine Sulfate," *JAMA* 113 (1939): 1022–23. For an authoritative version of the view that antidepressants were not just uninteresting to the pharmaceutical industry before the 1960s but actually inconceivable until the late 1950s, see David Healy, *The Antidepressant Era* (Cambridge, Mass.: Harvard University Press, 1996), chap. 2 and passim. Amphetamine is decribed as having antidepressant action in Anon., "Logical Therapy in the Menopause," Benzebar pamphlet, 1949, GAP, box 2, folder "Piness vs. Alles: Documents to be Returned."

53. Myerson, Loman, and Damashek, "Physiologic Effect of Benzedrine"; A. Myerson, Julius Loman, Max Rinkel, and Mark Lesses, "The Effect of Amphetamine (Benzedrine) Sulfate and Paredrine Hydrobromide on Sodium Amytal Narcosis," *New England Journal of Medicine* 221 (1939): 1015–19; A. Myerson, "The Reciprocal Pharmacologic Effects of Amphetamine (Benzedrine) Sulfate and the Barbiturates," *New England Journal of Medicine* 221 (1939): 561–64; Myerson, "The Rationale for Amphetamine Sulphate Therapy." Anon., "Research Meeting 8/7/42 #54," August 11, 1942, GAP, box 2, folder: "SKF vs. Alles: Documents Received from Alles Office."

54. Thompson to Alles, February 24, 1939; Alles, "Alles experiments with d and l a-methylphenethylamine and its salts," undated [1939]; both in GAP, box 2, folder "SKF vs. Alles: Documents Received from Alles Office.' Myron Prinzmetal and Gordon Alles, "The Central Nervous System Stimulant Effects of Dextroamphetamine," *Proceedings of the Society of Experimental Biology and Medicine* 42 (1939): 206–7.

Notes to Chapter 3

1. Robert M. Kennedy, *The German Campaign in Poland, 1939,* Department of the Army Pamphlet No. 20-255 (Washington, D.C.: Department of the Army, 1956) (http://www.ibiblio.org/hyperwar/USA/DAP-Poland/index .html; accessed December 7, 2006); L. F. Ellis, *The War in France and Flanders, 1939–1940* (London: HMSO, 1954) (http://www.ibiblio.org/hyperwar/UN/ UK/UK-NWE-Flanders/index.html; accessed December 7, 2006); Gerhard Weinberg, *A World at Arms* (Cambridge: Cambridge University Press, 1994), chap. 2–3. Newspaper quoted in William Sargant, *The Unquiet Mind: The Autobiography of a Physician in Psychological Medicine* (Boston: Little, Brown, 1967), 45–47.

2. Peter Steinkamp, "Pervitin Testing, Use and Misuse in the German Wehrmacht," in *Man, Medicine, and the State: The Human Body as an Object of Government Sponsored Medical Research in the 20th Century,* ed. Wolfgang Eckart, 61–71 (Stuttgart: Franz Steiner Verlag, 2006).

3. Steinkamp, "Pervitin Testing"; Wolf Kemper, "Pervitin—Die Endsieg-Droge," in *Nazis on Speed: Drogen im Dritten Reich,* ed. Werner Pieper, 122–33 (Lohrbach: Gruene Kraft, 2003); Hartmut Noeldeke, "Einsatz von Leistungssteigernden Medikamenten," in Pieper, *Nazis on Speed,* 134–42; Otto Graf, "Increase of Efficiency by Means of Pharmaceutics," in *German Aviation Medicine, World War II,* vol. 2. Prepared under the Auspices of the Surgeon General, U.S. Air Force (Washington, D.C.: Department of the Air Force, 1950), 1080–1103.

4. Steinkamp, "Pervitin Testing"; Anon., "Crank in Combat" (http:// speed-zonee.tripod.com/M4/Cases.html, accessed March 8, 2004).

5. The American scientists studying possible use of amphetamine knew of the German problems with methamphetamine. See, for instance, A. C. Ivy and F. R. Goetzl, "A Review of the Literature on Pervitin or Desoxyephedrine," Report #3, undated [1941?], NAS Archives, Abstracts and Reports, Subcommittee on Clinical Investigation; Robert S. Bigelow, "Benzedrine, Possible Operational Uses of in Navy and Marine Corps," Report #183, July 7, 1943, NAS Archives, folder "CAM Special Reports," Committee on Aviation Medicine files (hereafter, CAM).

6. The medical and historical literature on traumatic war neuroses is far too great to cite here. Secondary sources that I found particularly useful include Albert Cowdry, *Fighting for Life: American Military Medicine in World War II* (New York: Free Press, 1994), chap. 7; John Talbott, "Soldiers, Psychiatrists, and Combat Trauma," *Journal of Interdisciplinary History* 27 (1997): 437–54; Ben Shephard, *A War of Nerves: Soldiers and Psychiatrists in the Twentieth Century* (Cambridge, Mass.: Harvard University Press, 2001); Paula Schnurr, "PTSD

and Combat-Related Psychiatric Symptoms in Older Veterans," *PTSD Research Quarterly* 2, no. 1 (1991): 1–6. Thanks also to Hans Pols for occasional discussions of the subject.

7. C. N. Baganz, "The Importance of a Proper Psychiatric Survey in the Enrollment of the Personnel of Military Forces," *Military Surgeon* 86 (1940): 471–77; W. C. Porter, "The Military Psychiatrist at Work," *American Journal of Psychiatry* 98 (1941): 317–23; K. M. Bowan, "Psychiatric Examination in the Armed Forces," *War Medicine* 1 (1941): 213–18; William C. Menninger, "Condensed Neuropsychiatric Examination for Use by Selective Service Boards," *War Medicine* 1 (1941): 843–53; Ivan Berlein and Raymond Waggoner, "Selection and Induction," in *Neuropsychiatry in World War II*, vol. 1, ed. A. J. Glass, R. J. Bernucci, and R. S. Anderson, 153–91 (Washington, D.C.: Department of the Army, 1966); Robert Cardona and Elspeth C. Ritchie "Psychological Screening Recruits Prior to the U.S. Military," in *Recruit Medicine*, ed. B. L. DeKoning (Washington D.C.: Department of the Army, 2006) (available at http://bordeninstitute.army.mil/published_volumes/recruit_medicine/RM-ch16.pdf, accessed July 16, 2007), 297–309. On British military psychiatry, see Mark Harrison, *Medicine and Victory* (Oxford: Oxford University Press, 2007), 120–26, 170–83, and passim.

8. Roy Grinker et al., "A Study of Psychological Predisposition to the Development of Operational Fatigue. I. In Officer Flying Personnel," *American Journal of Orthopsychiatry* 16 (1946): 191–206, quote on 191; Spiegel quoted in David R. Jones, "The Macy Reports: Combat Fatigue in World War II Fliers," *Aviation, Space and Environmental Medicine* 58 (1987): 807–11; D. W. Hastings, D. G. Wright, and B. C. Glueck, *Psychiatric Experiences of the Eighth Air Force* (New York: Josiah Macy Jr. Foundation, 1944), 6.

9. Abraham Kardiner, *The Traumatic Neuroses of War* (Washington, D.C.: National Research Council, 1941), quote at 116. Abraham Kardiner and Herbert Spiegel, *War Stress and Neurotic Illness*, 2nd ed. (New York: Hoeber, 1947). For more background on Kardiner's insistence, despite his deeply Freudian perspective, on the neuro-endocrine basis of war neurosis see Talbott, "Soldiers, Psychiatrists, and Combat Trauma," and Allan Young, "Our Traumatic Neurosis and Its Brain," *Science in Context*, 14 (2001): 661–83. For the neuro-endocrine view of combat fatigue as related to both depression and the 'fight-or-flight' reaction among psychiatrists and medics at the front, see Roy Laver Swank, "Combat Exhaustion," *Journal of Nervous and Mental Diseases* 109 (1949): 475–508; Hastings, Wright, and Glueck, *Psychiatric Experiences of the Eighth Air Force*; David Wright, *Notes on Men and Groups Under Stress in Combat* (New York: Josiah Macy Jr. Foundation, 1945), esp. 9–10; Roy Grinker and John Spiegel, "Brief Psychotherapy in War Neuroses," *Psychosomatic Medicine* 6 (1944): 123–31; Dean Andersen, *Praise the Lord and Pass the Penicillin: Memoir of a Combat Medic in the Pacific in World War II* (Jefferson, N.C.: McFarland,

2003), 143, 169. The esteemed historian of military medicine Albert Cowdry (in *Fighting for Life,* 136), unconsciously adopts the "fight or flight" concept of the medical men he studied, illustrating the pervasiveness of the neuro-endocrinological concept in psychiatric thinking about war neurosis at the time.

10. Shephard, *War Of Nerves,* 224.

11. Julius Schreiber, "Morale Aspects of Military Mental Hygiene," *Diseases of the Nervous System* 4 (1943): 197–201; Herbert Spiegel, "Psychiatric Observations in the Tunisian Campaign," *American Journal of Orthopsychiatry* 14 (1944): 381–85.

12. Alfred Price, *Blitz on Britain 1939–45,* rev. ed. (Stroud, Gloucestershire: Sutton, 2000); Peter Townsend, *Duel of Eagles* (New York: Simon and Schuster, 1970), chap. 25 and passim, captures the atmosphere among Fighter Command airmen well. Given that the RAF's caffeine "wakey-wakey" tablets stirred complaints because they prevented a good night's sleep, it seems doubtful that amphetamine would have been popular in Fighter Command during the Battle of Britain. See Flying Personnel Research Committee (hereafter, FPRC), "Minutes of 11th meeting," June 28, 1940, 4, UKNA, AIR 57/41.

13. See FPRC, "Minutes," esp. 11th meeting of June 28, 1940, and 13th meeting of November 9, 1940, UKNA, AIR 57/40 and AIR 57/41. "Note by Sir Charles Wilson. Use of Benzedrine," undated, PREM 3/103/2, and RAMC Intelligence Officer, "Drugging and Doping of War Fliers," [May? 1942], UKNA, FD1/6380.

14. RAMC Intelligence Officer, "Drugging and Doping of War Fliers"; Ove Bøje, "Doping: A Study of the Means Employed to Raise the Level of Performance in Sport," *Bulletin of the World Health Organization* 8 (1939): 439–69.

15. D. R. Davis, "The Use of Benzedrine in Normal Subjects," [January 1941?], FPRC 234; D. R. Davis, "Investigation into the Psychological Effects of Benzedrine on Normal Adults," January 1941, FPRC 237; both in UKNA, AIR 57/3.

16. R. H. Winfield, "Report on the Factors Influencing the Onset and Production of Fatigue in Catalina Flying Boat Crews," August 18, 1941, FPRC 355, UKNA, AIR 57/6.

17. On Winfield, see T. M. Gibson and M. H. Harrison, *Into Thin Air: A History of Aviation Medicine in the RAF* (London: Robert Hale, 1984), 69–73 and passim.

18. R. H. Winfield, "The Use of Benzedrine to Overcome Fatigue in Operational Flights in Coastal Command," October 1941, FPRC 361, UKNA, AIR 57/6. Also see FPRC, "Minutes," April 6, 1941, 6; and August 20, 1941, 9–10, UKNA, AIR 57/42.

19. Charles Stephenson, "Minutes of the Committee on Medical Research," September 1941, 40, ANRP, box 12, folder 26.

20. Air Commodore H. E. Whittington, "Minutes of 18th FPRC Meeting," April 6, 1941, 2, UKNA, AIR 57/42. On the adrenal steroids as performance

enhancers in World War II, see Nicolas Rasmussen, "Steroids in Arms: Science, Government, Industry, and the Hormones of the Adrenal Cortex in the United States, 1930–1950," *Medical History* 46 (2002): 299–324. On the RAF's bombing campaign, see Max Hastings, *Bomber Command* (New York: Dial, 1979).

21. Flight Lieutenant W. K. Stewart, "Influence of Drugs on the Ability to Withstand Centrifugal Force," FPRC 338, AIR 57/6; "Minutes of 18th FPRC Meeting," April 6, 1941, 6, UKNA, AIR 57/42.

22. R. C. Browne, "The Influence of Oxygen Deficiency and Drugs on Flying the Link Trainer" [1941–42], FPRC 285, AIR 57/4; J. Argyll Campbell, "Effect of Drugs in Increasing Resistance to Oxygen Want," 1940, FPRC 141, AIR 57/1–2; D. Russell Davis, "The Use of Benzedrine in Normal Subjects," FPRC 234; and idem, "Investigation of the Psychological Effects of Benzedrine on Normal Adults," FPRC 237, UKNA, AIR 57/3. These studies by Davis are presumably those referred to as planned for January 1941 at Farnborough, in the minutes of 14th FPRC meeting, November 12, 1940, 6, UKNA, AIR 57/41. Browne's study, based on its file number, was probably completed in March.

23. In FPRC minutes, Winfield is first noted as studying the use of Methedrine in Bomber crews in August 1941 (Minutes of 20th meeting, August 20, 1941, 9–10, AIR 57/42). He may not yet have actually begun on that date. Winfield's raid on the Renault plant near Paris must have been that of March 3–4, 1942, and the "daylight attack on Lubeck" must have been the one conducted through cloud cover on July 17, 1942, unless it was the March 1942 incendiary attack on Lubeck, conducted in very bright moonlight and illuminated by firestorm. I thank Bob Baxter for his help with this problem, and highly recommend his Web site, http://www.bomber-command.info. See also Martin Middlebrook and Chris Everitt, *The Bomber Command War Diaries: An Operational Reference Book, 1939–1945* (New York: Viking, 1985), and Rob Davis's Web site, www.blueyonder.co.uk.

24. Winfield, "Use of Benzedrine to Overcome Fatigue on Operational Flights in Bomber Command," [mid 1942?], FPRC 493, UKNA, AIR 57/9.

25. Ibid.; Anon., "Minutes of 28th FPRC meeting," November 26, 1942, UKNA, AIR 57/42.

26. Roland Winfield, *The Sky Belongs to Them* (London: William Kimber, 1976), 122ff.

27. For evidence of Winfield's enduring influence, see Dan Wheeler, ed., *Warfighter Endurance Management: A Guide for the Air Force Community* (U.S. Air Force School of Aerospace Medicine, undated [2003?]); available at www.brooks.af.mil/web/enhance/cope/files/Warfighter%20Endurance%20 Management.pdf (accessed March 20, 2004).

28. Anon., "Minutes of 28th FPRC meeting." A. N. Richards to Col. James Simmons, March 16, 1942, ANRP, box 12, folder 6 ("CMR outgoing 1942–43").

Also Paul K. Smith memo, "Trip to Philadelphia," November 21, 1941, NAS, RG 341, box 123, folder "Benzedrine: AML Reports." It is not clear if British Benzedrine shipments consisted of medically standard 10mg or smaller 5 mg tablets typically dispensed by the Allied military services.

29. FPRC, Minutes of 20th Meeting, August 20, 1941, 9–10; and Minutes of 28th Meeting, November 26, 1942, 6–7, AIR 57/42; Churchill to Ismay, March 24, 1941, and Churchill to Ismay, "What about flying out some of this for the storm troops of MANDIBLES," March 29, 1941, UKNA, PREM 3/103/2.

30. Subcommittee on Analeptic Substances, Minutes of 1st Meeting, August 18, 1941; E. A. Carmichael to A. Landsborough Thomson, September 23, 1941; and Subcommittee on Analeptic Substances, Minutes of 3rd Meeting, October 21, 1941—all in UKNA, FD1/6380.

31. Subcommittee on Analeptic Substances, Minutes of 5th Meeting, February 28, 1942; D. P. Cuthbertson, "Summary of Tentative Conclusions Based on 42 Ergometer Studies on Six Army Subjects," May 12, 1942; Subcommittee on Analeptic Substances, Minutes of 6th Meeting, June 12, 1942; W. C. Wilson, "Trials of Analeptics," October 12, 1942; E. L. Davies (& W. Somerville), "The Effect of Benzedrine (Amphetamine) Sulphate on Marked Fatigue in Trained Troops," December 16, 1942. All in UKNA, FD1/6380.

32. E. Lloyd Davis (with Major W. Somerville, RAMC), "The Effect of Benzedrine (Amphetamine) Sulphate in Preventing Mental Fatigue in Officers Engaged in Staff Work," February 4, 1943, UKNA, FD1/6380.

33. Rick Atkinson, *An Army at Dawn: The War in Africa, 1942–1943* (New York: Henry Holt, 2002), 419 and passim; Jon Latimer, *Alamein* (Cambridge, Mass.: Harvard University Press, 2002), chap. 14.

34. A. M. Lester, "A Comparative Test of the Action and Relative Merits of Benzedrine and Pervitin," October 1942; and A. L. Chute, "The Action of Benzedrine on Fatigue," October 11, 1942—both in UKNA, FD1/6380. Also, [Anon.], "The Use of Benzedrine in War Operations," July 20, 1943, GAP, box 12, folder "The Tactical Importance of Benzedrine Sulfate." For official acknowledgment of the drug's use at Alamein, see Brigadier Q. V. B. Wallace, "The Battle of Alamein and the Campaign in Libya," *Inter-Allied Conferences on War Medicine: Active Operations, June 1943* (London: Staples, 1947), 312–19.

35. P. Jory, "Appendix B to O.R.G. Report No. 78 dated December 1942, Benzedrine," December 1942, UKNA, WO 203/691.

36. This account of the 24th Armoured Brigade at Alamein is taken from Sebastian Ritchie, *Our Man in Yugoslavia* (London: Frank Cass, 2004), chap. 1.

37. Ibid. Also see Ronald Walker, *Alam Halfa and Alamein* (Wellington: Historical Publications Branch [NZ Government], 1967), 3432–44; and Latimer, *Alamein*, 209–11.

38. F. A. E. Crew memo to E. A. Carmichael, January 25, 1944, UKNA, FD1/6380; P. Jory, "Appendix B to O.R.G. Report No. 78."

39. [Anon.], "Notes on the Use of Benzedrine in War Operations," attached to H. J. Bensted memo, December 23, 1942, UKNA, WO 222/9.

40. Body Protection Committee, Minutes of 19th Meeting, November 27, 1942, UKNA, FD1/5292. At least three million Benzedrine tablets were supplied by early 1942, according to sources: A. N. Richards to Col. James Simmons, March 16, 1942, ANRP, box 12, folder 6 (CMR outgoing 1942–43); cf. CAM Report #38, January 26, 1942, NAS. A higher 1941 figure of six million comes from Paul K. Smith memo, "Trip to Philadelphia," November 21, 1941, NAS, RG 341, box 123, folder "Benzedrine: AML Reports." W. R. Bett, L. H. Howells, and A. D. Macdonald report a total of seventy-two million tablets consumed by the U.K. military during the war (*Amphetamine in Clinical Medicine: Actions and Uses* [Edinburgh: Livingstone, 1955], 4). Beyond the RAF and the Eighth Army (who, between them, probably used the bulk of it) I have been unable to find details on how the services used the drug or on how much each service used.

41. [Anon.], "Notes on the Prevention of Fatigue in Flying Personnel," Air Ministry, June 1943 (reprinted September 1943), UKNA, AIR 57/10. Also see F. H. K. Green and Gordon Clovell, *History of the Second World War: Medical Research* (London: HMSO, 1953), 21–22, 38. On the declining enthusiasm toward Benzedrine in higher circles as the war went on, see D. Russell Davis, "Psychomotor Effects of Analeptics and Their Relation to 'Fatigue' Phenomena in Air-Crew," *British Medical Bulletin* 5 (1947): 43–45.

42. "Letter of Dr. Keys," August 1, 1940, Subcommittee on Clinical Investigation (hereafter, SCI) Bulletin, entry of August 14, 1940, NAS, Series 5, 10–11. See The Quartermaster School, "The History of Rations," Conference Notes Prepared for the Quartermaster General, January 1949, The Quartermaster Foundation, http://www.qmfound.com/history_of_rations.htm (accessed May 19, 2006); Gerald Peterson and Sam Kimpton, "World War Two Ration History," 2001 (http://www.ww2rationtechnologies.com/History.html, accessed December 7 2006); Patricia Sullivan, "Ancel Keys, K Ration Creator, Dies," *Washington Post*, November 24, 2004, A01.

43. Extracts from Ivy report of September 6, 1940, SCI Bulletin, NAS, Series 5, 48–49.

44. A. C. Ivy and L. R. Krasno "Amphetamine (Benzedrine) Sulfate: A Review of its Pharmacology," *War Medicine* 1 (1941): 15–42.

45. D. Bruce Dill, "The Harvard Fatigue Laboratory: Its Development, Contributions, and Demise," *Circulation Research* 20, Supp. 1 (1967): 161–70, quote at 164; the quote is anonymous but is probably Henderson, in 1935. Also see Carleton B. Chapman, "The Long Reach of Harvard's Fatigue Laboratory, 1926–1947," *Perspectives in Biology and Medicine* 34 (1990): 17–33.

46. Eliot Foltz, C. J. Barborka, and A. C. Ivy, "The Influence of Benzedrine and Pervitin upon Work Output and Recovery When Rapidly Exhausting Work Is Done by Trained Subjects," Report No. 3 ("Not an O.S.R.D. Project"), undated 1941–1942; Eliot Foltz, M. J. Schiffrin, and A. C. Ivy, "The Influence of Benzedrine and Caffeine on the Performance of Rapidly Exhausting Work Is by Untrained Subjects," Report No. 4 ("Not an O.S.R.D. Project"), undated 1941–1942. Both in NAS, Series 5, folder "Reports, Subcommittee on Clinical Investigation." For Abbott's interest, see E. H. Volwiler to A. B. Hastings, March 6, 1942, recorded in CAM Bulletin, March 1942, NAS, 490.

47. Anon., "Second Survey of the CAM," January 4–26, 1942, NAS, CAM Report #38, 17. See M. J. Schiffrin, A. C. Ivy, and L. Paskind, "The Effects of Benzedrine, Pervitin, and Caffeine on the Response of Human Subjects under Conditions of 'Anoxia' Produced by the Nitrogen Dilution Technique," CAM Report #10, undated 1942; H. F. Adler, W. L. Burkhardt, and A. C. Ivy, "Detailed Report on the Effect of Benzedrine, Pervitin, and Caffeine in Maintenance of Efficiency under Ordinary Conditions and Conditions of Anoxia (Decompression Tank). A Comparison between Nitrogen Dilution and Decompression Tank Techniques," CAM Report #9, undated [1942], NAS, Series 5, CAM Special Reports. On the research at the City College of New York, see "Extracts from the Diary of the Committee on Aviation Medicine of the National Research Council of U.S.A," May 28, 1941, FPRC 330, UKNA, AIR 57/5, "Reports, Flying Personnel Research Committee." A. C. Ivy et al., "The Effect of Various Drugs on Psychomotor Performance at Ground Level and at Simulated Altitudes of 18,000 feet in a Decompression Chamber," Report #14 (OEMcmr-72, final report), February 5, 1943, NAS, Series 5, SCI, folder "Reports." This work is described as already "completed" in SCI Bulletins, November 17, 1942, NAS, Series 5, SCI, folder "Bulletins."

48. A. C. Ivy et al., "The Effect of Various Drugs on Psychomotor Performance at Ground Level and at Simulated Altitudes of 18,000 ft. 'Decompression Chamber,'" Committee on Aviation Medicine Special Reports #58, July 14, 1942, NAS, Series 5, CAM Special Reports. Compare "Second Survey of the CAM," and Ivy et al., "The Effect of Various Drugs" (OEMcmr-72 Final Report); it is noteworthy that the final report stresses differences among the drugs and neglects statistics. On judgment, also see A. C. Ivy, "What Benzedrine Is or Does" (Report #2), undated [1942?], NAS, Series 5, SCI, folder "Reports." SKF sales of Benzedrine to the government begin in Q4 1942, in the amount of $14,000, a significant but not massive amount compared to the more than $800,000 spent by the U.S. military during the war; Alles to Piness, Alles handwritten accounting sheet attachment, February 15, 1946, GAP, box 6, folder "Correspondence and Other Documents Relating to Accountings 1945–1947."

49. A. C. Ivy et al., "Pertaining to the Effect of B2B (dextroamphetamine) and of Preoxygenation plus B2B on the Incidence of "Bends" and "Incapacitating Bends and Chokes" at 40,000 ft for One Hour," CAM Report #113, December 23, 1942; H. W. Ryder et al., "An Assay of Dextro-Amphetamine for Its Protective Value in Decompression Sickness," CAM Report #112, January 28, 1943. Both in NAS, Series 5, CAM Special Reports.

50. David Dill, memo "Conference on Pilot Fatigue and Related Problems," February 24, 1941; Paul K. Smith, report and memo "Studies of the Use of Drugs in Fatigue," December 15, 1941; Paul K. Smith, report and memo "Service Tests of the Use of Drugs in Fatigue," February 25, 1942; George Mason, report and memo "Fatigue Relieving Properties of Amphetamine Derivatives," October 31, 1942. All in USNA, RG 341, entry 44, box 123, folder "Fatigue: AML Reports."

51. Army Air Forces, "Report of the Commanding General of the Army Air Forces to the Secretary of War. Section Two: Building an Air Force," dated January 4, 1944; (http://www.wpafb.af.mil/museum/history/wwii/aaf/aaf2 .1.htm, accessed March 20, 2004).

52. Office of the Air Surgeon, "Benzedrine Alert," February 1944, *Air Surgeon's Bulletin* (no pagination); Welfred Lind, "With a B-29 over Japan—A Pilot's Story," *New York Times Sunday Magazine,* March 25, 1945, 5, 37–38. John Stuart, "Army Air Leaders Want U.S. on Guard for Sudden Attack," *New York Times,* February 10, 1945, 1, 3. Don Hart, memo "Fatigue and Morale Problem of Fighter Pilots," May 28, 1945, USNA, RG 341, entry 44, box 123, folder "Fatigue: AML Reports."

53. A. C. Ivy and R. H. Seashore, "The Effects of Analeptic Drugs in Relieving Fatigue from Prolonged Military Operations. An Advance Summary," undated [1943? stamped 26 January 1946], USNA, RG 227, entry 29, box 15, folder "OEMcmr-46." Office of the Surgeon General, War Department, Circular Letter No. 58, February 23, 1943; cited in Robert Bigelow, "Benzedrine, Possible Operational Uses of in Navy and Marine Corps," CAM Report #183, July 7, 1943, NAS, Series 5, CAM Special Reports.

54. Ivy, "What Benzedrine is or Does," ('Report No. 2'); Ivy and Seashore, "The Effects of Analeptic Drugs," recreational request at 5.

55. Office of the Surgeon General, Circular Letter No. 58. Anon., "Energy in Pills," *Business Week,* January 15, 1944, 40–46.

56. E. L. Corey and A. P. Webster, "Field Study of the Effects of Benzedrine on Small Arms Firing under Conditions of Acute Fatigue," June 2, 1943, USNA, RG 341, Series 44, box 123, folder "Benzedrine: NAVY Reports."

57. Ibid., 12.

58. The bulk of the description is drawn from Joseph H. Alexander, *Across the Reef: The Marine Assault of Tarawa* (Washington: U.S. Marine Corps/ Department of Defense, 1993) (http://www.ibiblio.org/hyperwar/USMC/

USMC-C-Tarawa, accessed November 5, 2005). Also see Charles T. Gregg, *Tarawa* (New York: Stein and Day, 1984); Dick Hannah, *Tarawa: Toughest Battle in Marine Corps History* (Washington, D.C.: U.S. Camera, 1944), quote at 13.

59. The public image of the battle was largely shaped by Norman Hatch's remarkable documentary; see Peter Neushul and James D. Neushul, "With the Marines at Tarawa," *US Naval Institute Proceedings* (April 1999), 74–79. After-battle reports of McLeod and Nelson in "Second Marine Division Report on Gilbert Islands Tarawa Operation," December 23, 1943, issued as U.S. Marine Corps FMFRP 12–90 (http://www.ibiblio.org/hyperwar/USMC/rep/Tarawa/2dMarDiv-AR.html, accessed November 5, 2005), 58, 75.

60. H. Brill and T. Hirose, "The Rise and Fall of a Methamphetamine Epidemic: Japan 1945–1955," *Seminars in Psychiatry* 1 (1969): 179–94; Hemmi Takemitsu, "How We Handled the Problem of Drug Abuse in Japan," in F. Sjoqvist and M. Tottie eds., *Abuse of Central Stimulants* (Stockholm: Almqvist and Wiksell, 1969), 147–53; M. Kato, "Epidemiology of Drug Dependence in Japan," in C. J. Zarafonetis ed., *Drug Abuse: Proceedings of the International Conference* (Philadelphia: Lea and Febiger, 1972), 67–70. The Japanese military use of methamphetamine in the war led to a severe amphetamine abuse epidemic afterward. I suggest in chapter 4 that much the same occurred in the United States, but the problem was not quickly acknowledged because it was driven by oral consumption of pills and inhalers rather than injection, which carries a greater stigma.

61. D. Russell Davis, "Psychomotor Effects of Analeptics and Their Relation to 'Fatigue' Phenomena in Aircrew," *British Medical Bulletin* 5 (1947): 43–45. R. B. Paine and G. T. Hauty, "The Effects of Experimentally Induced Attitudes upon Task Proficiency," *Journal of Experimental Psychology* 47 (1954): 265–73; idem, "Factors Affecting the Endurance of Psychomotor Skill," *Journal of Aviation Medicine* 26 (1955): 382–89.

62. D. B. Dill and A. C. Ivy, "'Acute Pilot's Fatigue' A Consideration and Analysis," CAM Report #29, October 20, 1941, NRC, Numbered Reports (#4); Anon., SCI Bulletin, November 17, 1941, 181; both in SCI, NAS, Series 5. J. N. DuBarry, "The Tactical Importance of Benzedrine Sulfate for the Ground Forces," December 4, 1942, GAP, box 12, folder "The Tactical Importance of Benzedrine Sulfate." "When the Going Gets Tough," Benzedrine advertisement, *Minnesota Medicine* 27 (October 1944): 799.

63. British military Benzedrine Sulfate consumption has been reported as totaling more than seventy-two million tablets in the course of the Second World War, in W. R. Bett, Leonard Howells and A. D. MacDonald, *Amphetamine in Clinical Medicine* (Edinburgh: E. & S. Livingstone, 1955), 4. According to SKF sales accounting, the U.S. military purchased $877,000 worth of Benzedrine Sulfate tablets in the course of the war. Further research is required to determine prices paid and quantities ordered by the various US military services. Wartime sales

figures from Alles to Piness, Alles handwritten accounting sheet attachment, February 15, 1946, GAP, box 6, folder "Correspondence and Other Documents Relating to Accountings 1945–1947." For McCloy's interference on behalf of SKF, see Francis Boyer to John McCloy, July 1, 1942; C. C. Hillman to McCloy, July 3, 1942 (two letters); Hillman to McCloy, memo re. "Benzedrine Sulfate," July 4, 1942; Boyer to McCloy, July 23, 1942; D. C. McDonald, "Memorandum for Dr. Vannevar Bush," July 31, 1942; McDonald, "Memorandum for Dr. Vannevar Bush," August 1, 1942; Bush to McDonald, August 3, 1942; E. C. Andrus to McDonald, August 5, 1942. All in USNA, RG 107, entry 180, box 45, folder 441.

64. Grinspoon and Hedblom, *The Speed Culture*, 18, suppose that 1.5 million U.S. servicemen consumed a total of 160 million tablets during the war, a mere guess given that it is plainly impossible that half of these were supplied by British personnel as these authors believe, because that number exceeds the total consumption of the British military. On servicemen helping themselves to pills stored in emergency kits, veteran Merchant Marineman Jim Higman, personal communication.

65. On 1945 amphetamine tablet production by SKF and its competitors, see chapter 4 below. "Milestone in Medical History," Benzedrine Sulfate advertisement, *California and Western Medicine* 59 (August 1943): 9.

Notes to Chapter 4

1. Alles, "B-Phenyl-isopropyl amine Action on circulation—Man—Oral Administration Hyman Miller"; "B-Phenyl-isopropyl amine Action on circulation—Man—Oral Administration Maxy Pope"; "B-Phenyl-isopropyl amine Action on circulation—Man—Oral Administration Burnett Wisegarver"; "B-Phenyl-isopropyl amine Action on circulation—Man—Oral Administration Gordon Alles"—all February 30, GAP, box 5, folder "SKF vs. Alles: Alles Lab Records." Abraham Myerson, "Effect of Benzedrine Sulfate on Mood and Fatigue in Normal and Neurotic Persons," *Archives of Neurology and Psychology* 36 (1936): 816–22; Eugene Davidoff, "A Clinical Study of the Effect of Benzedrine Sulfate on Self-Absorbed Patients," *Psychiatric Quarterly* 10 (1936): 652–59; E. Davidoff and E. C. Reifenstein, "The Stimulating Action of Benzedrine Sulfate," *JAMA* 108 (1937): 1770–76; P. Solomon, R. Mitchell, and M. Prinzmetal, "The Use of Benzedrine Sulfate in Postencephalitic Parkinson's Disease," *JAMA* 108 (1937): 1765–70; M. Nathanson, "The Central Action of Beta-Aminopropylbenzene (Benzedrine)," *JAMA* 108 (1937): 528–31; Anon., "Pep-Pill Poisoning," *Time*, May 10, 1937, 45.

2. Howard Becker, "Becoming a Marihuana User," *American Journal of Sociology* 59 (1953): 235–42. E. W. Anderson, "Further Observations on Benzedrine," *British Medical Journal* 2 (1938): 60–65; S. A. Peoples and E. Gutt-

man, "Hypertension Produced with Benzedrine," *Lancet* 1 (1936): 1107–9; E. Guttman, "The Effect of Benzedrine on Depressive States," *Journal of Mental Science* 82 (1936): 618–25; Editorial, "The Confidence Drug," *Pharmaceutical Journal* 138 (1937): 539; Paul Reiter, "Erfaringer om Benzedrin," *Ugeskrift for Laeger* 99 (1937): 459–60; see the review of prewar German literature in Otto Graf, "Increase of Efficiency by Means of Pharmaceutics," in *German Aviation Medicine, World War II,* vol. 2. Prepared under the Auspices of the Surgeon General, U.S. Air Force (Washington, D.C.: Department of the Air Force, 1950), 1080–1103. On British abuse in the 1960s, see chapter 6 in this volume.

3. R. R. Monroe and H. J. Drell, "Oral Use of Stimulants Obtained from Inhalers," *JAMA* 135 (1947): 909–15.

4. Ibid., 914.

5. "Jags from Inhalers," *Newsweek,* December 15, 1947, 54.

6. Tutty Clarkin in Robert Reisner, *Bird: The Legend of Charlie Parker* (New York: Citadel Bonanza, 1962), 67–68; here Parker is said to have used inhalers before he began using heroin. Parker had certainly begun using heroin by 1937, according to Carl Woideck, *Charlie Parker: His Music and Life* (Ann Arbor: University of Michigan Press, 1998), 10. Art Pepper, *Straight Life: The Story of Art Pepper* (New York: Schirmer, 1979), 43; Gene Lees, *Leader of the Band: The Life of Woody Herman* (New York: Oxford University Press, 1995), 104.

7. Lewis MacAdams, *Birth of the Cool* (New York: Free Press, 2001), 38 and passim; John Birks Gillespie and W. Alfred Fraser, *To Be, or Not . . . to Bop* (New York: Doubleday, 1979), esp. 107–13. Ross Russell, *Bird Lives! The High Life and Hard Times of Charlie (Yardbird) Parker* (New York: Charterhouse, 1973), 263; Clarkin in Reisner, *Bird,* 68. For more sophisticated histories of bebop, see Daniel Belgrad, *The Culture of Spontaneity: Improvisation and the Arts in Postwar America* (Chicago: University of Chicago Press, 1998), chap. 8 and passim; Scott Knowles DeVeaux, *The Birth of Bebop: A Social and Musical History* (Berkeley: University of California Press, 1997).

8. John Morton Blum, *V Was for Victory: Politics and American Culture during World War II* (New York: Harcourt Brace Jovanovich, 1976), 205–6; Stuart Cosgrove, "The Zoot Suit and Style Warfare," *History Workshop* 18 (1984): 77–91; Steve Chibnall, "Whistle and Zoot: The Changing Meaning of a Suit of Clothes," *History Workshop* 19 (1985): 56–81; Eric Lott, "Double V, Double Time: Bebop's Politics of Style," *Callaloo* 36 (1988): 597–605.

9. Anon., "Be-Bop Be-Bopped," *Time,* March 25, 1946, 52; DeVeaux, *Birth of Bebop.*

10. For the Beatniks' overall attitude toward drugs, see Jill Jonnes, *Hep-Cats, Narcs and Pipe Dreams: A History of America's Romance with Illegal Drugs* (New York: Scribner's, 1996), chap. 11.

11. Jack Kerouac, *Visions of Cody* (London: Deutsch, 1973), 193–95; Barry Miles, *Jack Kerouac: King of Beats: A Portrait* (New York: Henry Holt, 1998), 90–91.

12. Barry Miles, *Ginsberg: A Biography* (London: Viking, 1990), 78–79.

13. Jack Kerouac, interview with Ted Berrigan, *Paris Review* 43 (summer 1968), available at http://www.theparisreview.com/media/4260_KEROUAC .pdf (accessed December 7, 2006); Jack Kerouac, *Safe in Heaven Dead* (Madras: Hanuman Books, 1992), 81–82, cited and discussed in Belgrad, *The Culture of Spontaneity*, chap. 9. On Kerouac's craving for spontaneity, also see Dennis McNally, *Desolate Angel: Jack Kerouac, the Beat Generation, and America* (Cambridge, Mass.: Da Capo, 2003).

14. Ann Charters, *Kerouac: A Biography* (London: Deutsch, 1974), 52; McNally, *Desolate Angel*, 84.

15. Jack Kerouac, *Selected Letters, 1940–1956*, ed. Ann Charters (New York: Viking, 1995), 101.

16. Miles, *Ginsberg*, 99–104.

17. Miles, *Jack Kerouac*, chap. 5; John Clennon Holmes, *Go: A Novel* (New York: Thunder's Mouth, 1997), 143; David Halberstam, *The Fifties* (New York: Villard Books, 1993), 298–302.

18. Charters, *Kerouac*, 131–33; McNally, *Desolate Angel*, 133–34; Miles, *Jack Kerouac*, 147–49. *On the Road* is not the only product of this method; Kerouac apparently wrote *The Subterraneans* in three days of October 1953, entirely on Benzedrine (Kerouac, *Selected Letters*, 401).

19. Jack Kerouac, *On the Road* (New York: Viking, 1958), 37.

20. Carolyn Cassady, *Off the Road: My Years with Cassady, Kerouac, and Ginsberg* (New York: Morrow, 1990), 23–24.

21. Lawrence Lipton, *The Holy Barbarians* (New York: Messner, 1957), chap. 7; Seymour Fiddle, "Circles beyond the Circumference: Some Hunches about Amphetamine Abuse," in *Amphetamine Abuse*, ed. J. R. Russo, 149, chaps. 7–9 and passim (Springfield, Ill.: Charles C. Thomas, 1968).

22. Miles, *Kerouac*, 99; Barry Miles, *William Burroughs: El Hombre Invisible* (New York: Hyperion, 1993), 44; Miles, *Ginsberg*, 77.

23. Miles, *Ginsberg*, 88–89; Miles, *Burroughs*, 47–48; John Steinbeck Jr., afterword to William Burroughs Jr., *Speed* (Woodstock, N.Y.: Overlook, 1981), 168.

24. Kerouac, *On the Road*, 142; see MacAdams, *Birth of the Cool*, 140.

25. Sydney Waud, "The Effects of Toxic Doses of Benzyl Methyl Carbinamine (Benzedrine) in Man," *JAMA* 110 (1938): 206–7. Wallace memo, May 18, 1937; W. F. Thompson memo, "Low CNS Inhalers," March 28, 1942; Miles Valentine memo, "Benzedrine Inhaler Situtation in Canada," June 11, 1943 (which identifies Camp Horden as a base where soldiers might be abusing in-

halers); all in GAP, box 15, unlabeled folder. Theodore Wallace to Alles, June 22, 1943, GAP, box 7, folder "SKF vs. Alles: Documents Requested by SKF on Disclosure."

26. Charles O. Jackson, "The Amphetamine Inhaler: A Case Study of Medical Abuse," *Journal of the History of Medicine and Allied Sciences* 26 (1971): 187–96, and idem, "Before the Drug Culture: Barbiturate/Amphetamine Use in American Society," *Clio Medica* 11 (1976): 47–58; Paul Green, "The Barbiturate Time Bomb," *American Druggist* 112 (September 1945): 76ff.; Rita H. Kleeman, "Sleeping Pills Aren't Candy," *Saturday Evening Post* 217, February 24, 1945, 17, 85; Anon., "Sleep-Pill Curbs," *Business Week,* October 20, 1945, 36. The last of these items places daily U.S. consumption of barbiturates at seven million capsules in later 1945, and the previous one places it at around six million in the beginning of 1945. For a set of "typical" cases of barbiturate abuse in California, often in conjunction with amphetamine (tablets), see Memo from "Baes and Dowdy, Inspectors" to "Secretary and Members of the Callifornia State Board of Pharmacy," undated [1944], GAP, box 12, folder "California Board of Pharmacy Benzedrine Legislation A.B. 285—1945." There was not yet a strong consensus about the addictiveness of barbiturates at the beginning of the war (see Louis Goodman and Alfred Gilman, *The Pharmacological Basis of Therapeutics* [New York: Macmillan, 1941], chap. 9, esp. 135–36), but it seems to have solidified by 1945, when these contemporary articles appeared citing the U.S. Surgeon General as a source for the dangers of the barbiturates.

27. Jackson, "The Amphetamine Inhaler"; Peter Temin, *Taking Your Medicine: Drug Regulation in the United States* (Cambridge, Mass.: Harvard University Press, 1980); John Swann, "FDA and the Practice of Pharmacy: Prescription Drug Regulation before the Durham-Humphrey Amendment of 1951," *Pharmacy in History* 36 (1994): 55–70; Harry Marks, "Revisiting 'The Origins of Compulsory Drug Prescriptions,'" *American Journal of Public Health* 85 (1995): 109–15; John Swann, "The 1941 Sulfathiazole Disaster and the Birth of Good Manufacturing Practices," *Pharmacy in History* 41 (1999): 16–25.

28. R. Sharp memo, "Meeting of 4/28/44 on Benzedrine Inhaler for California, and Cedrinol," May 2, 1944, GAP, box 15, unlabeled folder. Alles handwritten record of conversations with Boyer, May 16, 1944, and May 18, 1944; Ray Warnack to O. J. May, September 25, 1944, GAP, box 12, folder "California Board of Pharmacy Benzedrine Legislation A.B. 285—1945."

29. John A. Foley to Alles, September 6, 1944, GAP, box 2, folder "SKF vs. Alles documents received from Alles Office." [Alles?] "Brief Presented to Mr Kraft," [January 1945], GAP, box 12, folder "California Board of Pharmacy Benzedrine Legislation A.B. 285 –1945." Alles to Affleck, December 29, 1944; and Alles to O. J. May, January 7, 1945—both in GAP, box 12, folder "California Board of Pharmacy."

30. Alles to O. J. May, January 7, 1945, GAP, box 12, folder "California Board of Pharmacy." Alles to O. J. May, July 17, 1945; and O. J. May to Alles, July 23, 1945 (quote)—both in GAP, box 4, folder "1945–1946." For a review of the legislation and its interpretation in enforcement, see William Whelan, "Dangerous and Hypnotic Drug Act," *California Medicine* 94, no. 1 (1961): 12–16.

31. A. J. Affleck to Alles, April 18, 1945 (quote); M. T. Rabbitt to Thompson, June 7, 1945; R. A. Wagner memo to May, "Benzedrine Inhaler Complaint," January 22, 1947—all in GAP, box 15, unlabeled folder. Alles typed record of phone call with O. J. May, April 1948, GAP, box 12, folder "California Board of Pharmacy"; Jackson, "The Amphetamine Inhaler."

32. Linn Walsh to Alles, November 8, 1948; and Alles to Walsh, November 12, 1948—both in GAP, box 12, folder "California Board of Pharmacy." Charles O. Jackson, "The Amphetamine Democracy: Medicinal Abuse in the Popular Culture," *Southern Atlantic Quarterly* 74 (1975): 308–23, quote at 313. "New Inhaler Is Tamper Proof," *New York Times,* August 5, 1949. Hannah Lees, "Farewell to Benzedrine Benders," *Colliers Magazine,* August 13, 1949, 32, 66. Gordon Alles, U.S. Patent 1,879,003, September 27, 1932, would expire in September 1949; Fred Nabenhauer, U.S. Patent 1,921,424, August 8, 1933, would expire in August 1950. See "Proved under actual practicing conditions," Benzedrex Inhaler advertisement, *California Medicine* 72 (January 1950): 13; also "rapid decongestion –no excitation no wakefulness," Benzedrex Inhaler advertisement, *California Medicine* 75 (August 1951): 8.

33. American Medical Association, *New and Useful Drugs* (Chicago: Lipincott, 1962), 258–74; Lester Grinspoon and Peter Hedblom, "Amphetamines Reconsidered," *Saturday Review,* July 8, 1972, 40; Vonedrine Inhaler advertisement, *American Journal of Psychiatry* 101, no. 4 (January 1945): v. On the old decongestant phenylpropylmethylamine as a "designer drug" today, see Drug Enforcement Administration (USA), "Phenylpropylmethylamine in Broward County, Florida," *Microgram Bulletin* 37, no. 12 (December 2004): 1.

34. Steve Turner, *A Hard Day's Write, Revised Edition: The Stories behind Every Beatles Song* (New York: Harper, 1999), 180–81.

35. Anon, "Research Staff Meeting," #35, May 16, 1947, GAP, box 2, folder "SKF vs. Alles: Documents Received From Alles Office." Here 150 mg/day is described as optimal for weight loss, whereas a whole Benzedrex Inhaler gives a dose of 250 mg. James Ellroy, *My Dark Places: An LA Crime Memoir* (New York: Vintage, 1997), chap. 10, quote at 163–64). This passage is cited and discussed in David T. Courtwright, *Forces of Habit: Drugs and the Making of the Modern World* (Cambridge Mass.: Harvard University Press, 2003), 79–80, although without apparent awareness that the drug in question is technically not an amphetamine.

36. R. Sharp memo, "New Research Ideas," January 13, 1943, GAP, box 15.

37. R. S. Fox memo, "Meeting on Patents—4/6/42," April 8, 1942, GAP, box 15, unlabeled folder.

38. Joel Lexchin, "Intellectual Property Rights and the Canadian Pharmaceutical Marketplace: Where Do We Go from Here?" *International Journal of the Health Services* 35 (2005): 237–56; Ray Moynihan, "U.S. Drug Industry's Claims of Other Countries 'Freeloading' Are a Myth," *British Medical Journal* 330 (January 22, 2005): 165. See Joseph Stiglitz, "Trade Agreements and Health in Developing Countries," *Lancet*, January 22, 2009, and other items in on-line symposium on Trade and Health CDOI:10.1016/50140-6736(08)61799-1 DOI:10.1016/50140-6736(08)61780-8.

39. R. S. Fox memo, "Meeting on Patents—4/6/42."

40. "Control Obesity" Clark-o-Tabs advertisement; "Accepted!" Profetamine advertisement; both from druggists's magazines (full citation not found), plaintiff's exhibits in *SKF vs. Clark & Clark* records. Opinion of Judge Forman, *SKF vs. Clark & Clark*, 62 F. Supp. 971 (New Jersey 1945).

41. Opinion of Judge Forman, *SKF vs. Clark & Clark.*

42. *Smith, Kline & French Laboratories vs. Clark & Clark et al.*, No. 9048, 157 F. 2d 725 (3rd Cir. 1946). Raiser memo to May, September 27, 1949, GAP, box 16, folder "Originals March–May 1949."

43. Affidavits of Addison Ellis and J. Burton Lord, January 9, 1946, *SKF vs. Clark & Clark* records.

44. Charles Morris to Marion Thomas, November 13, 1945, plaintiff's exhibit submitted in appeals proceeding; Affidavits of Addison Ellis and J. Burton Lord, January 9, 1946; Affidavit of William Irby, December 22, 1945; Affidavit of Elmer Miller, December 31, 1945; Affidavit of Charles Morris, January 7, 1946; all in *SKF vs. Clark & Clark* records.

45. A Clark & Clark executive produced evidence purporting to show fourth quarter 1945 sales around 23 million tablets of 10 mg Profetamine and Clark-o-Tabs combined, or on average about 8 million per month. Clark & Clark employee Theodore Coggin testified that the firm's daily production capacity was only a little greater than 500,000 tablets. However Coggin's insistence on 500,000 tablets per day as firm's limit hinges on the need to dry thyroid tablets overnight. Thus Clark & Clark could have been making 500,000 each of thyroid-amphetamine and plain amphetamine tablets daily, even according to the evidence of this defense witness. Affidavit of Albert Weber, January 7, 1946; deposition of Theodore Coggin, January 7, 1946; both in *SKF vs Clark & Clark* records. That Clark & Clark production typically extended into the weekends was alleged by SKF and denied by Clark & Clark in court; weekday operations only are conservatively assumed here for purposes of calculating amphetamine production rates.

46. November 1945 sales of 10 mg Benzedrine Sulfate tablets were reported in court by SKF as slightly less than 4 million units. Quarterly account-

ing for 1945 shows Benzedrine Sulfate domestic civilian sales to be fairly stable, so there is no reason to doubt the typicality of this sales figure. At the time SKF's Dexedrine Sulfate sales volume was exceeding half of 10 mg Benzedrine Sulfate sales in dollar value. Assuming conservatively that Dexedrine was priced twice as high as Benzedrine, then SKF's rate of civilian sales of both its main brands of oral amphetamine combined in the fourth quarter of 1945 was about 5 million tablets monthly. Affidavit of O. J. May, December 27, 1945; both in *SKF vs Clark & Clark* records; Anon., undated [1950], "Sales Records of 1-phenyl-2-aminopropane in Tablets," GAP box 11, binder "SKF Accounting to Alles on Products 1936 to date."

47. In any event, taking the lowest and highest figures derivable from opposing testimony in the *SKF vs Clark & Clark* case, in late 1945 the combined monthly sales of these two largest amphetamine manufacturers must have stood between 13 million tablets (5 million from SKF and 8 million from Clark & Clark) and 55 million tablets (5 million from SKF tablets and 50 million from Clark & Clark). Estimating the Clark & Clark production rate at one million per weekday fits with most of the evidence offered by both sides, and produces a conservative 'best guess' of late 1945 sales from the two firms combined, and thus civilian domestic amphetamine consumption, of 30 million tablets per month.

48. Opinion of Judge Biggs, *Smith, Kline & French Laboratories vs Clark & Clark et al.*, 157 F. 2d 725 (3rd Cir. 1946). *Clark & Clark vs. Smith, Kline & French Laboratories*, No. 708, 329 U.S. 796; 67 Sup. Ct. 482; 91 L. Ed. 681 (1946); *Clark & Clark vs. Smith, Kline & French Laboratories*, 329 U.S. 834; 67 Sup. Ct. 622; 91 L. Ed. 706 (1947).

49. Council on Pharmacy and Chemistry, "Drugs for Obesity," *JAMA* 134 (1947): 527–29.

50. SKF's amphetamine product sales in 1945 are recorded as $2,970,000, and in 1949 as $11,760,000, according to "Smith, Kline & French's Answers to Defendant's Interrogatories, First Set," filed February 26, 1968, Exhibit 32, *SKF vs. Alles* records. These figures include a small proportion of hydroxyamphetamine sales. See above for details of the national rate of amphetamine consumption in 1945.

Notes to Chapter 5

1. Anon., "How Is a Doctor's Time Apportioned?" *Medical Marketing* (July 1944): 3–7; Christopher Callahan and German Berrios, *Reinventing Depression: A History of the Treatment of Depression in Primary Care, 1940–2004* (Oxford: Oxford University Press, 2005), chaps. 2–3. For a discussion of recent figures and trends in psychosomatic complaints, see Arthur J. Barsky and Jonathan Borus, "Somatization and Medicalization in the Era of Managed Care," *JAMA* 274 (1995): 1931–34.

2. Callahan and Berrios, *Reinventing Depression*, chaps. 2–4; John Francis Marion, *The Fine Old House* (Philadelphia: SmithKline Corp., 1980), 76–77.

3. William Menninger, "The Problem of the Neurotic Patient," *Annals of Internal Medicine* 27 (1947): 487–93; William Drayton, "Recognition and Management of the Depressed Mental State," *Pennsylvania Medical Journal* 54 (1951): 949–53; Kenneth Appel, "Presidential Address: The Present Challenge of Psychiatry," *American Journal of Psychiatry* 111 (1954): 1–12.

4. Menninger, "The Problem of the Neurotic Patient"; Drayton, "Recognition and Management of the Depressed Mental State"; Callahan and Berrios, *Reinventing Depression*. Also see below. Although barbiturates in the hands of a properly trained psychiatrist had credibility as an aid to talking therapy, as did amphetamines employed in the same way, amphetamine was considered in itself to have specific action against a neurotic condition whereas barbiturates were not.

5. See "when persistent depression settles upon the aged patient," Benzedrine Sulfate advertisement, *California and Western Medicine* 63 (September 1945): 11; "to alleviate prolonged postpartum depression," Benzedrine Sulfate advertisement, *JAMA* 130 (April 27, 1946): 49; "to combat depression associated with persistent pain," Benzedrine Sulfate advertisement, *JAMA* 133 (April 26, 1947): 35. Benzedrine sales in 1947 were $2,163,000, according to J. Shade, undated sales chart, GAP, box 2, folder "220-13k SKF vs. Alles Business Items on SKF and Drug Industry."

6. Alles to Thompson, July 22, 1938; Alles to Wallace, February 23, 1939; Thompson to Alles, February 24, 1939; [Anon.], "Patent Memo," January 11, 1940; Alles to Thompson, March 22, 1940; Thompson to Alles, September 9, 1941; Alles to Thompson, October 24, 1941—all in GAP, box 2, folder "SKF vs. Alles: Documents Received from Alles Office." Thompson to Alles, June 22, 1939, GAP, box 2, folder: "SKF vs. Alles: Documents Requested by SKF on Discovery." Fred Nabenhauer, U.S. Patents 2,276,508 and 2,276,509, March 17, 1942. On dextroamphetamine rejections, see R. S. Fox memo "Meeting on Alles Patent Cases 7/28/42," July 30, 1942, GAP, box 15, unlabeled folder; R. S. Fox memo "Meeting on Patents with Dr. Alles," May 11, 1943, GAP, box 15, folder "1943 Originals"; and R. S. Fox memo "Decision of District Court on Patentablility of Dexedrine, Pervitin and Levedrine," February 10, 1944, GAP, box 4, folder "1944."

7. "To brighten the outlook in Menstrual Dysfunction," Dexedrine Sulfate advertisement, *Psychosomatic Medicine* 8, no. 4 (July/August 1946): unpaginated; "When mild depression develops . . . ," Dexedrine Sulfate advertisement, *Psychosomatic Medicine* 8, no. 5 (September/October 1946): unpaginated.

8. Alles went so far as to regard SKF's early development strategy of Dexedrine as deliberately counterproductive; Alles to Thompson, April 3, 1951, GAP, box 2, folder "Piness vs. Alles."

9. Hyman Segal to Robert Turner, May 26, 1941, CA 67-280-IH, Defendant's Interrogatories to Plaintiff, First Set, filed October 2, 1967, Exhibit A. R. S. Fox memo re "Meeting on Alles Patent Cases 7/28/42," July 30, 1942, GAP, box 15, unlabeled folder. Among the "obesity workers" referred to in 1942, and authors of SKF-supported studies, were N. H. Colton and associates at the Endocrine Research Institute in Philadelphia, and presumably also Philip Rosenberg of Philadelphia. See P. Rosenberg, "The Further Use of Amphetamine (Benzedrine) Sulfate and Dextro-Amphetamine in the Treatment of Obesity," *Medical World* 60 (1942): 210–27; N. H. Colton et al., "The Management of Obesity with Emphasis on Appetite Control," *American Journal of Medical Science* 206 (1943): 75–86. Henry Christian, *The Principles and Practice of Medicine, Originally Written by the Late Sir William Osler and Revised by the Late Thomas McCrae*, 13th ed. (Boston: Appleton, 1938), 545. The AMA Council's cautious opinion is spelled out in the Council's *New and Nonofficial Remedies* (Chicago: American Medical Association, 1946), 281.

10. Wallace to Research Staff, "Ivy Obesity Study," February 8, 1945; Anon., "Minutes of Research meeting of 6/29/45," July 5, 1945; both in GAP, box 15, folder "Originals 1945." Stanley Harris, A. C. Ivy, and Laureen Searle, "The Mechanism of Amphetamine-Induced Loss of Weight," *JAMA* 134 (1947): 1468–75.

11. S. Charles Freed, "Psychic Factors in the Development and Treatment of Obesity," *JAMA* 133 (1947): 369–373; Walter Hamburger, "Emotional Aspects of Obesity," *Medical Clinics of North America* 35 (1951): 483–99; George Bray, "Archeology of Mind: Obesity and Psychoanalysis," *Obesity Research* 5 (1997): 153–56. Council on Pharmacy and Chemistry, "Drugs for Obesity." On life insurance and the recognition of overweight as a serious health risk, see George Bray, "Life Insurance and Overweight," *Obesity Research* 3 (1995): 97–99. "For Medically Sound Reduction of Overweight," Benzedrine advertisement, *Minnesota Medicine* 31 (March 1948): 317; "The Liver of an Overweight Patient," Dexedrine advertisement, *California Medicine* 74 (August 1951): unpaginated; "The Happy Fat Man: A Popular Misconception," Benzedrine advertisement, *JAMA* 145 (July 2, 1951): 75; "one disease that doesn't hurt," Benzedrine advertisement, *JAMA* 151 (January 3, 1953): 41.

12. J. Shade, undated [1955?] sales charts, GAP, box 2, folder "220-13k SKF vs. Alles Business Items on SKF and Drug Industry." On the search for more diet drugs, see Anon., "Research Staff Meeting #35," May 16, 1947, GAP, box 2, folder "SKF vs. Alles: Documents Received from Alles Office."

13. Charles O. Jackson, "Before the Drug Culture: Barbiturate/Amphetamine Use in American Society," *Clio Medica* 11 (1976): 47–58, 50, 53, cites FDA documents in estimating national amphetamine production in 1949 at 16,000 pounds, 1952 production at 60,000 pounds, and 1958 production at 75,000 pounds. These figures almost certainly are significant underestimates of actual

production/consumption, because the FDA surveys would inevitably miss the output of specialist diet pill makers that succeeded Clark& Clark; in any case, assuming survey methodology was consistent, they indicate proportional change in production by major firms over time. SKF's amphetamine product sales remained roughly the same in 1949 and 1952, indicating that the near-quadrupling of production was mostly attributable to competitors. On Dexamyl's standing in the best-seller list, see National Prescription Audit, *General Information Report*, 14th ed. (IMS America, 1975), 42; ibid., 15th, 16th, and 17th eds. Anon., "Sales Record of 1-Phenyl-2-Aminopropane Sulfate in Tablets," undated, GAP, box 11, folder "SKF Accounting to Alles on Products 1936 to Date." Anon., "Summary of Royalties Payable and Amounts Paid 1948–1955," undated [1955], GAP, box 2, folder "SKF vs. Alles: Documents Received from Alles Office."

14. See Dexedrine advertisements, such as "The Patient Describes His Depression," *American Journal of Psychology* 107 (June 1951): vii; "Dexedrine— The Antidepressant of Choice, and the Most Effective Drug for Control of Appetite," *American Journal of Medicine* 11 (December 1951): 28; see also Dexedrine advertisment depicting William Pitt, *California Medicine* (April 1953): unpaginated. *Dexedrine Reference Manual*, 3rd ed., 1953, College of Physicians, Philadelphia, Trade Ephemera Collection, SKF, box 1, folder 22; also "Fat People Die First," SKF brochure, circa 1955, College of Physicians, Philadelphia, Trade Ephemera Collection, SKF, box 1, folder 24.

15. Melvin Thorner, *Psychiatry in General Practice* (Philadelphia: W. B. Saunders, 1948), 551–52 and passim.

16. Abraham Myerson, Julius Loman, and William Damashek, "Physiologic Effect of Benzedrine and Its Relationship to Other Drugs of the Autonomic Nervous System," *American Journal of Medical Science* 192 (1936): 560–74; A. Myerson et al., "The Effect of Amphetamine (Benzedrine) Sulfate and Paredrine Hydrobromide on Sodium Amytal Narcosis," *New England Journal of Medicine* 221 (1939): 1015–19.

17. A. Myerson, "The Reciprocal Pharmacologic Effects of Amphetamine (Benzedrine) Sulfate and the Barbiturates," *New England Journal of Medicine* 221 (1939): 561–64.

18. Ibid.; Benjamin Cohen, Nathaniel Showstack, and Abraham Myerson, "The Synergism of Phenobarbital, Dilantin Sodium and Other Drugs in the Treatment of Instutional Epilepsy," *JAMA* 114 (1940): 480–84; Abraham Myerson, "The Rationale for Amphetamine (Benzedrine) Sulphate Therapy," *American Journal of Medical Science* 199 (1940): 729–37; Eugene Davidoff and Gerald Goodstone, "The Amphetamine-Barbiturate Therapy in Psychiatric Conditions," *Psychiatric Quarterly* 16 (1942): 541–48. In the view of SKF research managers, the combination drug was "not basically [a] sound idea and can't be got at scientifically. However, might be good commercial proposition";

[Anon], "Research Meeting 8/7/42 #54," August 11, 1942, GAP, box 2, folder "SKF vs. Alles Documents Received from Alles Office."

19. The use of sedatives to facilitate talking therapy dates from the 1930s; thanks to Edward Shorter (personal communication) for pointing this out. D. W. Hastings, D. G. Wright, and B. C. Glueck, *Psychiatric Experiences of the Eighth Air Force* (New York: Josiah Macy Jr. Foundation, 1944); Roy R. Grinker and John P. Speigel, *Men under Stress* (New York: McGraw Hill, 1945).

20. "Release the Story," Methedrine (injection) advertisement, *American Journal of Psychiatry* 108 (June 1952): v; Joseph Schein and Paul Goolker, "A Preliminary Report on the Use of d-Desoxyephedrine Hydrochloride in the Study of Psychopathology and Psychotherapy," *American Journal of Psychiatry* 107 (1951): 850–55.

21. Drayton, "Recognition and Management of the Depressed Mental State," quote at 949. See also Menninger, "The Problem of the Neurotic Patient." Surgeon General Thomas Parran was widely quoted for such assertions.

22. Jack Pressman, *Last Resort: Psychosurgery and the Limits of Medicine* (Cambridge: Cambridge University Press, 1998); Paul Boyer, *By the Bomb's Early Light: American Thought and Culture at the Dawn of the Atomic Age* (New York: Pantheon, 1985); Spencer Weart, *Nuclear Fear: A History of Images* (Cambridge, Mass.: Harvard University Press, 1998). See Gerald Grob, "Creation of the National Insitute of Mental Health," *Public Health Reports* 111 (1996): 378–81; Mike Gorman, *Every Other Bed* (Cleveland: World Publishing, 1956). Also see a synopsis of the National Mental Health Act, as well as NIMH legislative and adminstrative history, available at http://www.nimh.nih.gov/about/history.cfm (accessed May 28, 2006). The theme of the American family, menaced by divorce and delinquency, as a bulwark against communism runs throughout political discourse on mental health in the United States during the 1950s; for instance, see "Statement of Charles Schlaifer," Hearings, House Committee on Interstate and Foreign Commerce, Subcommittee on Health, re H-1420-5-D, 83rd congress, 1st session, October 8, 1953, 1049–1050; also Appel, "Presidential Address."

23. Menninger, "The Problem of the Neurotic Patient"; S. Mouchly Small, "Psychotherapeutic Orientation for the General Practitioner," *Medical Clinics of North America* (May 1948, New York number), 695–706; Meyer Brown, "The Recognition and Management of Depressed Mental States," *Illinois Medical Journal* 92 (1947): 95–98. See Callahan and Berrios, *Reinventing Depression*, chap. 2.

24. Anon., minutes of "Research Meeting December 21, 1945," December 27, 1945, minutes, Defendant's Answers to Plaintiff's Interrogatories, First Set, filed October 2, 1967, Exhibit G (first quote), *SKF vs. Alles* records; Anon., "Operating Committee—New Products" Meeting NP 28, October 5, 1950, GAP, box 16, folder "Originals July–December 1950" (second quote).

25. On consumerism in the war years and early postwar era, see John Morton Blum, *V Was for Victory: Politics and American Culture during World War II* (New York: Harcourt Brace Jovanovich, 1976), esp. chap. 3, jeweler quote at 97; see also Jeffrey Hart, *When the Going Was Good: American Life in the Fifties* (New York: Crown, 1982); Lynn Spigel, *Make Room for TV: Television and the Family Ideal in Postwar America* (Chicago: University of Chicago Press, 1992); David Halberstam, *The Fifties* (New York: Villard Books, 1993).

26. Myerson, "The Rationale for Amphetamine Sulphate Therapy"; W. Furness Thompson to Myerson, April 7, 1947, GAP, box 14, folder "Originals 1947"; R. L. Saville memo, April 23, 1947, GAP, box 2, folder "Pinness vs. Alles: Documents to be Returned" (Myerson quote); Edwin Maclean to Alles, January 22, 1948, GAP, box 15, folder "Originals January 1948"; E. A. Kimes memo, "Amphetamine with Sedative Summary," August 31, 1950, GAP, box 16, folder "Originals July–December 1950."

27. Alles to Piersol, October 20, 1947; Piersol to Alles, October 27, 1947— both in GAP, box 15, folder "Originals October–December 1947." Alles to Long, May 26, 1948, GAP, box 15, folder "Originals May 1948"; Alles to Long, November 8, 1948, Defendant's Interrogatories to Plaintiff, First Set, filed October 2, 1967, Exhibit D, *SKF vs. Alles* records. Swain to Alles, March 21, 1949, and Swain to Alles, October 17, 1949; GAP, box 4, folder "1949–1950."

28. [Anon], "Research Meeting 8/7/42" #54, August 11, 1942, GAP, box 2, folder "SKF vs. Alles: Documents Received from Alles Office"; G. Morris Piersol Jr. to Alles, October 13, 1947, GAP, box 15, folder "Originals October–December 1947."

29. Benzebar publicity mailing, "Logical Therapy in the Menopause," dated August 8, 1949, GAP, box 2, folder "Piness vs. Alles Documents to be Returned"; "Emotional Equilibrium for the Geriatric Patient," Benzebar advertisement, *American Journal of Medicine* 8 (June 1950): 16.

30. Thompson memo to Research Staff, "Research Division Committee System," April 5, 1946, GAP, box 15, unlabeled folder; [Anon.], "June 1947," "Dexam" mimeo, GAP, box 15, folder "Originals October–December 1947"; G. F. Miller memo to Operating Advisory Board re "Dexam," April 19, 1948, GAP, box 15, folder "Originals April 1948." C. M. N. Killen memo to Development Committee re "Amphetamine with Sedative ('DEXAM')," January 11, 1949, GAP, box 16, folder "Originals January–February 1949."

31. G. F. Miller memo to Operating Advisory Board, April 19, 1948, GAP, box 15, folder "Originals April 1948."

32. Memo from G. F. Miller to Longnecker re "DEXAM," April 9, 1948, GAP, box 14, folder "Originals 1946"; G. F. Miller memo to Operating Advisory Board re "Dexam," April 19, 1948, GAP, box 15, folder "Originals April 1948"; Herbert Gaskill (Penn Hosp) to Killen, October 18, 1948, GAP, box 15, folder "Originals October–November 1948"; Henry Grahn to Killen, Decem-

ber 15, 1948, GAP, box 15, folder "Originals October–November 1948"; Henry Grahn, "The Depressed Patient: Management with the Aid of a New Medication," *American Practitioner* 1 (1950): 795–97.

33. C. M. N. Killen, phone notes of conversation with Dr. Ella Roberts, November 13, 1947, GAP, box 15, folder "Originals October–December 1947." C. M. N. Killen to Ella Roberts, March 10, 1948, GAP, box 15, folder "Originals March 1948." C. M. N. Killen to Medical Committee, "Grant for Proposed Study of Dexam by Dr. Ella Roberts," February 25, 1948, GAP, box 15, folder "Originals March 1948" (quotes), and attached proposal by Roberts, "Proposed Study of the Use of #4713 (DEXAM) in the Treatment of Obesity in Diabetics and Non-Diabetics." We must keep in mind that the late 1940s were also a transitional period for relations between firms and medical scientists, as well as between firms and the government. What was once a mutually understood gentleman's arrangement was increasingly specified in writing, even if not yet in the form of a legal contract; this is helpful to the historian, who relies on written evidence.

34. C. M. N. Killen memo to Development Committee re "Amphetamine with Sedative ('DEXAM')," January 11, 1949, GAP, box 16, folder "Originals January–February 1949" (quotes).

35. Anon., "New Products Committee Meeting," March 9, 1949; GAP, box 16, folder "Originals March–May 1949." E. A. Kimes memo "Amphetamine with Sedative Summary," August 31, 1950, GAP, box 16, folder "Originals July–December 1950."

36. Raiser to May, September 27, 1949; both in GAP, box 16, folder "Originals March–May 1949."

37. Operating Committee—New Products Meeting 28, October 5, 1950; GAP, box 16, folder "Originals July–December 1950." On technology as social engineering, see Thomas Hughes, "The Seamless Web: Technology, Science, Etcetera, Etcetera," *Social Studies of Science* 16 (1986): 281–92. There is a very large literature in the history of technology on this topic.

38. Frank Boyer, "Dear Doctor" letter announcing "Dexamyl," with sample packet, undated [1950–51] (quotes), GAP, box 2, folder "Piness vs. Alles Documents to be Returned."

39. Anon., brochure, "For the Management of Everyday Mental and Emotional Distress—Dexamyl Tablets and Elixir," [circa 1951], College of Physicians Library, Philadelphia, Medical Ephemera Collection, TEC SKF, box 2, envelope 29. Ironically, some modern critics, as if nostalgic for Dexamyl, castigate the drug industry for modern antidepressants like Prozac, designed for depression without regard to the anxiety that often accompanies it. See Edward Shorter and Peter Tyrer, "Separation of Anxiety and Depressive Disorders: Blind Alley in Psychopharmacology and Classification of Disease," *British Medical Journal* 327 (2003): 158–60.

40. Henry Grahn to Killen, December 15, 1948, GAP, box 15, folder "Originals October–November 1948"; Grahn, "The Depressed Patient."

41. Ella Roberts, "The Treatment of Obesity with an Anorexigenic Drug," *Annals of Internal Medicine* 34 (1951): 1324–30. C. M. N. Killen to Medical Committee, "Grant for Proposed Study of Dexam by Dr. Ella Roberts," February 25, 1948, GAP, box 15, folder "Originals March 1948" (quotes), and attached proposal by Roberts, "Proposed Study of the Use of #4713 (DEXAM) in the Treatment of Obesity in Diabetics and Non-Diabetics." As we shall see, tolerance and return of lost weight were the reasons, in the late 1960s, that the National Academy of Sciences ultimately advised the FDA that amphetamine weight loss products were not very effective.

42. See, for example, "When Psychic Distress is the Cause of Overeating," Dexamyl advertisement, *American Journal of Medical Science* 223 (March 1952): 27; "When Obesity is an Expression of Mental and Emotional Distress," Dexamyl advertisement, *California Medicine* (May 1955): 69.

43. "5 Dexamyl Case Histories with 30 Photographs," GAP, box 16, folder "Originals 1952."

44. "A new case history with photographs" (patient C. P.), unpaginated Dexamyl advertisement, *California Medicine* (May 1953); "A Dexamyl Case History" (patient B. H.), unpaginated Dexamyl advertisement, *California Medicine* (August 1951); "A New Case History with Picture" (patient T. H.), unpaginated Dexamyl advertisement, *California Medicine* (December 1951).

45. In 1959, 2.5 percent of British prescriptions were for amphetamines, according to P. H. Connell ("Amphetamine Dependence," *Proceedings of the Royal Society of Medicine* 61 [1968]: 178–81), whereas the Newcastle studies described below found that about 3 percent of all prescriptions were for amphetamines in the study period. Details of inclusion criteria were given in neither case. As for U.S. consumption rates, in 1962, 0.9 percent of new retail prescriptions were for amphetamine "pyschostimulants," 1.9 percent for amphetamine weight loss drugs, and 0.7 percent for "non-amphetamine" weight loss drugs, adding to 3.5 percent; as with most psychotropics, about double this quantity of repeat prescriptions in all three categories were also filled (*National Prescription Audit*, College ed. [Baltimore, Md.: Gosselin, 1962], 6–15).

46. In other words, 85 –33 percent, or 52 percent, of the amphetamine patients were females with presumed psychiatric prescriptions as compared to the 15 percent of amphetamine patients who were males with presumed psychiatric prescriptions, a ratio of 3.5 to 1. L. G. Kiloh and S. Brandon, "Habituation and Addiction to Amphetamines," *British Medical Journal* 2 (1962): 40–43; S. Brandon and D. Smith, "Amphetamines in General Practice," *Journal of the College of General Practitioners* 5 (1962): 603–6.

47. Brandon and Smith, "Amphetamines in General Practice," 604. John Fry found that women accounted for up to 50 percent more consultations per

year per person than men ("Five Years of General Practice: A Study in Simple Epidemiology," *British Medical Journal* 2 [December 21, 1957]: 1453–57). To accommodate this factor, in our calculation we divide the female to male ratio of presumed psychiatric prescriptions by the ratio of office visits, obtaining 3/1.5, or 2 times as many amphetamine prescriptions per office visit for females.

48. One of these British studies found that Drinamyl (SKF's British brand name for Dexamyl) accounted for a remarkable 53 percent of all amphetamine products prescribed, whereas the other study found that the figure was 35 percent (Kiloh and Brandon, "Habituation and Addiction to Amphetamines"; Brandon and Smith, "Amphetamines in General Practice").

49. Frederick Lemere, "Treatment of Mild Depression in General Office Practice," *JAMA* 164 (1957): 516–18; John Fry, *Common Diseases: Their Nature, Incidence, and Care* (Lancaster, Pa.: Medical and Technical Publishing, 1974); C. A. H. Watts and B. M. Watts, *Psychiatry in General Practice* (London: Churchill, 1952), cited and quoted in Callahan and Berrios, *Reinventing Depression,* chap. 3. Another authoritative source recommending reassurance and sympathy for neurotic complaints is Stephen Taylor, *Good General Practice* (London: Oxford University Press, 1954), 415–23.

50. Callahan and Berrios, *Reinventing Depression.*

51. Kiloh and Brandon, "Habituation and Addiction to Amphetamines."

52. Kiloh and Brandon conclude that over 500 patients in Newcastle were addicted or habituated to amphetamines at time of writing, establishing that nearly 0.2 percent of the total population of 270,000, over one-fifth of the patients receiving amphetamines in the audit period, were dependent ("Habituation and Addiction to Amphetamines"). The annual number of patients receiving amphetamine prescriptions is the sum of these 0.2 percent dependent in the three-month audit, who may be assumed to remain on the pills throughout the year, plus the product of the remaining 0.6 percent (i.e.. 0.8 percent – 0.2 percent) and the number of times this group turns over each year, which is a function of the average duration in which they took amphetamines by prescription. Thus, assuming that those not dependent averaged four months of amphetamine therapy, one-third of a year (and also that 0.2 percent, being habituated, received the drugs throughout the year), then 2 percent of the population (3 × 0.6 percent + 0.2 percent) received an amphetamine prescription in the year. This further implies a rate of dependency around 10 percent (0.2 percent ÷ 2.0 percent) of all patients receiving amphetamine prescriptions during that year. Setting the annual prevalence of amphetamine prescription near its plausible maximum for the time, 3 percent rather than 2 percent, yields a dependency rate of 6.7 percent (0.2 percent ÷ 3.0 percent), and implies a plausible if low average duration of amphetamine therapy for those not dependent of between two and three months.

53. C. W. M. Wilson and S. Beacon, "An Investigation into the Habituating Properties of an Amphetamine-Barbiturate Mixture," *British Journal of Addiction* 60 (1964): 81–92. Kiloh and Brandon found that 53 percent of amphetamine prescriptions filled in Newcastle during their audit period were for Drinamyl ("Habituation and Addiction to Amphetamines").

54. D. Young and W. B. Scoville, "Paranoid Psychoses in Narcolepsy and Possible Danger of Benzedrine Treatment," *Medical Clinics of North America* (Boston number) (1938): 637–46.

55. Jacob Norman and John Shea, "Acute Hallucinations as a Complication of Addiction to Amphetamine Sulfate," *New England Journal of Medicine* 233 (1945): 270–71; F. A. Freyhan, "Craving for Benzedrine," *Delaware State Medical Journal* 21 (1949): 151–56; Peter Knapp, "Amphetamine and Addiction," *Journal of Nervous and Mental Diseases* 115 (1952): 406–32; A. H. Chapman, "Paranoid Psychosis Associated with Amphetamine Usage," *American Journal of Psychiatry* 111 (1954): 43–45.

56. P. H. Connell, *Amphetamine Psychosis* (London: Oxford University Press, 1958).

57. Knapp, "Amphetamine and Addiction"; Henry Grahn, "Amphetamine Addiction and Habituation," *American Practitioner* 9 (1958): 387–89.

58. Expert Committee on Addiction-Producing Drugs, Seventh Report, World Health Organisation Technical Reports series, no. 116 (1957): 9–10; see also Harris Isbell, personal communication cited in Knapp, "Amphetamine and Addiction." Expert Committee on Dependence-Producing Drugs, Fourteenth Report, World Health Organization Technical Reports series, no. 312 (1965).

59. Sidney Friedenberg, "Addiction to Amphetamine Sulfate," *JAMA* 114 (1940): 956; L. J. Hahne, "Addiction to Amphetamine (Benzedrine) Sulfate," *JAMA* 115 (1940): 1568; Freyhan, "Craving for Benzedrine"; Knapp, "Amphetamine and Addiction"; Morris Herman and Simon Nagler, "Psychoses Due to Amphetamine," *Journal of Nervous and Mental Disease* 120 (1954): 268–72; Charles Brown, "Benzedrine Habituation," *Military Surgeon* 104 (1949): 365–70.

60. "for your many patients lost in the maze of mild depression," Benzedrine advertisement, *JAMA* 144 (December 30, 1950): 15; "now, more than ever —Benzedrine Sulfate in mild depression," Benzedrine advertisment, *JAMA* 146 (August 25, 1951): 13. For a sanguine view of the medical value of the drugs in the late 1950s, see Chauncey Leake, *The Amphetamines: Their Actions and Uses* (Springfield, Ill.: C. Thomas, 1958).

61. Marion, *The Fine Old House*, 152–67; Judith Swazey, *Chlorpromazine in Psychiatry* (Cambridge, Mass.: MIT Press, 1974), chaps. 5–8.

62. Swazey, *Chlorpromazine in Psychiatry*, chaps. 6, 8. On the rise and fall of the lobotomy, see Pressman, *Last Resort*.

63. Marion, *The Fine Old House*, 170; C. M. Kline & Francis Boyer, *Smith, Kline & French Annual Report*, 1956. For annual amphetamine product sales, see "Smith, Kline & French's Answers to Defendant's Interrogatories, First Set," filed February 26, 1968, Exhibit 32, *SKF vs. Alles* records.

64. Anon., "Excerpts from Minutes of Management-Research Policy Committee Meeting #54-5," June 1, 1954, ANRP, box 16, folder 45; Dickinson Richards to A. N. Richards, August 12, 1954, ANRP, box 16, folder 22.

65. Mickey Smith, *Small Comfort: A History of the Minor Tranquilizers* (New York: Praeger, 1985); Susan Speaker, "From 'Happiness Pills' to 'National Nightmare': Changing Cultural Assessment of Minor Tranquilizers in America, 1955–1980," *Journal of the History of Medicine and Allied Sciences* 52 (1997): 338–76. On the discovery of Miltown, see Frank Berger, "Anxiety and the Discovery of the Tranquilizers," in *Discoveries in Biological Psychiatry*, ed. Frank Ayd and Barry Blackwell, 115–29 (Philadelphia: Lippincott, 1970). On the fit between minor tranquilizers and both Freudian psychiatry and the exigencies of general practice, respectively, see Jonathan Metzl, *Prozac on the Couch: Prescribing Gender in the Era of Wonder Drugs* (Durham, N.C.: Duke University Press, 2003); Callahan and Berrios, *Reinventing Depression*. However, the authors even of these worthy books mistakenly see Miltown as the "first drug for pimary care use with mild emotional disorders" (Callahan and Berios, *Reinventing Depression*, 107). For an example of psychiatric advice to general practitioners in the early 1960s, see Ronald Koegler, "Drugs, Neurosis, and the Family Physician," *California Medicine* 102, no. 1 (1965): 5–8. On the proportion of psychotropic drug prescribing in the United States attributable to primary care physicians, see Mitchell Balter and Jerome Levine, "The Nature and Extent of Psychotropic Drug Usage in the United States," *Psychopharmacology Bulletin* 5 (1969): 3–13; for the decline below 65 percent since 1980, see Mark Olfson and Gerald Klerman, "Trends in the Prescription of Psychotropic Medications: The Role of Physician Specialty," *Medical Care* 31 (1993): 559–64. I am unable to confirm that family practitioners accounted for 85 percent of psychotropic prescriptions in the 1950s, as I once stated (in "Making the First Antidepressant: Amphetamine in American Medicine, 1929–1950," *Journal of the History of Medicine and Allied Sciences* 61 [2006]: 288–323).

66. Speaker, "From 'Happiness Pills,'" 34.

67. Smith, *Small Comfort*. From about $5 million in domestic sales of Dexamyl tablets and spansules in 1953 and $7 million in 1955 (see Figure 5.8b), SKF's Dexamyl sales reached about $10 million in 1958 (based on Q1 accounting) and rose to more than $12 million in 1962 (based on Q3 accounting) through 1965 but declined sharply to $9 million in 1966. See Anon., "Smith Kline & French Laboratories, Dr Alles' Royalties on Sales . . . for the Quarter ended 3/31/58," p. 1, GAP, box 7, folder "1958–1959 Accounting"; Anon., "Smith Kline & French Laboratories, Dr Alles' Royalties on Sales . . . for the

Quarter ended September 30, 1962," p. 1, GAP, box 4, folder "220-13F-28"; M. E. Parkhurst to H. E. Morgan, "Estimated Royalties—Alles Estate," January 17, 1967, GAP, box 14, folder "Originals 1967." On Dexamyl's standing on the best-seller list in the mid-1970s, see *National Prescription Audit, General Information Report*, 14th ed. (Ambler, Pa.: IMS America, 1975), 42; ibid., 15th, 16th, and 17th eds.

Notes to Chapter 6

1. Edward Shorter, *A History of Psychiatry from the Era of the Asylum to the Age of Prozac* (New York: Wiley, 1997), chaps. 6–7, is a widely cited source stressing the benzodiazepine tranquilizers of the 1960s. For the similar notion that it was the first minor tranquilizers like Miltown that created a psychotropic culture from the mid-1950s, see Jonathan Metzl, *Prozac on the Couch: Prescribing Gender in the Era of Wonder Drugs* (Durham, N.C.: Duke University Press, 2003); and Christopher Callahan and German Berrios, *Reinventing Depression: A History of the Treatment of Depression in Primary Care 1940–2004* (Oxford: Oxford University Press, 2005), chap. 8. A more nuanced though still mistaken notion is that pharmaceutical marketing influence on psychiatric diagnosis began with the introduction of monoamine oxidase inhibitors and tricyclic antidepressants at the end of the 1950s; see David Healy, *The Antidepressant Era* (Cambridge, Mass.: Harvard University Press, 1996), 59 and passim.

2. Walter Sneader, *Drug Discovery: The Evolution of Modern Medicines* (Chichester, N.Y.: Wiley, 1985); idem, *Drug Discovery: A History* (Hoboken, N.J.: Wiley, 2005); Miles Weatherall, *In Search of a Cure: A History of the Pharmaceutical Industry* (Oxford: Oxford University Press, 1990); Philippe Pignarre, *Le grand secret de l'industrie pharmaceutique* (Paris: Éditions la Découverte, 2003); Robert Bud, *Penicillin: Triumph and Tragedy* (Oxford: Oxford University Press, 2007). For a glimpse of how marketing estimates were first formalized as a part of the new products development process, see Anon., "Sales Estimates for New Products," *Medical Marketing* (July 1945): 9, 12–15, 21. On test marketing, see Anon., "What's Needed to Give New Proprietaries & Toiletries a Chance to Succeed?" *F-D-C Reports* (May 25, 1959): 8–12.

3. Gordon Alles, "Some Relations between Chemical Structure and Physiological Action of Mescaline and Related Compounds," in *Neuropharmacology: Transactions of the Fourth Conference of September 25, 26, and 27, 1957*, ed. H. A. Abramson, 181–269, 187–88, and passim (New York: Macy Foundation, 1959). Healy, *Creation of Psychopharmacology*.

4. The other major biochemical screening method was to look for chemicals that reversed the adrenaline- and serotonin- depleting effects of reserpine on animal brain tissue. For a published description of how the drug firm CIBA used drug antagonism and conditioned behavior assays in tandem for screen-

ing new mental health drugs in 1956, see Jurg A. Schneider, "General Pharmacological and Toxicological Considerations in the Screening of Candidate Drugs for Use in Psychiatry," in *Psychopharmacology: Problems in Evaluation,* ed. Jonathan Cole and Ralph Gerard, 307–12 (Washington, D.C.: National Academy of Sciences/National Research Council, 1959). For government research, see Bernard Brodie, "Some Relations between Chemical Structure and Physiological Action of Mescaline and Related Compounds," in *Neuropharmacology: Transactions of the Third Conference of May 21, 22, and 23, 1956,* ed. H.A. Abramson, 323–41 (New York: Macy Foundation, 1957). On mental health drug discovery generally in the period, see Healy, *Creation of Psychopharmacology.*

5. Daniel Bjork, *B. F. Skinner: A Life* (New York: Basic Books, 1993); Marc Richelle, *B. F. Skinner: A Reappraisal* (Hove, U.K.: Lawrence Erlbaum, 1993); William O'Donohue and Kyle E. Ferguson, *The Psychology of B. F. Skinner* (London: Sage, 2001). On the controversial air crib and Skinner's ideas in the context of 1950s American culture, see Alexandra Rutherford, "B. F. Skinner's Technology of Behavior in American Life: From Consumer Culture to Counterculture," *Journal of the History of the Behavioral Sciences* 39 (2003): 1–23.

6. On the development and uses of the Skinner box, see Richelle, *B. F. Skinner: A Reappraisal,* chap. 3; Bjork, *B.F. Skinner: A Life,* chap. 5. B. F. Skinner and W. T. Heron, "Effects of Caffeine and Benzedrine upon Conditioning and Extinction," *Psychological Record* 1 (1937): 340–48.

7. W. K. Estes and B. F. Skinner, "Some Quantitative Properties of Anxiety," *Journal of Experimental Psychology* 29 (1941): 390–400; B. F. Skinner, "Some Contributions of an Experimental Analysis of Behavior to Psychology as a Whole," *American Psychologist* 8 (1953): 69–78; Joseph Brady, "Procedures, Problems and Perspectives in Animal Behavioral Studies of Drug Activity," in *Psychopharmacology: Problems in Evaluation,* ed. Jonathan Cole and Ralph Gerard, 255–63 (Washington, D.C.: National Academy of Sciences/National Research Council, 1959). B. F. Skinner, comments, in Cole and Gerard, *Psychopharmacology,* quote at 243. Karl Beyer to Max Tishler, October 17, 1956, ANRP, carton 21, folder 2.

8. Molitor to Major, January 20, 1955, ANRP, carton 17, folder 20 ("Merck: third party memoranda 1955, M-T"). John Boren (Walter Reed) to B. F. Skinner, June 27, 1955; Skinner, handwritten notes, labeled "Boren," June 1955; J. Boren & R. T. Ford (Merck?), memo on psychopharmocology meeting, November 25, 1955; V. G. Vernier to K. H. Beyer, "Summary of Consultant Meetings—December 20, 1955," February 2, 1956; Boren, "Summary of Consultant Meetings," December 20, 1955; Skinner, notes on Boren, September 17, 1956; Boren to Skinner, November 30, 1956—all in BFSP, box 4, folder "F1 2 Drugs."

9. Some behavioral tests were repeated with monkeys for confirmation, and there was also a test of drug influence on free, unconditioned behavior. See Clement Stone, "MK-202 Preclinical Evaluation," January 25, 1960, ANRP, carton 20, folder 4 "Merck: MK-202."

10. Albert Kurland, Luis Arbona, and Kenneth McCusker, "Clinical Trial of Methastyridone (MK-202) with Chronic Schizophrenics," *Journal of Nervous and Mental Disease* 133 (1961): 174–75.

11. J. Boren to C. A. Winter, re: "Discussion with Dr. Skinner," September 15, 1958, ANRP, box 17, folder 22; D. W. Richards, memo, "Mental Health Program," October 17, 1961, ANRP, box 21, folder 11.

12. On Elavil and animal behavior screening, see the description of the testimony by Edward L. Engelhardt in "Opinion of Justice Davis," *Merck & Co. Inc.*, No. 85-2740 (Fed. Cir. September 8, 1986), 800 F.2d 1091; 231 U.S.P.Q. (BNA) 375, September 8, 1986; also see D. W. Richards, "Preliminary Draft Report of Merck Institute Scientific Advisors, Meeting of October 16–17, 1961," ANRP, box 16, folder 49. Note that the version of amitriptyline's discovery as an antidepressant that emerges from the corporate documents cited here differs somewhat from that offered by its chemical discoverer, Edward Engelhardt, who claimed that he had asked the drug to be retried in depression after he heard about imipramine's successful use by Roland Kuhn. On Kuhn's role in the discovery of imipramine's antidepressant action, see Healy, *The Antidepressant Era*, chap. 2.

13. Pignarre, *Le grand secret.*

14. Linford Rees, "Treatment of Depression by Drugs and Other Means," *Nature* 186 (1960): 114–20; Healy, *The Antidepressant Era*, chap. 2.

15. ". . . if the individual is depressed," Benzedrine advertisement, *California and Western Medicine* 62 (April 1945): 33; also found in *American Journal of Psychology* 101 (March 1945): xiii. For other wartime examples of anhedonia-promoting Benzedrine advertisements, see "When Apathy Prolongs Convalescence," Benzedrine advertisement, *California and Western Medicine* 61 (August 1944): 43; "Simple Depression . . . 'the Most Favorable of All Disorders for Benzedrine Therapy,'" Benzedrine advertisement, *California and Western Medicine* 61 (December 1944): 35.

16. John Dewan, "Mild Depression," *Medical Clinics of North America* (March 1952): 527–37, quote at 530. In this and similar authoritative pieces from the 1950s, amphetamine is described as effective in depression only for milder cases in the short term. See Max Hamilton and Jack White, "Clinical Syndromes in Depressive States," *Journal of Mental Science* 105 (1959): 985–98, esp. 985 and passim; Max Hamilton, "A Rating Scale for Depression," *Journal of Neurology, Neuroscience and Psychiatry* 23 (1960): 56–62. Also see reviews of diagnostic and rating instruments in C. G. Watson, W. G. Klett, and T. W. Lorei, "Toward an Operational Definition of Anhedonia," *Psychological Reports* 26 (1970): 371–76; Donald Klein, "Endogenomorphic Depression: A Conceptual and Terminological Revision," *Archives of General Psychiatry* 31 (1974): 447–54. Nothing corresponding to Myerson's anhedonia can be found in the American Psychiatric Association's canonical *Diagnostic and Statistical Manual*

published in 1952 (widely known as *DSM-I*) in the definitions of depressions, whether reactive or endogenous. However, it is firmly in place by the influential 1980 edition, *DSM-III*. See American Psychiatric Association, *Diagnostic and Statistical Manual*, 3rd ed. (Washington, D.C.: American Psychiatric Association, 1980), 213–14, and American Psychiatric Association Committee on Nomenclature, *Diagnostic and Statistical Manual* (Washington, D.C.: American Psychiatric Association, 1952); also see Gerald Grob, "Origins of *DSM-I*: A Study in Appearance and Reality," *American Journal of Psychiatry* 148 (1991): 421–31.

17. Rees, "Treatment of Depression"; Donald Klein and Max Fink, "Psychiatric Reaction Patterns to Imipramine," *American Journal of Psychiatry* 119 (1962): 432–38; Donald Klein, "Anxiety Reconceptualized," in D. F. Klein and J. Rabkin, eds., *Anxiety: New Research and Changing Concepts* (New York: Raven, 1981), 235–63, quote at 235. Vivek Singh and Donald A. Malone Jr., "Should Amphetamines Be Added to SSRI Therapy to Enhance the Antidepressant Effect?" *Cleveland Clinic Journal of Medicine* 68 (2001): 748–49.

18. Rees, "Treatment of Depression"; Klein and Fink, "Psychiatric Reaction Patterns"; Klein, "Endogenomorphic Depression"; and idem, "Depression and Anhedonia," in *Anhedonia and Affect Deficit States*, ed David C. Clark and Jan Fawcett, 1–14 (New York: PMA Publishing, 1987). For the Freudian Otto Fenichel's views, see *The Psychoanalytic Theory of Neurosis* (New York: Norton, 1945). Singh and Malone Jr., "Should Amphetamines Be Added to SSRI Therapy?" On Kline's theories, see Healy, *The Antidepressant Era*, chap. 2.

19. Rees, "Treatment of Depression"; D. A. Slattery, A. L. Hudson, and D. J. Nutt, "The Evolution of Antidepressant Mechanisms," *Fundamental and Clinical Pharmacology* 18 (2004): 1–21; Healy, *The Antidepressant Era*, chap. 2; also see American Medical Association, *New and Non-Official Drugs* (Chicago: American Medical Association, 1962): 495–98, 500–502.

20. D. M. Shaw, "Anti-Depressant Drugs," *Practitioner* 192 (1964): 23–29, quote at 28.

21. The first proper double-blind RCT comparing old and new antidepressant therapies in neurotic depression was not published until 1964, and that study found imipramine to be no better than Dexamyl in improving core depressive symptoms. See E. H. Hare, C. McCance, and W. O. McCormick, "Impiramine and 'Drinamyl' in Depressive Illness: A Comparative Trial," *British Medical Journal* (March 28, 1964): 818–20; and Shaw, "Anti-Depressant Drugs," 28. There was an earlier Veterans Adminstration study, meeting fairly high standards as an RCT, that found imipramine better than placebo or Dexamyl after three weeks of therapy, but these subjects were an inpatient population so severely depressed that about one-third were classed as psychotic. Furthermore, differences between the treatment groups disappeared after three weeks; J. E. Overall et al., "Drug Therapy in Depressions: Controlled

Evaluation of Imipramine, Isocarboxazide, Dextroamphetamine-Amobarbital, and Placebo," *Clinical Pharmacology and Therapeutics* 3 (1962): 16–22.

22. Healy, *The Antidepressant Era*, 59.

23. Ronald R. Koegler, "Drugs, Neurosis, and the Family Physician," *California Medicine* 102 (January 1965): 5–8, quote at 7. In other words, the use of an amphetamine-barbiturate combination for commonplace depression was the acknowledged standard practice of the 1950s; see Callahan and Berrios, *Reinventing Depression*, 38.

24. Bernadine Z. Paulshock, "Coping on Amphetamines," *New England Journal of Medicine* 282 (1970): 346–51.

25. Prescription figures for 1963 in Morton Mintz, *The Therapeutic Nightmare* (Boston: Houghton Mifflin, 1965), 185; sales figures from the U.S. Census Bureau as reported in *F-D-C Reports* (November 9, 1964): 26–27; consumption survey data from Hugh Parry, "Use of Psychotropic Drugs by U.S. Adults," *Public Health Reports* 83 (1968): 799–810; Hugh Parry et al., "National Patterns of Psychotherapeutic Drug Use," *Archives of General Psychiatry* 28 (1973): 769–83. James Goddard, in "The Medical Business," *Scientific American* 229 (September 1973): 161–75, presents a graph indicating $500 million as the retail value of prescription mental health drugs consumed in 1963. This twofold discrepancy over the U.S. Census figures may reflect the difference between wholesale and retail drug sales prices. Dexamyl sales from H. E. Morgan to M. E. Parkhurst, "Estimated Royalties—Alles Estate," January 17, 1967, GAP, box 14, folder "Originals—1967."

26. In *JAMA*, the highest-circulation U.S. medical journal, in four randomly chosen consecutive weeks late in 1960, I counted twelve full-page tranquilizer advertisements for six different tranquilizer products. By contrast, the same issues carried four full-page advertisements for three different antidepressant drugs. Repeating the one-month survey of *JAMA* from late 1963, I found sixteen tranquilizer ads describing eight different products, and six ads for three different antidepressant products. The absence in these samples of full-page ads for amphetamine-based antidepressants, now off patent and less profitable, can explain why the ratio of full-page tranquilizer advertisements to antidepressant advertisements stands closer to three-to-one than two-to-one. See *JAMA* 174, November 26 through December 17, 1960; and *JAMA* 186, October 5 through October 26, 1963.

27. "Now You Can Treat the Underlying Cause of Many Imaginary Ills," unpaginated Niamid advertisement, *California Medicine* 92 (July 1960), and *JAMA* 173 (July 9, 1960); "You Can Often Treat the Underlying Cause of Chronic Fatigue," unpaginated Niamid advertisement, *California Medicine* 92 (May 1960, July 1960).

28. "When DEPRESSION Underlies Physical Complaints," Elavil advertisement, *JAMA* 186 (1963): 248–49; cf. Anon., "For the Management of Every-

day Mental and Emotional Distress—Dexamyl Tablets and Elixir," sales brochure, circa 1951, College of Physicians Library, Philadelphia, Medical Ephemera Collection, TEC SKF box 2, envelope 29.

29. Charles Bradley, "The Behavior of Children Receiving Benzedrine," *American Journal of Psychiatry* 94 (1937): 577–85; Katherine Cutts and Herbert Jasper, "Effect of Benzedrine Sulftae and Phenobarbital on Behavior Problem Children with Abnormal Electroencephalograms," *Archives of Neurology and Psychiatry* 41 (1939): 1138–45. For further details about Bradley and research at the Bradley Home, see Ilina Singh, "Bad Boys, Good Mothers, and the 'Miracle' of Ritalin," *Science in Context* 15 (2002): 577–603; and Elizabeth Bromley, "Stimulating a Normal Adjustment: Misbehavior, Amphetamines, and the Electroencephalogram at the Bradley Home for Children," *Journal of the History of the Behavioral Sciences* 42 (2006): 379–98. Bradley's work is listed among studies other than those sponsored by SKF in Wallace, "Research Memo," August 3, 1937, GAP, box 15, unlabeled folder.

30. Singh, "Bad Boys, Good Mothers."

31. "For Emotionally Disturbed Children," Deaner advertisement, *Journal of the American Women's Medical Association* 14, no. 2 (1959): 90; "Psychonormalizing Deaner," advertisement, *New England Journal of Medicine* 261 (September 19, 1959): ii; "Do Not Confuse It with Tranquilizers," Deaner advertisement, *Journal of the American Women's Medical Association* 14, no. 6 (1959): 464; "Rehabilitation of the disturbed child," Deaner advertisement, *Journal of the American Medical Association* 173, no. 10 (1960): 32; Linford Rees, "Treatment of Depression"; Donna Sy, "From Science to Quackwatch: The Discovery, Development, and Demedicalization of Deanol," unpublished paper written at University of California, Berkeley, for History 103, spring semester 2000.

32. "Lift the Depressed Patient up to Normal," Ritalin advertisement, *California Medicine* (March 1956): 1; Linford Rees, "Treatment of Depression"; Lester Grinspoon and Peter Hedblom, *The Speed Culture: Amphetamine Use and Abuse in America* (Cambridge, Mass.: Harvard University Press, 1975), chap. 9; Singh, "Bad Boys, Good Mothers"; Elizabeth Bromley, "Stimulating a Normal Adjustment."

33. In 1962, Northern British general practitioners wrote 52 percent of their amphetamine prescriptions for depression and broadly related mental health purposes, according to S. Brandon and D. Smith, "Amphetamines in General Practice," *Journal of the College of General Practitioners* 5 (1962): 603–6. However, U.S. prescription audits in the early 1960s indicate that "psychostimulants" accounted for about 1 percent of prescriptions, and amphetamine anti-obesity drugs about 2 percent (and "non-amphetamine" anti-obesity drugs a little less than 1 percent). The 1:1 versus 2:1 discrepancy can be reconciled by supposing either that weight loss was really less important in the United Kingdom or that many amphetamine prescriptions in the United

States were meant to affect weight and mood simultaneously, the majority of which were coded as "anti-obesity" in prescription audits; see *National Prescription Audit*, College ed. (Baltimore, Md.: Gosselin, 1962); and *National Prescription Audit, General Information Report*, 5th ed. (Baltimore, Md.: Gosselin, 1966), Table 13.

34. "DESOXYN Gradumet," advertisement, *JAMA* 174 (1960): 272–73; "Tight Squeeze?" unpaginated Ambar advertisement, *JAMA* 174 (December 3, 1960); "For the COMPENSTORY OVEREATER," unpaginated Biphetamine and Ionamin advertisement, *JAMA* 174 (December 10, 1960). For other advertising linking mood and appetite effects of amphetamines, see "Establish Desired Eating Patterns," Obedrin advertisment, *California Medicine* 83 (July 1955): 22; "For the Patient Who Really ~~Wants~~ Needs to Lose Weight," Obedrin-LA advertisement, *California Medicine* 102 (March 1965), 45; "When Obesity is an Expression of Mental or Emotional Distress. . . ," Dexamyl advertisement, *California Medicine* 82 (May 1955): 69.

35. John Swann, "Rainbow Diet Pills in Medical Practice, Industry, and Regulation 1938 to 1968," paper presented at the conference "Drugs Trajectories: Historical Studies of Biology, Medicine, and Industry," Max Planck Institute for History of Science, Berlin, June 7–8, 2002).

36. "MASS SUICIDE WEAPON," unpaginated Tepanil advertisement, *JAMA* 174 (November 26, 1960); "Look at All the People Who Can Use TENUATE," unpaginated advertisement, *JAMA* 174 (December 3, 1960); "For the COMPENSTORY OVEREATER," Biphetamine and Ionamine advertisement. "Preludin reduces the problems of overeating," unpaginated Preludin advertisement, *California Medicine* 92 (June 1960); "an oxazine . . . not an amphetamine," unpaginated Preludin advertisement, *New England Journal of Medicine* 258 (January 9, 1958). Compare, e.g., "When obesity is an expression of mental or emotional distress . . . ," Dexamyl advertisement, *California Medicine* 82 (May 1955): 69.

37. American Medical Association, *New and Nonofficial Drugs* (Phildelphia: Lippincott, 1962), 248–49, 267–69; L. G. Kiloh and S. Brandon, "Habituation and Addiction to Amphetamines," *British Medical Journal* 1 (1962): 40–43; Ian Oswald and V. R. Thacore, "Amphetamine and Phenmetrazine Addiction," *British Medical Journal* 2 (1963): 427–31.

38. James N. Giglio, *The Presidency of John F. Kennedy* (Lawrence: University Press of Kansas, 1991), 262–63; Robert Dallek, *An Unfinished Life: John F. Kennedy, 1917–1963* (Boston: Little, Brown, 2003), 394–408; Nina Burleigh, *A Very Private Woman* (New York: Random House, 1999), 212–13; Richard Reeves, "History Denied: Restricting Access to Presidential Records," March 15, 2003, First Amendment Center, http://www.firstamendmentcenter.org/commentary.aspx?id=6325 (accessed August 19, 2004).

39. Steven Suskin, *Broadway Yearbook* (Oxford and New York: Oxford University Press, 2002), 145; Max Wilk, *Schmucks with Underwoods: Conversations*

with America's Classic Screenwriters (New York: Applause Books, 2004), 157; Stephen Davis, *Old Gods Almost Dead: The 40-Year Odyssey of the Rolling Stones* (New York: Random House, 2001), 169. Quotes from Boyce Rensberger, "Amphetamines Used by a Physician to Lift Moods of Famous Patients," *New York Times*, December 4, 1972, section 1, 1, 34.

40. Rensberger, "Amphetamines Used by a Physician," 1, 34; Lawrence Altman, "Amphetamine and Ethics," *New York Times*, December 5, 1972, section 1, 35; Jane E. Brody, "Patient and His Doctor: Quandary for Medicine," *New York Times*, January 16, 1973, 1, 22; Lawrence Altmann, "Medical Society Faces Discipline Issues," *New York Times*, February 25, 1973, 1, 48; Boyce Rensberger, "Two Doctors Here Known to Users as Sources of Amphetamines," *New York Times*, March 25, 1973, 48; Iver Peterson, "Regents' Vote Unanimous," *New York Times*, April 26, 1975, 1, 23. American Medical Association Council on Scientific Affairs, "Council Report: Clinical Aspects of Amphetamine Abuse," in *Amphetamine Use, Misuse, and Abuse*, ed. David E. Smith, 11–17 (Boston: G. K. Hall, 1979).

41. Caroline Jean Acker, *Creating the American Junkie: Addiction Research in the Classic Era of Narcotic Control* (Baltimore, Md.: Johns Hopkins University Press, 2002).

42. The FDA conducted a voluntary survey of importers and manufacturers in 1962, and had arrived at a figure of 45 billion mg of amphetamine salts; but this excluded the production of the two largest manufacturers. Including their output, FDA estimated a total of more than 80 billion mg, one-half to two-thirds of which was diverted into illegal channels, according to FDA official Lewis Lasher in Bernie Sewart and Jack Lyndall, Hearings of Subcommittee on Health, Senate Committee on Labor and Public Welfare, *Hearings on S. 2628*, 88th Congress, 2nd session, March 12, 1964 (hereafter, *Hearings on S. 2628*), 23–24. Thus, the estimated quantity diverted translates to at least 4 billion 10 mg tablets per year. A standard dose of methamphetamine and dextroamphetamine was 5 mg. The entire U.S. population in 1962 was 187 million (http://www.census.gov/population/estimates/nation/popclockest.txt, accessed 7 January 2005).

43. Andy Warhol and Pat Hackett, *Popism: The Warhol Sixties* (Orlando, Fla.: Harcourt, 1980), 33. Victor Bockris, *The Life and Death of Andy Warhol* (New York: Bantam, 1989), 132, 144–47 and passim.

44. Geldzahler, quoted in Victor Bockris, *Warhol* (New York: Da Capo, 1997), 139.

45. Bockris, *Life and Death of Andy Warhol*, 225; Gary Comenas, "Sleep (1963)," Warholstars site (www.warholstars.org/filmch/sleep.html, accessed October 17, 2004). Formulation for Obetrol 20 from "Obetrol for Weight Control," advertisement, *California Medicine* 112 (April 1970): 14. On Warhol's pref-

erences in pills, see Comenas, http://www.warholstars.org/warhol/warhol1/andy/warhol/can/solanas17.html (accessed October 17, 2004); Bob Colacello, *Holy Terror: Andy Warhol Close Up* (New York: HarperCollins, 1990), 50, cites Brigid Berlin as his information source.

46. P. H. Connell, "Adolescent Drug Taking," *Proceedings of the Royal Society of Medicine* 58 (1965): 409–12; P. H. Connell, "Clinical Manifestations and Treatment of Amphetamine Type of Dependence," *Journal of the American Medical Association* 196 (1966): 718–23.

47. P. H. Connell, "What to Do about the Pep Pills," *New Society*, February 20, 1964, 6–8; Neale Pharaoh, "He Gets Out of It," *New Society*, February 20, 1964, 8.

48. Bruce Jackson, "White Collar Pill Party," *Atlantic Monthly* 218 (August 1966): 35–40. Seymour Fiddle, "The Case of the Peak User John," in *Amphetamine Abuse*, ed. J. R. Russo, 119–44 (Springfield, Ill.: Charles C. Thomas, 1968).

49. For a nice example of the way anthropological insight into drug use began to weaken the distinction between medical and nonmedical use, even in mainstream medical consciousness, see Edmund Pellegrino, "Prescribing and Drug Ingestion Symbols and Substances," *Drug Intelligence and Clinical Pharmacy* 10 (1976): 624–30. It is worth noting that this line of argument, by shifting attention from drug suppliers to the cultural determinants of demand, is friendly to drug industry interests.

50. Susan Speaker, "From 'Happiness Pills' to 'National Nightmare': Changing Cultural Assessment of Minor Tranquilizers in America, 1955–1980," *Journal of the History of Medicine and Allied Sciences* 52 (1997): 338–76.

51. The *locus classicus* for the "pharmacological Calvinism" concept is G. Klerman, "Drugs and Social Values," *International Journal of the Addictions* 5 (1970): 313–19; however, Margaret Mead's nuanced discussion in 1969 congressional hearings bears at least equal attenton; cited and exerpted in Mickey Smith, *Small Comforts* (New York: Praeger, 1985), 180.

52. Speaker, "From 'Happiness Pills' to 'National Nightmare.' " On the history of this type of cultural critique, see Robert Nye, "The Evolution of the Concept of Medicalization in the Late Twentieth Century," *Journal of the History of the Behavioral Sciences* 39, no. 2 (2003): 115–29.

53. For instance, Nikolas Rose considers the 2000 rate of 6.5 million annual "standard doses" of psychiatric drugs per 100,000 population, or 65 pills per person, extraordinary and noteworthy, and likewise the nearly 18 percent of the U.S. pharmaceutical market devoted to psychotropics. In 1964, the U.S. was consuming nearly as many if not more standard doses per person per year of amphetamines and minor tranquilizers alone, taking into account only the minor tranquilizers sold on prescription by retail pharmacies (45 million prescriptions, or 2.7 billion pills at 60 pills per precription, 14 per person) and

the entire 8 billion amphetamine pills produced by U.S. manufacturers according to FDA production surveys (42 per person). Indeed, by Rose's definition of
"standard dose" as the lowest dose commonly prescribed and made as a single pill, for amphetamine 5 mg, the U.S. in the mid-1960s was consuming 16
billion such units or 84 "doses" per person per year *in amphetamine alone*, one-
third more than *all psychotropics* today. (On the other hand, if the psychiatric
purpose rather than the psychotropic effect of drug use is paramount, perhaps
42 doses per person per year is the right measure of amphetamine consumption in the 1960s, since around half was taken for weight loss.) Taking into account the tranquilizers (major and minor) dispensed by hospitals in 1964, and
the hypnotics and sedatives dispensed both at hospitals and pharmacies,
would likely increase these numbers by another 15–20 doses per person, not
to mention MAOI and tricyclic antidepressants. Counting these all would add
up to consumption of about twice as many "standard doses" of psychotropics
per person per year in the mid-1960s as Rose finds in 2000, defining terms
comparably. In 1967, psychotropics comprised 17 percent of the U.S. pharmaceutical market, almost the same as in 2000. Thus, the cost per unit of drug is
rising, but any recent growth in the volume of psychotropic drug consumption has not yet surpassed the outrageous levels of the last generation. See
Nikolas Rose, "Becoming Neurochemical Selves," in *Biotechnology: Between
Commerce and Civil Society*, ed. Nico Stehr (New Brunswick, N.J.: Transaction,
2004). On the retail psychotropics market in the 1960s, see Mitchell Balter and
Jerome Levine, "The Nature and Extent of Psychotropic Drug Usage in the
United States," *Psychopharmacology Bulletin* 5 (1969): 3–13. On tranquilizer prescription rates, see Mitchell Balter, "Coping with Illness: Choices, Alternatives,
and Consequences," in *Drug Development and Marketing*, ed. Robert Helms,
27–46, esp. Table 1 (Washington, D.C.: American Enterprise Institute, 1975).
These last two retail audit-based sources seriously underestimate amphetamine consumption, because the bulk of amphetamines was evidently not dispensed at retail pharmacies in the 1960s. It should be noted that in this period,
when nonmedical amphetamine consumption outweighed minor tranquilizer
consumption, the vast quantities of barbiturates being consumed medically
and nonmedically were classed as hypnotics.

    54. The 1962 production survey as described by FDA official Lewis
Lasher in *Hearings on S. 2628*, 23–24. Several informed commentators in congressional hearings in 1969 understood that production then stood as high as
10 billion 10 mg units of amphetamine salts, such as Edward Wolfson of the
American Public Health Association, in *Diet Pill (Amphetamines) Traffic,
Abuse, and Regulation*, Hearings before the Subcommittee to Investigate Juvenile Delinquency, Senate Committee on the Judiciary, 92nd Congress, 1st session, February 7, 1972 [hereafter, *Diet Pill (Amphetamines) Traffic, Abuse, and
Regulation*], 105–9; also see submission of National Institute of Mental

Health Director Sidney Cohen, Hearings of Senate Committee on Crime, 99th Congress, 1st session, November 18, 1969, 353. A flat level of about 28 million retail prescriptions per year from 1964 to 1970 appears in Figure 1 and Table 1 in Balter, "Coping with Illness." This prescription rate, obtained by an audit of retail pharmacy sales, implies annual consumption of only about 1.7 billion tablets; however, it cannot serve in itself as a measure of national amphetamine consumption when billions of tablets were being dispensed directly, and billions more diverted from manufacturers for sale without medical intervention.

55. Under these conditions, where their records were open to investigation by law enforcement, only manufacturers able to account for their output through legitimate channels reasonably well would be likely to report. In fact, two different sets of production figures were reported to the Bureau of Narcotics. One set, based in a voluntary survey of firms, yielded 1969 production figures equivalent to 3.4 billion 10 mg tablets of amphetamine salts, and 1.2 billion 10 mg methamphetamine salts; the other, based on legally required reporting by firms requesting production quotas, yielded a 1969 production equivalent to 1.7 billion 10 mg units of amphetamine base, and 0.8 billion 10 mg units methamphetamine base. These figures are not as inconsistent as they might appear, because the base requires conversion to heavier salts to represent 10 mg dosage units as dispensed. Applying the multiplier of 1.7 to amphetamine, to account for conversion to monobasic amphetamine sulphate, and the multiplier of 1.2 to methamphetamine, for conversion to the hydrochloride salt, yields estimates of about 3 billion amphetamine tablets and 1 billion methamphetamine tablets. Even 4 billion is a conservative estimate of actual pill production, since 5 mg is a more typical dose of both dextroamphetamine and methamphetamine. See "Amphetamines and Methamphetamine, Notice of Proposed Production Quotas"; query of Birch Bayh, February 16, 1972, Exhibit 10; and submission of John Ingersoll, April 5, 1972, Exhibit 11, all in *Diet Pill (Amphetamines) Traffic, Abuse, and Regulation*, 91–95.

56. About 5 percent of U.S. adults reported taking stimulant drugs medically in 1969–70; see Parry, "Use of Psychotropic Drugs"; Parry et al., "National Patterns of Psychotherapeutic Drug Use," esp. Table 5.

57. Kiloh and Brandon, "Habituation and Addiction to Amphetamines"; Brandon and Smith, "Amphetamines in General Practice"; C. W. M. Wilson and S. Beacon, "An Investigation into the Habituating Properties of an Amphetamine-Barbiturate Mixture," *British Journal of Addiction* 60 (1964): 81–92. It can be argued that Dexamyl was more addictive than other amphetamine preparations because of the barbiturate content. However, a very high proportion of the amphetamines prescribed in primary care were, in fact, Dexamyl (over 50 percent in one of the British studies) and similar combination products. See chapter 5 above.

58. James Inciardi and Carl Chambers, "The Epidemiology of Amphetamine Use in the General Population," *Canadian Journal of Criminology and Corrections* 14 (1972): 166–72; see also Carl Chambers, "Differential Drug Use in the New York State Labor Force" (1971), in *Diet Pill (Amphetamines) Traffic, Abuse, and Regulation,* Hearings before the Subcommittee to Investigate Juvenile Delinquency, Senate Committee on the Judiciary, 92nd Congress, 1st session, February 7, 1972, 288–337.

59. The data from the New York survey (based on an order of magnitude more complete sampling than the national study) indicate past six-month medical amphetamine usage of state residents over age eighteen at 4.6 percent. This figure is derived by the following procedure from the findings of Chambers and collaborators. In 1970, 375,000 New York residents over age fourteen reported using "pep pill" (antidepressant-type) pharmaceutical amphetamines either occasionally or regularly in the past six months, 55 percent, or 206,000 of them, partially or wholly by prescription. A total of 543,000 reported using "diet pill" (amphetamines plus sedative or tranquilizer) amphetamines either occasionally or regularly in the past six months. Subtracting the 13 percent that also used "pep pills" to avoid double counting leaves 472,000 using diet pills only. Of all "diet pill" users, 78 percent obtained their drugs partially or wholly by prescription, leaving 368,000 past six month medical users of "diet pills." Assuming that all who obtained either pep pills or diet pills by prescription were adults (reasonable at a time when childhood prescription for hyperkinesis or enuresis was rare), 574,000 (206,000 + 368,000) adults used prescription-type amphetamines medically in the six months prior to the New York survey. This represents 4.6 percent of New York's 12,359,000 adult population at the time, consistent with the comparable national past year medical amphetamine use among U.S. adults of 5 percent. See Inciardi and Chambers, "The Epidemiology of Amphetamine Use in the General Population"; and Chambers, "Differential Drug Use in the New York State Labor Force."

60. Applying the New York rates to the entire 1970 U.S. population over age fourteen of 149,352,000, 6.5 percent, or 9.7 million Americans, would have used amphetamines medically or nonmedically in the past six months, almost 3.8 million would have used the drugs nonmedically at least some of the time, and more than 2.1 million would have "abused" them by the New York definition of the term. This extrapolation counts only pharmaceutical-type amphetamines ("pep pills" and "diet pills") and leaves out all users of methamphetamine, presumed to be high-dose injectors (because of the study design and timing) and likely to be over-represented in New York. This extrapolation also assumes that medical and nonmedical amphetamine use *combined* were equal throughout the U.S. but allows the proportion of medical and nonmedical use to vary locally. It similarly assumes that "abuse" rates were independ-

ent of whether some drugs were obtained by prescription, not an unreasonable assumption when pharmaceutical amphetamines could be obtained so easily with or without one. For estimates of past-year consumption of medical and nonmedical use, these figures must be adjusted upward. To compensate for the difference between past-year and past-six-month usage, the 9 percent difference between 4.6 percent and 5 percent adult medical usage might be assumed to apply independent of age and whether drugs are obtained by prescription. Thus increasing the above figures by 9 percent yields a 1970 national past-year nonmedical and medical usage of 10.6 million, nonmedical "misuse" of 4.1 million, and "abuse" by New York definitions of 2.3 million. Age-specific 1970 national and New York population figures obtained from the Statistical Abstract of the United States, 1971; available at http://www2.census.gov/prod2/statcomp/documents/1971-02.pdf, accessed December 20, 2006.

61. As noted, the extrapolation to national figures deliberately excluded methamphetamine injectors, the numbers of which, in any case, were presumably atypical in New York, and also underestimated by the New York survey's reliance on fixed addresses. In addition, from 1969 to 1970, the reported legal manufacture of amphetamine and methamphetamine base declined by 17 percent, reflecting reduced consumption because of new legal controls on prescription ("Statement of John E Ingersoll, Director, Bureau of Narcotics and Dangerous Drugs," February 1, 1972, in *Diet Pill (Amphetamines) Traffic, Abuse, and Regulation*, 226–32.).

62. The higher figure would be more likely because, even though on these calculations little more than 2 percent of the total population was taking amphetamines in a given year, the addiction rate among an American population including large numbers of purely recreational amphetamine users circa 1970 surely must exceed that of a strictly medical northern English user population circa 1960. Also, as noted above, as a measure of the amphetamine epidemic's peak circa 1969, the estimate of total past-year users has a low bias. A further reason to consider the higher figure more likely is that population-level amphetamine dependency rate in the U.K. in 1966 was estimated at 0.4 percent, and it should have been lower than the American rate, considering the much greater supply of illicitly distributed pharmaceutical amphetamines in the U.S. Thus, about 800,000 dependent amphetamine users in the U.S. (implying a dependency rate equivalent to the U.K.'s 0.4 percent) should be regarded as an absolute minimum (U.K. figure from Thomas Bewley, "Recent Changes in the Pattern of Drug Abuse in the United Kingdom," *Bulletin on Narcotics* 18, no. 4 (1966): 1–9).

63. Nikolas Rose, *Inventing Our Selves: Psychology, Power, and Personhood* (Cambridge and New York: Cambridge University Press, 1996), esp. chap. 7; Jeffrey Hart, *When the Going Was Good: American Life in the Fifties* (New York: Crown, 1982); Ruth Schwartz Cowan, *More Work for Mother: The Ironies of*

Household Technology from the Open Hearth to the Microwave (New York: Basic Books, 1983); Lynn Spigel, *Make Room for TV: Television and the Family Ideal in Postwar America* (Chicago: University of Chicago Press, 1992); Kristin Ross, *Fast Cars, Clean Bodies: Decolonization and the Reordering of French Culture* (Cambridge, Mass.: MIT Press, 1996); Victoria de Grazia, *Irresistable Empire: America's Advance through 20th Century Europe* (Cambridge, Mass: Harvard University Press, 2005).

64. On the "fun morality" concept (attributed to Reisman), see Jean Baudrillard, *The Consumer Society: Myths and Structures,* trans. Chris Turner (London: Sage, 1998), 80, 156.

65. It might seem paradoxical at first that amphetamine could be viewed as a drive booster for work and pursuit of pleasure but a drive limiter when applied to eating. The paradox is resolved if one supposes that more than one type of drive implicitly shapes the thinking of amphetamine prescribers. For eating, consumption must be *limited* by an amphetamine-reinforcable drive. This may be related to what Baudrillard calls the special "double solicitude" toward the body required of the modern consumer, one type of "solicitude" or drive (linked to the Freudian death drive by Baudrillard) working puritanically toward physical perfection. See Baudrillard, *Consumer Society,* chap. 8. There is a strong resonance here with Harry Levine's interpretation of the construction of alcoholism; see "The Discovery of Addiction: Changing Conceptions of Habitual Drunkenness in America," *Journal of Studies on Alcohol* 15 (1978): 493–506.

66. Paulshock, "Coping on Amphetamines."

Notes to Chapter 7

1. *LA Free Press* interview with Ginsberg, December 1965, reproduced in Allen Ginsberg and Anonymous, "A 19 Year-Old-Girl and Poet Allen Ginsberg Talk about Speed," Do It Now Foundation; http://www.doitnow.org/pages/ginsberg.html, accessed December 21, 2004.

2. Ibid.

3. Huncke, extract from his "Underground Journal," quoted in Jonathan Black, "The 'Speed' that Kills or Worse," *New York Times Sunday Magazine,* June 21, 1970, 15–24.

4. J. F. Shick, D. E. Smith, and F. H. Meyers, "Patterns of Drug Use in the Haight-Ashbury Neighborhood," *Clinical Toxicology* 3 (1970): 19–56; D. E. Smith, "Speed Freaks vs. Acid Heads," *Clinical Pediatrics* 8, no. 4 (1969): 185–88.

5. Shick, Smith, and Meyers, "Patterns of Drug Use"; Roger Smith, "Traffic in Amphetamines: Patterns of Illegal Manufacture and Distribution," *Journal of Psychedelic Drugs* 2, no. 2 (1969): 20–27.

6. John Kramer, Vitezslav Fischman, and Don Litlefield, "Amphetamine Abuse: Patterns and Effects of High Doses Taken Intravenously," *JAMA* 201 (1967): 305–9; B. M. Angrist and Samuel Gershon, "Amphetamine Abuse in New York, 1966–1968," *Seminars in Psychiatry* 1 (1969): 195–207, quote at 204.

7. Smith, "Traffic in Amphetamines"; J. W. Rawlin, "Street Level Abusage of Amphetamines," in J. R. Russo, ed., *Amphetamine Abuse* (Springfield, Ill.: Charles Thomas, 1966), chap. 6.

8. Smith, "Traffic in Amphetamines"; New York narcotics official Michael Costello estimated that 80 percent of the amphetamines sold on the street were pharmaceutical ("Highlights of Testimony at the Hearings on Amphetamines, April 14 and 15, 1971, New York City," in *Diet Pill (Amphetamines) Traffic, Abuse, and Regulation,* Hearings before the Subcommittee to Investigate Juvenile Delinquency, Senate Committee on the Judiciary, 92nd Congress, 1st session, February 7, 1972 (hereafter, *Diet Pill (Amphetamines) Traffic, Abuse, and Regulation*), 204–6; according to the Federal Narcotics chief John Ingersoll, an estimated two-thirds of the speed seized on the street is amphetamine, and seven out of eight illicit laboratories were making methamphetamine; "Statement of John E Ingersoll, Director, Bureau of Narcotics and Dangerous Drugs," February 1, 1972, in *Diet Pill (Amphetamines) Traffic, Abuse, and Regulation,* 226–32, 229. Elsewhere in the hearings, Ingersoll estimated that 75–95 percent of the amphetamines sold on the street were manufactured by U.S. pharmaceutical firms; James Graham, "Amphetamine Politics on Capitol Hill," *Trans-Action Magazine,* January 1972, in *Diet Pill (Amphetamines) Traffic, Abuse, and Regulation,* 185–95, 191.

9. Smith, "Traffic in Amphetamines," 21.

10. John P. Morgan and Doreen Kagan, "Street Amphetamine Quality and the Controlled Substances Act of 1970," in David E. Smith, ed., *Amphetamine Use, Misuse, and Abuse* (Boston: G. K. Hall, 1979), 73–91. For a glimpse of the Hells Angels and their involvement with speed in the era, see Hunter S. Thompson, *Hells Angels* (New York: Random House, 1966), 212–13 and passim.

11. Shick, Smith, and Meyers, "Patterns of Drug Use"; Fred Davis and Laura Munoz, "Heads and Freaks: Patterns and Meanings of Drug Use among Hippies," *Journal of Health and Social Behavior* 9 (1968): 156–64; James Carey and Jerry Mandel, "A San Francisco Area 'Speed' Scene," *Journal of Health and Social Behavior* 9 (1968): 164–74; Roger Smith, "The World of the Haight-Ashbury Speed Freak," *Journal of Psychedelic Drugs* 2, no. 2 (1969): 77–83; Smith, "Speed Freaks vs. Acid Heads"; David E. Smith, "The Characteristics of Dependency in High-Dose Methamphetamine Abuse," *International Journal of Addictions* 4, no. 3 (1969): 453–59.

12. Shick, Smith, and Meyers, "Patterns of Drug Use"; Carey and Mandel, "A San Francisco Area 'Speed' Scene"; Roger Smith, "The World of the

Haight-Ashbury Speed Freak"; D. E. Smith, "Speed Freaks vs. Acid Heads"; D. E. Smith and John Luce, *Love Needs Care* (Boston: Little, Brown, 1971); discussed in Lester Grinspoon and Peter Hedblom, *The Speed Culture: Amphetamine Use and Abuse in America* (Cambridge, Mass.: Harvard University Press, 1975), chap. 7.

13. Charles Fischer et al., "Behavioral Mediators in the Polyphasic Mortality Curve of Agregate Amphetamine Toxicity," *Journal of Psychedelic Drugs* 2, no. 2 (1969): 28–36; D. E. Smith, "Speed Freaks vs. Acid Heads."

14. Roger Smith, "The World of the Haight-Ashbury Speed Freak." Also quoted in Edward Brecher, *The Consumers Union Report on Licit and Illicit Drugs* (Boston: Little, Brown, 1972), 288.

15. Do It Now Foundation, "Flashbacks: Early PSA's"; http://www .doitnow.org/pages/psas.html, accessed October 25, 2006).

16. Anon., "The Religious Significance of Psychedelic Drugs," conference program, June 24, 1967; Anon, "Speed Kills" "Program—November 2, 1968" —both in UCSF-PH, folder 3:1. Albert Rosenfeld, "Drugs That Even Scare Hippies," *Life Magazine,* October 27, 1967, 81–82; Jack Shepherd, "The Cruel Chemical World of Speed," *Look Magazine,* March 5, 1968, 53–59; Black, "The 'Speed' That Kills or Worse."

17. H. Brill and T. Hirose, "The Rise and Fall of a Methamphetamine Epidemic: Japan 1945–1955," *Seminars in Psychiatry* 1 (1969): 179–94; Hemmi Takemitsu, "How We Handled the Problem of Drug Abuse in Japan," in F. Sjoqvist and M. Tottie, eds., *Abuse of Central Stimulants* (Stockholm: Almqvist and Wiksell, 1969), 147–53; M. Kato, "Epidemiology of Drug Dependence in Japan," in *Drug Abuse: Proceedings of the International Conference,* ed. C. J. Zarafonetis, 67–70 (Phildelphia: Lea and Febiger, 1972).

18. Anne C. Gay and George R. Gay, "Haight-Ashbury: Evolution of a Drug Culture in an Age of Mendacity," *Journal of Psychedelic Drugs* 4, no. 1 (1971): 81–90.

19. Submission of David E. Smith, undated [late 1970?], in *Diet Pills (Amphetamines) Traffic, Abuse, and Regulation,* Exhibit 6, 86–91.

20. General Curtis E. LeMay, with MacKinley Kantor, *Mission with LeMay: My Story* (New York: Doubleday, 1965), 565; cited in *Respectfully Quoted: A Dictionary of Quotations,* 1989, Bartleby.com, http://www.bartleby.com/73/127 .html, accessed August 21, 2006.

21. D. Bentel, D. Crim, and D. E. Smith, "Drug Abuse in Combat: The Crisis of Drugs and Addiction among American Troops in Vietnam," *Journal of Psychedelic Drugs* 4, no. 1 (1971): 23–30; these authors cite personal communication from Army doctors that 10 percent of enlisted men returning with honorable discharges through Oakland had used heroin in Vietnam. Congressmen Murphy and Steele, "The World Heroin Problem," Report of a Special Study Mission, May 27, 1971, Washington, GPO, placed the prevalence of heroin ad-

diction among returning veterans at 10 percent, implying that upward of three hundred thousand veterans of the conflict were addicts at some point (cited in Bentel, Crim, and Smith, "Drug Abuse in Combat"). On field survey evidence, see Jerome Char, "Drug Abuse in Viet Nam," *American Journal of Psychiatry* 129 (1972): 463–65. Two overdose deaths per day in 1970 is noted in the statement of Jon Mitchell Steinberg, *Diet Pills (Amphetamines) Traffic, Abuse, and Regulation*, 480–86. On the political importance of the Vietnam heroin problem, see Jill Jonnes, *Hep-Cats, Narcs and Pipe Dreams: A History of America's Romance with Illegal Drugs* (New York: Scribner's, 1996), chap. 14.

22. Lester Grinspoon and Peter Hedblom, *The Speed Culture: Amphetamine Use and Abuse in America* (Cambridge, Mass.: Harvard University Press, 1975), 19. Samuel Black, Kenneth Owens, and Ronald Wolff, "Patterns of Drug Use: A Study of 5,482 Subjects," *American Journal of Psychiatry* 127 (1970): 420–23; Bentel, Crim, and Smith, "Drug Abuse in Combat"; Morris D. Stanton, "Drug Use in Vietnam: A Survey among Army Personnel in the Two Northern Corps," *Archives of General Psychiatry* 26 (1972): 279–86. Former Cobra helicopter pilot Lance McElhiney quoted in Rhonda Cornum, John Caldwell, and Kory Cornum, "Stimulant Use in Extended Flight Operations," *Aerospace Power Journal* (spring 1997); http://www.airpower.maxwell.af.mil/airchronicles/apj/apj97/spr97/cornum.html, accessed December 7, 2006.

23. G. F. Solomon et al., "Three Psychiatric Casualties from Vietnam," *Archives of General Psychiatry* 25 (1971): 522–24. Mike Beamon in *Everything We Had: An Oral History of the Vietnam War by Thirty-Three American Soldiers Who Fought It*, ed. Al Santoli (New York: Random House, 1981), 180; the night patrol man is described by Michael Herr, "Dispatches," in *Reporting Vietnam: America Journalism 1969–1975*, vol. 2 (New York: Library of America, 1998), 556–57.

24. Bentel, Crim, and Smith, "Drug Abuse in Combat," 27. The full quote, from a soldier who preferred heroin, explains that with the right drug regimen "you don't shit in your pants . . . [and] get so scared out there that you could blow it and get everybody killed. It like makes you more alert and more aware, even more paranoid. When you walk point, man, you get sharp or you get blown away. When you are high, you don't miss snake eyes [hidden Vietnamese signs for mined trails] or miss picking up the vibes if the village people who know something is coming down."

25. D. Russel Davis, "Psychomotor Effects of Analeptics and Their Relation to 'Fatigue' Phenomena in Aircrew," *British Medical Bulletin* 5 (1947): 43–45.

26. G. T. Hauty and R. B. Payne, "Mitigation of Work Decrement," *Journal of Experimental Psychology* 49 (1955): 60–67; R. B. Payne and G. T. Hauty, "The Effects of Experimentally Induced Attitudes upon Task Proficiency," *Journal of Experimental Psychology* 47 (1954): 267–73; idem, "Factors Affecting the En-

durance of Psychomotor Skill," *Journal of Aviation Medicine* 25 (1955): 380–89; R. B. Payne, G. T. Hauty, and E. W. Moore, "Restoration of Tracking Efficiency as a Function of Amount and Delay of Analeptic Medication," *Journal of Comparative and Physiological Psychology* 50 (1957): 146–49; also see review of Air Force and other literature in Bernard Weiss and Victor Laties, "Enhancement of Human Performance by Caffeine and the Amphetamines," *Pharmacological Reviews* 14 (1962): 1–36.

27. G. T. Hauty and R. B. Payne, "Effects of Dextro-Amphetamine upon Judgment," *Journal of Pharmacology and Experimental Therapeutics* 120 (1957): 33–36; S. Goldstone, W. K. Boardman, and W. T. Lhamon, "Effect of Quinal Barbitone, Dextroamphetamine, and Placebo on Apparent Time," *British Journal of Psychology* 49 (1958): 324–28; P. B. Dews and W. H. Morse, "Some Observations on an Operant in Human Subjects and Its Modification by Dextroamphetamine," *Journal of the Experimental Analysis of Behavior* 1 (1958): 359–64; G. M. Smith and H. K. Beecher, "Amphetamine, Secobarbital, and Athletic Performance, III. Quantitative Effects on Judgment," *JAMA* 172 (1960): 1623–29; Weiss and Laties, "Enhancement of Human Performance." Anon., "Summary of Royalties Payable and Amounts Paid," 1955, GAP, box 2, folder " SKF vs. Alles: Documents Received from Alles Office."

28. A case in point are the Canadian troops killed by an American pilot on amphetamine in 2002—a judgment error caused by the amphetamine which, according to him, he was compelled to take. The arguments and evidence made by those in the military who brought back amphetamine during the 1990s was largely old and feeble. There was the shopworn argument, for example, that "air crews are a well-screened, intelligent, motivated and mentally healthy population" with a "remarkably low incidence of any sort of addictive behavior or other mental pathology." Clean-cut aviators presented little risk of abuse. (The same arguments were made during the Second World War but did not prevent what seems to have been widespread amphetamine abuse.) There were anecdotes that many pilots liked the drug and even considered it "essential" during the first war against Iraq, although there seemed little interest in why these combat pilots could not have carried out their orders without being drugged. The perfectly good argument was made that pilots and other men forced to stay in combat for a long time were better off awake than asleep. It is one thing, however, to provide amphetamine to soldiers whose special duties allow them no other option but to stay awake, for instance, paratroops or commandos far behind enemy lines. This is something the German military continued to do through the end of the Second World War, and post-Vietnam experiments with flight simulators and simple tests confirmed that exhausted soldiers pay better attention and suffer fewer lapses, or "microsleeps," on amphetamine. But it is quite another matter to give men amphetamine rather allowing needed rest, simply to accelerate military oper-

ations on the assumption that pharmacologically extended performance is fully competent and "normal," both physically and mentally. See Cornum, Caldwell, and Cornum, "Stimulant Use in Extended Flight Operations"; Rene Spiegel, "Effects of Amphetamines on Performance and on Polygraphic Sleep Parameters in Man," *Advances in Biosciences* 21 (1979): 189–201; Paul Newhouse et al., "The Effects of d-Amphetamine on Arousal, Cognition, and Mood after Prolonged Total Sleep Deprivation," *Neuropsychopharmacology* 2 (1989): 153–64; John Caldwell, J. Lynn Caldwell, and Kecia Darlington, "The Utility of Dextroamphetamine for Attenuating the Impact of Sleep Deprivation in Pilots," *Aviation, Space and Environmental Medicine* 74 (2003): 1125–34. On the Afghanistan incident, the pilot's claim that amphetamine impaired his judgment, and the U.S. Military reaction, see Elliot Borin, "The U.S. Military Needs Its Speed," *Wired Magazine,* February 10, 2003 (http://www.wired.com/news/medtech/0,1286,57434,00.html, accessed September 4, 2004); Ian Sample, "Sleepless Troops May Be Sent into Battle on a High," *Sydney Morning Herald,* July 31, 2004, A20.

29. Anon., "Alleges Stimulation of Olympic Athletes," *New York Times,* October 1, 1948, 36. On Coppi's open admissions, see Gazzetta, "Doping" (http://www.cycling4fans.de/index.php?id=1361, accessed October 25, 2006); this source and many others cite a 1998 documentary on Italian television (RAI Tre) by Giancarlo Governi.

30. Les Woodland, *Dope: The Use of Drugs in Sport* (Sydney: Reed, 1980), chap. 1.

31. Allan Ryan, "Guest Editorial: Use of Amphetamines in Athletics," *JAMA* 170 (1959): 562.

32. L. A. Johnson, "Amphetamine Use in Professional Football," Ph.D. diss., U.S. International University, San Diego, California, 1972); cited in Arnold Mandell, "The Sunday Syndrome: A Unique Pattern of Amphetamine Abuse Indigenous to American Professional Football," *Clinical Toxicology* 15 (1979): 225–32.

33. Mandell, "The Sunday Syndrome: A Unique Pattern"; A. Mandell, Kim D. Stewart, and Patrick Russo, "The Sunday Syndrome: From Kinetics to Altered Consciousness," *Federation Proceedings* 40 (1981): 2693–98, 2697.

34. Mandell, Stewart, and Russo, "The Sunday Syndrome," 2697.

35. Ibid., passim; Johnson, "Amphetamine Use in Professional Football"; *Ridge v. Woodward et al.,* San Diego Superior Court, Civil Action No. 317816, 1973.

36. Brosman quoted in Bil Gilbert, "Drugs in Sport, Part 2: Something Extra on the Ball," *Sports Illustrated,* June 30, 1969, 30–42, quote at 30.

37. Jim Bouton, *Ball Four* (New York: World, 1970), 157.

38. Bil Gilbert, "Drugs in Sport, Part 1: Problems in a Turned-On World," *Sports Illustrated,* June 23, 1969, 64–72; idem, "Drugs in Sport, Part 2: Some-

thing Extra on the Ball," *Sports Illustrated,* June 30, 1969, 30–42, football quote at 37; idem, "Drugs in Sport, Part 3: High Time to Make Some Rules," *Sports Illustrated,* July 7, 1969, 30–35; Robert Baxley, "The Mandell Case and Proceedings for Revocation or Suspension of a Physician's and an Attorney's License," in David E Smith, ed., *Amphetamine Use, Misuse, and Abuse* (Boston: G. K. Hall, 1979), 303–17.

39. Ryan, "Use of Amphetamines in Athletics"; Gene M. Smith and Henry K. Beecher, "Amphetamine Sulfate and Athletic Performance. I. Objective Effects," *JAMA* 170 (1959): 542–57. For subsequent controversy over the significance of this study, see William Pierson, "Amphetamine Sulfate and Performance: A Critique," *JAMA* 177 (1961): 345–47; and William Cochran, Gene Smith, and Henry Beecher, "A Reply," *JAMA* 177 (1961): 347–49.

40. NFL Commissioner Paul Tagliabue, "Leading the Fight against Steroids," *New York Times,* February 24, 2004 (http://www.nfl.com/news/story/7132443, accessed October 25, 2006); quote from Peter Gent, "Are Teams Doing Enough in NFL Drug Cases," *New York Times,* July 31, 1983, S2; Tyler Kepner, "MLB gets Tougher on Steroid Use," *Santa Barbara News Press,* January 14, 2005, C1, C9; Michael Sokolove, "Sports Desk; Hot Topic," *New York Times Magazine,* February 5, 2006, section 6, 24.

41. Kramer, Fischman, and Litlefield, "Amphetamine Abuse"; Ian Oswald and V. R. Thacore, "Amphetamine and Phenmetrazine Addiction," *British Medical Journal* 2 (1963): 427–31.

42. R. T. Willey, "Abuse of Methylphenidate (Ritalin)," *New England Journal of Medicine* 285 (1971): 464.

43. W. P. Martin et al., "Physiologic, Subjective, and Behavioral Effects of Amphetamine, Methamphetamine, Ephedrine, Phenmetrizine, and Methylphenidate in Man," *Clinical Pharmacology and Therapeutics* 12 (1971): 245–58; Marian Fischman, "Cocaine and the Amphetamines," in Herbert Meltzer, ed., *Psychopharmacology: The Third Generation of Progress* (New York: Raven, 1987), 1543–53; D. Sulzer, M. Sonders, N. W. Poulsen, and A. Galli, "Mechanisms of Neurotransmitter Release by Amphetamines: A Review," *Progress in Neurobiology* 75 (2005): 406–33.

44. D. E. Smith and R. B. Seymour, "Addiction Medicine and the Free Clinic Movement," *Journal of Psychoactive Drugs* 29, no. 2 (1997):155–60; David C. Lewis, "The Role of Internal Medicine in Addiction Medicine," *Journal of Addictive Diseases* 15, no. 1 (1996): 1–17; David E. Smith, interview with author, December 29, 2004. See William White, *Slaying the Dragon: The History of Addiction Treatment and Recovery in America* (Bloomington, Ind.: Lighthouse Institute, 1998), 272–73, 287–90; American Society of Addiction Medicine, "History" (http://www.asam.org/info/history.htm, accessed February 7, 2006).

45. Maurice H. Seevers, "Drugs, Monkeys, and Men," *Michigan Quarterly Review* 8, no. 1 (1969): 3–14; Gerald Denau, Tomoji Yanagita, and Maurice

Seevers, "Self-Adminstration of Psychoactive Substances by the Monkey," *Psychopharmacologia* 16 (1969): 30–48; N. B. Eddy et al., "Drug Dependence: Its Significance and Characteristics," *Bulletin of the World Health Organization* 32 (1965): 721–33. In such experiments, it is worth noting, amphetamines are more addicting when the dose per lever press is higher, even when there is no limit on the rate or total quantity of drug consumption; this suggests why eating inhalers or injecting high doses is more addictive than low-dose pills. See, for example, the methamphetamine results in J. R. Weeks and R. J. Collins "Screening for Drug Reinforcement Using Intravenous Self-Administration in the Rat," in *Methods of Assessing the Reinforcing Properties of Abused Drugs,* ed. M. A. Bozarth, 35–43 (New York: Springer-Verlag, 1987).

46. Abraham Myerson, "Anhedonia," *American Journal of Psychiatry* 79 (1922): 87–103, quote at 91. Amphetamine withdrawal anhedonia is now a model system for discovering new antidepressants; see Mark Geyer and Athina Markou, "Animal Models of Psychiatric Disorders," in *Psychopharmacology: The Fourth Generation of Progress,* ed. Floyd Bloom and David Kupfer, 787–98 (New York: Raven, 1995). On dopamine and depression today, also see D. A. Slattery, A. L. Hudson, and D. J. Nutt, "The Evolution of Antidepressant Mechanisms," *Fundamental and Clinical Pharmacology* 18 (2004): 1–21. Perhaps dopamine mechanisms will be central to Klein's "atypical" depression, the type responsive to amphetamine but not tricyclics.

47. R. A. Wise and M. A. Bozarth, "Brain Substrates for Reinforcement and Drug Self-Administration," *Progress in Neuro-Psychopharmacology and Biological Psychiatry* 5 (1981): 467–74; idem, "A Psychomotor Stimulant Theory of Addiction," *Psychological Review* 94, no. 4 (October 1987): 469–92; Barry J. Everitt, Anthony Dickinson, and Trevor W. Robbins, "The Neuropsychological Basis of Addictive Behaviour," *Brain Research Reviews* 36 (2001): 129–38; Sulzer et al., "Mechanisms of Neurotransmitter Release by Amphetamines."

48. Julius Axelrod, "Biogenic Amines and Their Impact in Psychiatry," *Seminars in Psychiatry* 4 (1972): 199–211; P. M. Groves and G. V. Rebec, "Biochemistry and Behavior: Some Central Actions of Amphetamine and Antipsychotic Drugs," *Annual Review of Psychology* 27 (1976): 91–127; Lewis Seiden, Karen Sabol, and George Ricuarte, "Amphetamine: Effects on Catecholamine Systems and Behavior," *Annual Review of Pharmacology and Toxicology* 32 (1993): 639–77; Slattery, Hudson, and Nutt, "The Evolution of Antidepressant Mechanisms"; Sulzer et al., "Mechanisms of Neurotransmitter Release by Amphetamines."

49. Groves and Rebec, "Biochemistry and Behavior"; Solomon Snyder, "A 'Model Schizophrenia' Mediated by Cathecholamines," *American Journal of Psychiatry* 130 (1973): 61–67; Geyer and Markou, "Animal Models of Psychiatric Disorders"; Alan Baumeister and Jennifer Francis, "Historical Development of the Dopmaine Hypothesis of Schizophrenia," *Journal of the History of the Neurosciences* 11 (2002): 265–77.

50. Eddy et al., "Drug Dependence"; David Wilkie, "Addiction to Amphetamine," *British Medical Journal* 2 (September 15, 1962): 730; P. H. Connell, "Adolescent Drug Taking," *Proceedings of the Royal Society of Medicine* 58 (1965): 409–12; P. D. Scott and D. R. C. Willcox, "Delinquency and the Amphetamines," *British Journal of Psychiatry* 111 (1965): 865–75; D. S. Nachsen, "Amphetamine," *Lancet* (August 7, 1965): 289; P. H. Connell, "Clinical Manifestations and Treatment of Amphetamine Type of Dependence," *JAMA* 196 (1966): 718–23.

51. Editor, "Freedom from Amphetamines," *British Medical Journal* (July 17, 1971): 133–34; Frank Wells, "The Effects of a Voluntary Ban on Amphetamine Prescribing by Doctors on Abuse Patterns—Experience in the United Kingdom," in *Amphetamines and Related Stimulants: Chemical, Biological, Clinical and Social Aspects*, ed. John Caldwell (Boca Raton, Fla.: CRC Press, 1980), 189–92, quote at 192.

52. David Hawks et al., "Abuse of Methylamphetamine," *British Medical Journal* (21 June, 1969): 715–21; J. Strang, "Crack, Cocaine, and Amphetamines: Extent and Nature of Abuse in the UK," *Proceedings of the Royal College of Physicians of Edinburgh* 22 (1992): 8–12. In 1959, more than 5.5 million prescriptions for amphetamines were filled through the National Health Service, while, in 1968, that number had declined to about 4 million. See P. H. Connell, "Amphetamine Dependence," *Proceedings of the Royal Society of Medicine* 61 (1968): 178–81; Sir Denick Dunlop, "The Use and Abuse of Psychotropic Drugs," *Proceedings of the Royal Society of Medicine* 63 (1970): 1279–82; and Joy Mott, "The Epidemiology of Self-reported Drug Misuse in the United Kingdom," *Bulletin on Narcotics* 28, no. 1 (1976): 43–54. It is unclear how to square Dunlop's estimate that amphetamines accounted for 4 million NHS prescriptions, or about 1 percent of all such prescriptions, with the Newcastle studies' finding that amphetamine prescriptions ran closer to 3 percent in 1960; presumably, the lower figure does not include as many products, for example, diet pills. The doctor's prescribing moratorium was ultimately quite effective in reducing both medical and street speed use, presumably because Britain had much less pharmaceutical amphetamine flowing direct from manufacturers to the street without prescription than the U.S. did.

53. American Medical Association Council on Drugs, "New Drugs and Developments in Therapeutics," *JAMA* 183 (1963): 362–63; American Medical Association Committee on Alcoholism and Addiction and Council on Mental Health, "Dependence on Amphetamines and Other Stimulant Drugs," *JAMA* 197 (1966): 1023–27, quotes at 1023, 1027.

54. American Medical Association Council on Scientific Affairs, "Clinical Aspects of Amphetamine Abuse," *JAMA* 240 (1978): 2317–19; idem, "Drug Abuse Related to Prescribing Practices," *JAMA* 247 (1982): 864–66.

55. FDA History, "Interview with William W. Goodrich, Office of the General Counsel, 1939–1971," U.S. Food and Drug Administration (http://www.fda.gov/oc/history/oralhistories/goodrich/default.htm, accessed August 24, 2004).

56. Morton Mintz, "Still Hard to Swallow," *Washington Post,* November 2, 2001, B1; Louis Lasagna, "Congress, the FDA, and New Drug Development: Before and After 1962," *Perspectives in Biology and Medicine* 32 (1989): 322–43.

57. Lasagna, "Congress, the FDA, and New Drug Development"; Philip Hilts, *Protecting America's Health: The FDA, Business, and One Hundred Years of Regulation* (New York: Knopf, 2003), chap. 9; John Francis Marion, *The Fine Old House* (Philadelphia: SmithKline Corporation, 1980), 186.

58. Lasagna, "Congress, the FDA, and New Drug Development." Kennedy, in his State of the Union Address of January 1962, called for new FDA powers "halting unsafe and worthless products, preventing misleading labels, and cracking down on the illicit sale of habit-forming drugs" (http://www.geocities.com/americanpresidencynet/1962.htm, accessed September 1, 2006).

59. Morton Mintz, "Heroine of FDA Keeps Bad Drug off Market," *Washington Post,* July 15, 1962, A1. Lasagna, "Congress, the FDA, and New Drug Development"; Hilts, *Protecting America's Health,* chap. 10; Donna Hamilton, "A Brief History of the Center for Drug Evaluation and Research," U.S. Food and Drug Administration (http://www.fda.gov/cder/about/history/Histext.htm, accessed October 25, 2006).

60. Some analysts believe that this construction of barbiturates and amphetamines as "dangerous drugs" in the 1950s represented an FDA strategy for acquiring more regulatory power. Certainly, the FDA Commissioner testified extensively in favor of legislation to impose severe restrictions on these drugs, but industry and medical lobbies successfully blocked such measures in 1951 and 1956, as well as in 1961. See Rufus King, *The Drug Hang-Up: America's Fifty Year Folly* (Springfield, Ill.: Charles Thomas, 1972), chaps. 25–26 and passim. Also available online at Schaffer Library of Drug Policy, http://www.druglibrary.org/special/king/dhu/dhumenu.htm, accessed October 26, 2006.

61. Statement of George P. Larrick, Hearings of Subcommittee on Health, Senate Committee on Labor and Public Welfare, *Hearings on S. 2628,* 88th Congress, 2nd session, March 12, 1964 (hereafter, *Hearings on S. 2628*), 16–22; Statement of Senator Thomas Dodd, ibid., 46–49.

62. *Hearings on S. 2628,* 49–50 (AMA), 54–56 (NARD), 59–66 (APA); King, *The Drug Hang-Up,* chap. 26.

63. *Hearings on S. 2628,* 2–3; Anon., "Only Brief Discussion on Tranquilizers at One-Day Senate Subcommittee Hearing," *F-D-C Reports* (August 24,

1964): 31; Anon., "Hearings Needed on 'Psychotoxic' Drug Coverage," *F-D-C Reports* (September 7, 1964): 3–8.

64. Statements of Jay McMullen, February 9, 1965, and transcripts of *CBS Evening News* of September 2 and 3, 1964, in *Drug Abuse Control Amendments of 1965*, Hearings of the House Committee on Interstate and Foreign Commerce, 89th Congress, 1st session, January 27–28 and February 2, 9, and 10, 1965, 271–83, 283–87 (quote at 83). Anon., "Rep. Harris' Interstate Cmte. Leaning to Barb-Amphet Bill with Provision for Later FDA Listing of Drugs with a Potential for Abuse," *F-D-C Reports* (February 15, 1965): 12–15; Anon., "Bill Retains Counterfeit Drug Section, Adds H-E-W Proposed 'Cop' Amendments," *F-D-C Reports* (March 1, 1965): 13; Anon., "Brown Suggests Surveying Congressmen on Their Consumption of 'Goof balls and Pep Pills,'" *F-D-C Reports* (August 3, 1965): 19; King, *The Drug Hang-Up*, chap. 26.

65. For instance, *Smith, Kline & French v. Heart Pharmaceutical Corporation et al.*, Civil Action 57-341, U.S. District Court, Southern District of New York, 90 F Supp. 976 (1950); "Counterfeit Dexedrine and Dexamyl Operation," *F-D-C Reports* (November 2, 1964): 3.

66. King, *The Drug Hang-Up*, chap. 26.

67. "Pharmacist Rules Outlined on Refilling Stimulants and Depressants," *F-D-C Reports* (June 28, 1965): 20; John Swann, "Drug Abuse Control under FDA, 1938–1968," *Public Health Reports* 112 (November/December 1996): 83–86; *Crime in America—Why 8 Billion Amphetamines?* Hearings of the Select House Committee on Crime, 91st Congress, 1st session, November 18, 1969 (hereafter, *Why 8 Billion Amphetamines?*).

68. Susanna McBee, "The End of the Rainbow May Be Tragic: Scandal of the Diet Pills," *Life Magazine* 64 (January 26, 1968), in *Diet Pill (Amphetamines) Traffic, Abuse, and Regulation*, 245–51. Anon, "Pill Popping," *Vogue* (15 November, 1969): 104–5, and much related literature, is cited and discussed by Susan Speaker, "From 'Happiness Pills' to 'National Nightmare': Changing Cultural Assessment of Minor Tranquilizers in America, 1955–1980," *Journal of the History of Medicine and Allied Sciences* 52 (1997): 338–76. Quote from James Graham, "Amphetamine Politics on Capitol Hill," *Trans-Action Magazine*, January 1972, in *Diet Pill (Amphetamines) Traffic, Abuse, and Regulation*, 185–95, quote at 186.

69. Graham, "Amphetamine Politics on Capitol Hill."

70. Ibid. (Dodd quote at 188, Graham quote at 193, Ingersoll quote at 191). I must disagree with Susan Speaker, who has perceptively analyzed shifting popular views of tranquilizers from the 1950s through the 1970s, that the link between street drug abuse and medical overprescription represents any confusion or conflation. Rather, with Dodd I would argue that it was the drug industry that constructed the link as "confusion," at least as far as amphetamines are concerned.

71. On hyperkinesis prevalence and the need for amphetamines, see testimony of Dr. Sidney Cohen, *Why 8 Billion Amphetamines?* 2–4, 7, 12; Statement of Dr. John D. Griffith, ibid., 14–30. Also see James Graham, "Amphetamine Politics on Capitol Hill."

72. On Jacobson and Pepper, see Boyce Rensberger, "Amphetamines Used by a Physician to Lift Moods of Famous Patients," *New York Times,* December 4, 1972, sec. 1, 1, 34.

73. Graham, "Amphetamine Politics on Capitol Hill," 195.

74. The retrospectively reported production of amphetamine and methamphetamine base in 1968 was 24,992 kg, and in 1970 was 20,662 kg; "Statement of John E. Ingersoll, Director, Bureau of Narcotics and Dangerous Drugs," February 1, 1972, in *Diet Pill (Amphetamines) Traffic, Abuse, and Regulation,* 226–232, statistics at 231.

75. See, for instance, R. Maynard, "Omaha Pupils Given 'Behavior Drugs,'" *Washington Post,* June 29, 1970; Anon, "Pep Pills for Pupils," *Newsweek,* July 13, 1970; J. M. Rogers, "Drug Abuse: Just What the Doctor Ordered," *Psychology Today,* September 1971, 16–24; see also Office of Child Development, "Report of the Conference on the Use of Stimulant Drugs in Treatment of Behaviorally Disturbed Children," Washington D.C., Department of Health, Education, and Welfare, January 11–12, 1971. All reproduced in *Federal Involvement in the Use of Behavior Modification Drugs on Grammer School Children of the Right to Privacy Inquiry,* Hearing Before a Subcommittee of the House Committee on Government Operations, 91st Congress, 2nd session, September 29, 1970, Appendix II. See Carl Chambers and Dodi Schultz, "Women and Drugs: A Startling Journal Survey, The Drugs Women Use," *Ladies Home Journal,* November 1971; Carl Chambers and Dodi Schultz, "Housewives and the Drug Habit: What They Take—And Why," *Ladies Home Journal,* December 1971, both reproduced in *Diet Pill (Amphetamines) Traffic, Abuse, and Regulation.*

76. U.S. Food and Drug Administration, "George P. Larrick," http://www.fda.gov/oc/commissioners/larrick.html (accessed August 11, 2006); idem, "James L. Goddard," http://www.fda.gov/oc/commissioners/goddard .html (accessed October 26, 2006). See Hilts, *Protecting America's Health,* chap 11.

77. On RCTs, see Abraham Lilienfeld, "Ceteris Paribus: The Evolution of the Clinical Trial," *Bulletin of the History of Medicine* 56 (1982): 1–18; Ted J. Kaptchuk, "Intentional Ignorance: A History of Blind Assessment and Placebo Controls in Medicine," *Bulletin of the History of Medicine* 72 (1998): 389–433; Harry M. Marks, *Progress of Experiment: Science and Therapeutic Reform in the United States, 1900–1990* (Cambridge: Cambridge University Press, 1997); idem, "Rigorous Uncertainty: Why R. A. Fisher Is Important," *International Journal of Epidemiology* 32 (2003): 932–37; Iain Chalmers, "Fisher and Bradford Hill: Theory and Pragmatism?" *International Journal of Epidemiology* 32 (2003): 922–24.

78. U.S. Food and Drug Administration, "Herbert Ley, Jr.," http://www .fda.gov/oc/commissioners/ley.html (accessed October 26, 2006).

79. Center for Devices and Radiological Health, "Code of Federal Regulations, Title 21, Volume 4, "Subchapter C—Food and Drugs; Part 201—Labeling," U.S. Food and Drug Administration, http://www.accessdata.fda .gov/scripts/cdrh/cfdocs/cfcfr/CFRSearch.cfm?CFRPart=201&showFR=1& subpartNode=21:4.0.1.1.2.6 (accessed October 27, 2006). National Academy of Sciences, *Drug Efficacy Study: A Report to the Commissioner of Food and Drugs from the National Academy of Sciences* (Washington, D.C., 1969): the example quoted is from the evaluation of "NDA 12-415 E-01" on "Delfetased Stedy Tabs" (a methamphetamine-amobarbital combination), in *Diet Pills (Amphetamines) Traffic, Abuse, and Regulation*, 88–90; studies cited here include General Practitioner Research Group, "Dexamphetamine Compared with an Inactive Placebo in Depression," *Practitioner* 192 (1964): 151–54; J. E. Overall et al., "Drug Therapy in Depressions: Controlled Evaluation of Imipramine, Isocarboxazide, Dextroamphetamine-Amobarbital, and Placebo," *Clinical Pharmacology and Therapeutics* 3 (1962): 16–22.

80. Statement of Charles Edwards, *Diet Pill (Amphetamines) Traffic, Abuse, and Regulation*, 9–13. Center for Drug Evaluation and Research, Medical Review of Application Number 83-900, http://www.fda.gov/cder/foi/nda/ pre96/83-900_Amphetamine.htm (accessed August 17, 2004).

81. Claude Pepper, comment in *Why 8 Billion Amphetamines?* 8–9. Statement of John Ingersoll, February 1, 1972, in *Diet Pill (Amphetamines) Traffic, Abuse, and Regulation*, 226–32, esp. 228–29.

82. Statement of Charles Edwards, *Diet Pill (Amphetamines) Traffic, Abuse, and Regulation*, 9–13.

83. John Ingersoll, "Amphetamines and Methamphetamines, Aggregate Production Quotas," February 10, 1972, in *Diet Pill (Amphetamines) Traffic, Abuse, and Regulation*, 171–73.

84. On the 1971 UN Psychotropics Convention, see Claude Pepper, *Diet Pills (Amphetamines) Traffic, Abuse, and Regulation*, Exhibit 16, 116–18; see also King, *The Drug Hang-Up*, chap. 21; Jay Sinha, "The History and Development of the Leading International Drug Control Conventions," February 21, 2001 (prepared for the Senate Special Committee on Illegal Drugs, Library of Parliament, Canada, http://www.parl.gc.ca/37/1/parlbus/commbus/senate/com -e/ille-e/library-e/history-e.htm#B.percent20Conventionpercent20onpercent 20Psychotropicpercent20Substances (accessed September 5, 2006). Rush Loving Jr., "Putting Some Limits on 'Speed,'" *Fortune* (March 1971): 99, 127–28.

85. Birch Bayh, October 27, 1971, "Statement on the Transfer of Ritalin and Preludin to Schedule II," Hearings Before the Subcommittee to Investigate Juvenile Delinquency, 474–79. On Dexamyl's standing in the best-seller

list, see *National Prescription Audit, General Information Report*, 14th ed. (IMS America, 1975), 42; ibid., 15th, 16th, and 17th eds.

86. Wallace, research memo, March 23, 1937, GAP, box 15, unlabeled folder; Nabenauer to Alles, July 7, 1938, GAP, box 16, folder "Correspondence Not Listed in Card File"; Alles to Thompson, October 24, 1941, GAP, box 2, folder "SKF vs. Alles documents requested by SKF on discovery"; Anon., "Research Meeting April 16, 1942," April 21, 1942, GAP, box 2, folder "SKF vs. Alles: documents received from Alles Office."

87. Gordon Alles, "Some Relations between Chemical Structure and Physiological Action of Mescaline and Related Compounds," in *Neuropharmacology: Transactions of the Fourth Conference of September 25, 26, and 27, 1957*, ed. H. A. Abramson (New York: Macy Foundation, 1959), 181–269. David Dill to Alles, October 2, 1959; Alles, "Proposal to U.S. Army Chemical Center Procurement Agency for contract . . . in reponse to CMLMC-PA-213 RFP-61," December 1959; Alles to David McCurdy, January 25, 1961; and Alles, "Progress Report of Animal Studies on MDA and Its Analogs," [December 1961?]—all in GAP, box 11, folder "Army Chemical Warfare Laboratories." Mahlon David Fairchild, "Some Central Nervous System Effects of Four Phenyl-Substituted Amphetamine Derivatives," Ph.D. diss., Department of Pharmacology, University of California, Los Angeles, 1963.

88. Alles, laboratory notebook and records of expedition to Ethiopia beginning November 26, 1955, circa 1955–56, GAP, box 12, folder "Khat Experiments–GAA & MDF–1958." "Gordon A. Alles [obituary]," *Engineering and Science* (February 1963): 18–19; also David Fairchild, personal communication.

Notes to Chapter 8

1. J. Gfroerer and M. Brodsky, "The Incidence of Illicit Drug Use in the United States, 1962–1989," *British Journal of Addiction* 87 (1992): 1345–51.

2. Joseph Spillane, *Cocaine: From Medical Marvel to Modern Menace in the United States, 1884–1920* (Baltimore, Md.: Johns Hopkins University Press, 2000); Stephen Snelders, Charles Kaplan, and Toine Pieters, "On Cannabis, Chloral Hydrate, and Career Cycles of Psychotrophic Drugs in Medicine," *Bulletin of the History of Medicine* 80 (2006): 95–114; Charles O. Jackson, "Before the Drug Culture: Barbiturate/Amphetamine Abuse in American Society," *Clio Medica* 11 (April 1976): 47–58 (this last piece is interesting in that it reflects the perception that amphetamine was dead as a pharmaceutical, which it virtually was in the mid-1970s).

3. Christina Dye, "Crystal's Comeback," *Newservice* (July/August 1989): 1–3; Arthur Cho, "Ice: A New Form of an Old Drug," *Science* 249 (1990): 631–34; Arthur Hughes, "Epidemiology of Amphetamine Use in the United

States," in Arthur Cho and David Segal eds., *Amphetamine and Its Analogs* (San Diego: Academic Press, 1994), 439–57.

4. Numbers of past year users of amphetamine (including methamphetamine) from National Drug Use and Health surveys are available at www.drugabusestatistics.samhsa.gov, and Anon., "Primary Methamphetamine/Amphetamine Treatment Admissions: 1992–2002," DASIS report, September 17, 2004, Office of Applied Studies, Substance Abuse and Mental Health Services Administration (SAMHSA), available at http://www.oas.samhsa.gov (accessed September 15, 2006). Also see Janet C. Greenblatt and Joseph C. Gfroerer, "Methamphetamine Abuse in the United States (1997)," Office of Applied Studies, Substance Abuse and Mental Health Services Administration (SAMHSA), and Anon., "Methamphetamine Use, Abuse, and Dependence: 2002, 2003 and 2004," NSDUH Report, September 16, 2005, available at www.oas.samhsa.gov/2k5/meth/meth.htm (accessed September 15, 2006). In 2005, there were more than twice as many Americans over the age of twelve reporting past month use of illicit amphetamines compared to heroin, and twice as many classed with "abuse or dependence"; Substance Abuse and Mental Health Services Administration, Office of Applied Studies, "Results from the 2005 National Survey on Drug Use and Health: National Findings," Department of Health and Human Services, available at http://oas.samhsa.gov/NSDUH/2k5NSDUH/2k5results.htm (accessed September 15, 2006).

5. Roger Smith, "Traffic in Amphetamines: Patterns of Illegal Manufacture and Distribution," *Journal of Psychedelic Drugs* 2, no. 2 (1969): 20–27; U.S. Drug Enforcement Administration, "Methamphetamine" update, 2006, available at http://www.usdoj.gov/dea/concern/meth.html (accessed December 15, 2006); Dye, "Crystal's Comeback"; Cho, "Ice: A New Form of an Old Drug"; Hughes, "Epidemiology of Amphetamine Use."

6. Jessica McBride, "Crank, The 'Rural Crack,' Hits the Heartland— Hard," *Milwaukee Journal Sentinel,* November 8, 1998, available for download at http://www.mapinc.org/drugnews/v98/n1021/a08.html; Dye, "Crystal's Comeback"; for Oklahoma City and speed, see, for example, "The Oklahoma City Bombing Case: The Second Trial," Court TV Online, available at http://www.courttv.com/archive/casefiles/oklahoma/nichols/week2.html; full transcripts available at CNN Interactive, http://edition.cnn.com/US/9703/okc.trial/transcripts/ (accessed December 15, 2006).

7. Dirk Johnson, *Meth: America's Home-Cooked Menace* (Center City, Minn.: Hazelden, 2005), 9. Peter Kramer, *Listening to Prozac* (New York: Viking, 1993), 7–10, 219.

8. The problem of temperament or original mood disorder and drug abuse is fraught with the chicken/egg problem, but some evidence nevertheless exists to support the notion that many people become drug abusers in an effort to adjust their abnormal moods; see D.A. Regier et al., "Comorbidity of

Mental Disorders with Alcohol and Other Drug Abuse: Results from the Epidemiologic Catchment Area (ECA) Study," *JAMA* 264 (1990): 2511–18; Alvaro Camacho and Hagop Askisal, "Proposal for a Bipolar-Stimulant Spectrum: Temperament, Diagnostic Validation and Therapeutic Outcomes with Mood Stabilizers," *Journal of Affective Disorders* 85 (2005): 217–30.

9. Shulgin's qualitative experiences with the two drugs are described in extremely similar terms. Shulgin judges, however, that the drugs probably work differently on the mind, because they exhibit little cross-tolerance in terms of subjective effects. Alexander and Ann Shulgin, *PIHKAL: A Chemical Love Story* (Berkeley: Transform Press, 1991), 715–16, 736–37.

10. A. S. Roberts and F. Alexander, "Report on Clinical Evaluation of SKF #5 (amphedoxamine)," Smith, Kline & French Laboratories, August 21, 1957. PDF available from Erowid References Database, http://www.erowid.org/references/refs_view.php?ID=1076 (accessed September 17, 2006); also cited and described by Richard Yensen et al., "MDA-Assisted Psychotherapy with Neurotic Outpatients: A Pilot Study," *Journal of Nervous and Mental Disorders* 163 (1976): 233–45. Paul Thiessen and David A. Cook, "The Properties of 3,4-methylenedioxyamphetamine (MDA). I. A Review of the Literature," *Clinical Toxicology* 6, no. 1 (1973): 45–52. This source cites the following patents on MDA: E. J. Fellows and L. Cook, "MDA as Anorexigenic," U.S. Patent 2,974,148, 1961; SKF Laboratories, "MDA as Ataractic," British Patent 82880, 1960; H. D. Brown, "MDA as Antitussive," U.S. Patent 2,820,739, 1958. Untoward CNS effects at 120mg/day in obesity trials with MDA were reported in a personal communication from SKF personnel, cited in C. Naranjo, A. T. Shulgin, and T. Sargent, "Evaluation of 3,4-methylenedioxyamphetamine (MDA) as an Adjunct to Psychotherapy," *Medicina et Pharmacologia Experimentalis (International Journal of Experimental Medicine)* 17, no. 4 (1967): 359–64.

11. Quote from Alexander Shulgin, "Psychotomimetic Agents Related to the Catecholamines," *Journal of Psychedelic Drugs* 2, no. 2 (1969): 14–9, quote at 16.

12. Frederick Meyers, Alan Rose, and David E. Smith, "Incidents Involving the Haight-Ashbury Population and Some Uncommonly Used Drugs," *Journal of Psychedelic Drugs* 1, no. 2 (1968): 139–46; David E. Smith, "The Psychotomimetic Amphetamines with Special Reference to DOM (STP) Toxicity," *Journal of Psychedelic Drugs* 2, no. 2 (1969): 37–42; Lester Grinspoon and Peter Hedblom, *The Speed Culture: Amphetamine Use and Abuse in America* (Cambridge, Mass.: Harvard University Press, 1975), 56–57; see also Shulgin and Shulgin, *PIHKAL*, 715–16, 736–37. On the plausibility of rumors about MDA's escape from an armory, David E. Smith, interview with author, December 29, 2004.

13. Naranjo, Shulgin, and Sargent, "Evaluation of 3,4-Methylenedioxyamphetamine"; Claudio Naranjo, *The Healing Journey: New Approaches to Con-*

sciousness (New York: Pantheon Books, 1974); Yensen et al., "MDA-Assisted Psychotherapy with Neurotic Outpatients"; Nicholas Saunders, *E for Ecstasy* (London: N. Saunders, 1993), chap. 3, available at http://www.ecstasy.org/ books/e4x/e4x.ch.03.html (accessed October 27, 2006); Anon., "Claudio Naranjo, Pioneer of the Feeling Enhancers," BLTC Research, http://mdma.net/ claudio-naranjo (accessed August 2, 2004); Anon., "Utopian Pharmacology: Mental Health in the Third Millennium; MDMA and Beyond," BLTC Research, http://www.hedweb.com/ecstasy (accessed August 2, 2004). Evidence for the continued recreational use of MDA includes D. Reed, R. H. Cravey, and P. R. Sedgwick, "A Fatal Case Involving Methylenedioxyamphetamine," *Clinical Toxicology* 5 (1972): 3–6; T. Lukaszewski, "3,4-Methylenedioxyamphetamine Overdose," *Clinical Toxicology* 15 (1979): 405–9; A. Poklis, M. A. Mackell, and W. K. Drake, "Fatal Intoxication from 3,4-Methylenedioxyamphetamine," *Journal of Forensic Science* 24, no. 1(1979): 70–75.

14. Anon., "U.S. Will Ban 'Ecstasy,' A Hallucinogenic Drug," *New York Times,* June 1, 1985, 6; Bruce Eisner, *Ecstasy: The MDMA Story* (Berkeley: Ronin, 1994), chap. 1.

15. Eisner, *Ecstasy,* prologue, xiv and passim. Lisa Foderaro, "Psychedelic Drug Called Ecstasy Gains Popularity in Manhattan Nightclubs," *New York Times,* December 11, 1988, 58; Office of Applied Studies, Substance Abuse, and Mental Health Services Administration (SAMHSA), "2003 National Survey on Drug Use & Health: Results," available at http://oas.samhsa.gov/nhsda/ 2k3nsduh/2k3Results.htm (accessed January 22, 2006).

16. SAMHSA, "2003 National Survey on Drug Use & Health: Results"; Raymond Hernandez, "In New Drug Battle, Use of Ecstasy among Young Soars," *New York Times,* August 2, 2000, A21.

17. SAMHSA, "2003 National Survey on Drug Use & Health: Results"; Jane Carlisle Maxwell, "Patterns of Club Drug Use in the U.S., 2004," Gulf Coast Addiction Technology Transfer Center, University of Texas at Austin, http://www.utexas.edu/research/cswr/gcattc/Trends/ClubDrug-2004-web .pdf (accessed January 22, 2006).

18. James Inciardi and Carl Chambers, "The Epidemiology of Amphetamine Use in the General Population," *Canadian Journal of Criminology and Corrections* 14 (1972): 166–72; also see chapter 6 above.

19. On the history of Attention Deficit Disorder, see Peter Conrad, "The Discovery of Hyperkinesis: Notes on the Medicalization of Deviant Behavior," *Social Problems* 23 (1975): 12–21; Lawrence Diller, "The Run on Ritalin: Attention Deficit Disorder and Stimulant Treatment in the 1990s," *Hastings Center Report* 26 (1996): 12–19; Peter Conrad and Deborah Potter, "From Hyperactive Children to ADHD Adults: Observations on the Expansion of Medical Categories," *Social Problems* 47 (2000): 559–82; Andrew Lakoff, "Adaptive Will: The Evolution of Attention Deficit Disorder,"*Journal of the History of the Behavioral*

Sciences 36 (2000): 149–69. Precise estimates of total numbers of people using AD/HD medication are not available to me, but commercial analysts place the number of children who used Attention Deficit medications in 2000 at 3–4 million, and the number of adults using them in 2005 at 600,000, making 5 million a reasonable estimate for the total number of current-year U.S medication users (this assumes that users under seventeen years of age have increased to 4.5 million since 2000); Cheryl Barton, "CNS Drug Discoveries: What the Future Holds. Attention Deficit Hyperactivity Disorder (ADHD)," 2005, Espicom Business Intelligence, http://www.espicom.com/prodcat.nsf/Product_ID_Lookup/00000160?OpenDocument (accessed October 16, 2006). These estimates exceed the 2.5 million children said *currently* to be using medications in 2003, according to a large national survey; S. N. Visser and C. A. Lesesne, "Mental Health in the United States: Prevalence of Diagnosis and Medication Treatment for Attention-Deficit/Hyperactivity Disorder—United States, 2003," *Morbidity and Mortality Weekly Report* 54, no. 34 (September 2, 2005): 842–47, available at http://www.cdc.gov/mmwr/preview/mmwrhtml/mm5434a2.htm (accessed October 16, 2006). The two figures may easily be reconciled, however, by noting that the national survey evidently asked a question about "current" use, which would probably be interpreted by many respondents as past-month use, whereas the commercial analysis appears to be referring to past-year use. On recent prevalence estimates, especially in adults, see Joseph Biederman, "Attention-Deficit/Hyperactivity Disorder: A Selective Overview," *Biological Psychiatry* 57, no. 11 (2005): 1215–20.

20. For current arguments on whether Attention Deficit is a real disease, along with debate about what causes and defines Attention Deficit as a disease (if it is one), see Sami Timimi and Eric Taylor, "ADHD is Best Understood as a Cultural Construct," *British Journal of Psychiatry* 184 (2004): 8–9, along with subsequent responses, and also articles in *Biological Psychiatry* 57, no. 11 (June 1, 2005). For sociological and historical purposes, the fact that many doctors treat it as a medical condition makes it one, so we need not venture here into problems of defining "disease."

21. Ronald Koegler, "Drugs, Neurosis, and the Family Physician," *California Medicine* 102, no. 1 (1965): 5–8, estimated that one-third of general medical practice consisted of psychosomatic complaints that were really neuroses and problems of living. For more recent sensitivity, see Arthur J. Barsky and Jonathan Borus, "Somatization and Medicalization in the Era of Managed Care," *JAMA* 274 (1995): 1931–34.

22. Mary Eberstadt, "Why Ritalin Rules," *Policy Review* 94 (1999): 24–40, quote at 34.

23. Conrad, "The Discovery of Hyperkinesis"; Diller, "The Run on Ritalin"; Conrad and Potter, "From Hyperactive Children to ADHD Adults"; Henrikje Klasen, "A Name, What's in a Name? The Medicalization of Hyperactiv-

ity, Revisited," *Harvard Review of Pyschiatry* (2000): 334–44. On local overdiagnosis and overprescription, as well as the role of patient advocacy groups, see testimony of Terrance Woodworth, Hearing Before the Subcommittee on Early Childhood, Youth and Families, Committee on Education and the Workforce, House of Representatives, 106th Congress, 2nd session, Serial No. 106-109, May 16, 2000, available at http://www.dea.gov/pubs/cngrtest/ct051600.htm (accessed January 21, 2006).

24. L. S. Goldman et al., "Diagnosis and Treatment of Attention Deficit–Hyperactivity Disorder in Children and Adolescents," *JAMA* 279 (1998): 1100–1107; D. Sulzer, M. Sonders, N. W. Poulsen, and A. Galli, "Mechanisms of Neurotransmitter Release by Amphetamines: A Review," *Progress in Neurobiology* 75 (2005): 406–33.

25. Diller, "The Run on Ritalin," 17–18.

26. U.S. Department of Justice, Drug Enforcement Administration, "Controlled Substances: Final Revised Aggregate Production Quotas for 2005," *Federal Register* 70, no. 216 (November 9, 2005), available at Office of Diversion Control, http://www.deadiversion.usdoj.gov/fed_regs/quotas/2005/fr1109 .htm (accessed January 27, 2006); see chapter 6 of this volume for 1969 consumption estimates. Note that 10 mg amphetamine base is equivalent to 12–20 mg amphetamine salt, the typical form in which the drug is taken as pills and the dose that is usually stated on drug labels. Furthermore, 5 mg methamphetamine or dextroamphetamine salts are the typical content of pills, although some pharmaceutical amphetamines contain much higher levels of active drug.

27. Anon., "Shire: No Kidding Around with Adderall XR," InPharm.com, November 12, 2004, http://www.inpharm.com/External/InpH/1,2580,1-4-0-0-inp_intelligence_news-0-257065,00.html (accessed November 23, 2004). See testimony of Terrance Woodworth, *Hearing Before the Subcommittee on Early Childhood, Youth and Families*, May 16, 2000; Anon., "NIDA Infofax," http://www.nida.nih.gov:80/Infofax/ritalin.html; Anon., "NIDA InfoFacts: Methylphenidate (Ritalin)," National Institute on Drug Abuse, http://www.nida .nih.gov:80/Infofax/ritalin.html; Anon., "Ritalin Abuse: Statistics," Frontline, http://www.pbs.org/wgbh/pages/frontline/shows/medicating/drugs/ ritalinstats.html (all accessed November 29, 2004). Christiane Poulin, "Medical and Nonmedical Stimulant Use among Adolescents: From Sanctioned to Unsanctioned Use," *Canadian Medical Association Journal* 165 (2001): 1039–44; S. E. McCabe, C. J. Teter, C. J. Boyd "The Use, Misuse, and Diversion of Prescription Stimulants among Middle and High School Students," *Substance Use and Misuse* 39 (2004):1095–1116

28. Christopher Tennant, "The Ritalin Racket," undated, http://articles .student.com/article/ritalin (accessed November 29, 2004); Anon, "NIDA InfoFacts"; Anon, "Ritalin Abuse: Statistics"; S. E. McCabe, J. R, Knight, C. J.

Teter, H. Wechsler, "Non-Medical Use of Prescription Stimulants among U.S. College Students: Prevalence and Correlates from a National Survey," *Addiction* 100 (2005): 96–106, and erratum in *Addiction* 100 (2005): 573; B. C. Carroll, T. J. McLaughlin, and D. R. Blake, "Patterns and Knowledge of Nonmedical use of Stimulants among College Students," *Archives of Pediatrics and Adolescent Medicine* 160 (2006): 481–85; K. M. Hall, M. M. Irwin, K. A. Bowman, W. Frankenberger, and D. C. Jewett, "Illicit Use of Prescribed Stimulant Medication among College Students," *Journal of American College Health* 53, no. 4 (2005):167–74; Elizabeth Wurtzel, *More, Now, Again: A Memoir of Addiction* (New York: Simon and Schuster, 2001), 33–35, 42, and passim.

29. Office of Applied Studies, Substance Abuse and Mental Health Services Administration (SAMHSA), "2005 National Survey on Drug Use & Health: Results," U.S. Department of Health and Human Services, http://oas .samhsa.gov/NSDUH/2k5NSDUH/2k5results.htm (accessed September 20, 2006).

30. L. A. Kroutil et al., "Nonmedical Use of Prescription Stimulants in the United States," *Drug and Alcohol Dependence* 84 (September 15, 2006): 135–43

31. Birch Bayh, Exhibit 10, and John Ingersoll, Exhibit 11, *Diet Pill (Amphetamines) Traffic, Abuse and Regulation,* Hearings before the Subcommittee to Investigate Juvenile Delinquency, Senate Committee on the Judiciary, 92nd Congress, 1st session, February 7, 1972 (hereafter *Diet Pill (Amphetamines) Traffic, Abuse and Regulation*), 90–95. Here 2.5 billion doses is the 1969 production of amphetamine and methamphetamine base, reported by firms applying for quotas, divided in 10 mg units. The active ingredient in most pills actually weighs 1.5–2.5 times the base depending on the particular salt form, translating this quantity to about 4 billion 10 mg doses of amphetamine salts. In reasonably good agreement, manufacturers voluntarily reported production of amphetamine and methamphetamine equivalent to 4.5 billion 10 mg (salts) tablets in 1971 in a different context (ibid.). Both numbers are serious underestimates of actual production, since not all producers reported in either context.

32. On 1969–70 amphetamine usage, 5 percent of the U.S. population, in 1970, was estimated to have used the drugs medically in the previous year, and, depending on the source, one-half or three-quarters of these were using the drugs for weight loss (these figures are not necessarily inconsistent, since overweight was seen as a result of mood disorders and many people would have been prescribed amphetamine for depression and weight loss together); see Hugh Parry et al., "National Patterns of Psychotherapeutic Drug Use," *Archives of General Psychiatry* 28 (1973): 769–83.

33. In the early 1990s, for instance, 2 million Americans were taking prescription diet pills, and then 10 million in the mid-1990s when "Phen-Fen" became popular, and then down to 4 million in the late 1990s when this medica-

tion fell out of favor and certain nonprescription pills became more popular (see below).

34. Alan S. Levy and Alan W. Heaton, "Weight Control Practices of U.S. Adults Trying to Lose Weight," *Annals of Internal Medicine* 119 (1993): 661–66; Mary Serdula et al., "Weight Control Practices of U.S. Adolescents and Adults," *Annals of Internal Medicine* 119 (1993): 667–71; Randall Stafford and David Radley, "National Trends in Antiobesity Medication Use," *Archives of Internal Medicine* 163 (2003): 1046–50; Heidi M. Blanck, Laura K. Khan, and Mary K. Serdula, "Prescription Weight Loss Pill Use among Americans: Patterns of Pill Use and Lessons from the Fen-Phen Market Withdrawal," *Preventive Medicine* 39 (2004): 1243–48. Stafford and Radley report that, based on doctor visit surveys by IMS, in 1996–97 about 10 million Americans were using prescription diet pills, up from 2 million in 1994, a number that plunged to below 4 million in 1998, after the Phen-Fen withdrawal. Blanck et al. have evidence, based on user survey data, that perhaps 10 million (i.e. 2.5 percent of the population over 12) took prescription diet pills in the peak period of Phen-Fen popularity, and this is reasonable agreement. They also found that a third of these took nonprescription diet pills as well. The early 1990s survey data of Levy and Heaton, and Serdula et al., suggest that 7 or 8 million American women and 1 or 2 million men were taking weight-loss drugs, either prescription or nonprescription, at a time when Stafford and Radley place prescription diet pill users at fewer than 5 million. Thus, at least 10 million Americans take diet pills at any one time and switch readily between prescription and nonprescription pills, sometimes taking both.

35. "MASS SUICIDE WEAPON," unpaginated Tepanil advertisement, *JAMA* 174 (November 26, 1960); "Look At All the People Who Can Use TENUATE," unpaginated advertisement, *JAMA* 174 (December 3, 1960); AMA Council, *New and Nonofficial Drugs* (Philedelphia: Lippincott, 1962), 248–49, 267–69; "Reducing the Problems of Reducing," Preludin advertisement in *American Practitioner* 12 (August 1961): 27a; "Preludin Reduces the Problems of Reducing," unpaginated Preludin advertisement in *JAMA* 174 (December 3,1960); E. M. Brecher, *Licit and Illicit Drugs* (Boston: Little, Brown, 1973), chap. 39, 294–98.

36. Alexander M. Walker, "Aminorex," Harvard School of Public Health, http://www.hsph.harvard.edu/Organizations/DDIL/amino.html (accessed December 10, 2004); Alfred Fishman, "Aminorex to Fen/Phen: An Epidemic Foretold," *Circulation* 99 (1999): 156–61; H. P. Gurtner et al., "Häufen sich die primär vasculären Formen des chronischen Cor pulmonale?" *Journal Suisse de Médicine* 41 (1968): 1579–89; 43 (1968):1695–1707; H. Voss and H. Harms, "Epidemiologie und Klinik der primär vaskulären pulmonalen Hypertonie," *Zeitschrift für Kreislaufforschung* 59 (1970): 887–91; F. Follath, F. Burkhart, and W. Schweizer, "Drug-Induced Pulmonary Hypertension?" *British Medical Jour-*

nal 1 (1971): 265–66; Editorial, "An Epidemic of Pulmonary Hypertension," *Lancet* 252 (1971): ii; Arthur Hadler, "Studies of Aminorex, A New Anorexigenic Agent," *The Journal of Clinical Pharmacology and the Journal of New Drugs* 7 (1967): 296–302.

37. Lindsey Gruson, "A Controversy over Widely Sold Diet Pills," *New York Times*, February 13, 1982, 52; Jane Brody, "Pills to Aid the Dieter: How Safe Are They?" *New York Times*, November 9, 1983, C1; Edward Steinberg, "Diet Stand Disputed," Letters to the Editor, *New York Times*, November 30, 1983, C11; N. R. Kleinfeld, "The Ever-Fatter Business of Thinness," *New York Times*, September 7, 1986, F1, F28. For examples of medical reports describing PPA's amphetamine-like dangers, see G. Norvenious, E. Widerlov, and G. Lonnerholm, "Phenylpropanolamine and Mental Disturbances," *Lancet* 2 (1979): 1367–68; A. Blum, "Phenylpropanolamine: An Over-the-Counter Amphetamine," *JAMA* 245 (1981): 1346–47; A. J. Dietz, "Amphetamine-Like Reactions to Phenylpropanolamine," *JAMA* 245 (1981): 601–2; F. H. Lovejoy Jr., "Stroke and Phenylpropanolamine," *Pediatric Alert* 12 (1981): 45; E. Bernstein and B. Diskant, "Phenylpropanolamine, a Potentially Hazardous Drug," *Annals of Emergency Medicine* 11 (1982): 311–15; S. M. Mueller, "Phenylpropanolamine, a Non-Prescription Drug with Potentially Fatal Side Effects," *New England Journal of Medicine* 308 (1983): 653; Roberta Glick et al., "Phenylpropanolamine: An Over-the-Counter Drug Causing Central Nervous System Vasculitis and Intracerebral Hemorrhage," *Neurosurgery* 20 (1987) : 969–74.

38. Marian Burros, "Children are Focus of Diet Pill Issue," *New York Times*, October 3, 1990, C1, C4; Barry Meier, "Diet-Pill Death Raises Questions on FDA Role," *New York Times*, August 4, 1990, 48; Anon., "FDA Curbs Diet Drugs," *New York Times*, August 8, 1991, D8; Sarah Lueck, "FDA Officials Suspected PPA Link to Higher Stroke Risk Since '80s," *Wall Street Journal*, November 8, 2000, B6; Jeff Gerth and Sheryl Gay Stolberg, "Another Part of the Battle: Keeping a Drug on the Shelves of Stores," *New York Times*, December 13, 2000, A31; Editorial, "A Prescription for Peril," *Los Angeles Times*, March 30, 2004, B12; Kevin Sack and Alicia Mundy, "Over-the-Counter Peril," *Los Angeles Times*, March 28, 2004, A1; Anon., "Chattem Says Judge Approved Dexatrim Settlement," *New York Times*, August 28, 2004, C4.

39. R. Langreth, "Critics Claim Diet Clinics Misuse Obesity Drugs," *Wall Street Journal*, March 31, 1997, B8; L. Abenheim et al., "Appetite-Supressant Drugs and the Risk of Primary Pulmonary Hypertension," *New England Journal of Medicine* 335 (1996): 609–16; H. M. Connoly et al., "Valvular Heart Disease Associated with Fenfluramine-Phentermine," *New England Journal of Medicine* 337 (1997): 581–88; L. Cannistra, "Valvular Heart Disease Associated with Dexfenfluramine," *New England Journal of Medicine* 337 (1997): 636; D. J. Graham and L. Green, "Further Cases of Valvular Heart Disease Associated with Fenfluramine-Phentermine," *New England Journal of Medicine* 337 (1997): 635;

E. J. Mark et al., "Fatal Pulmonary Hypertension Associated with Short-Term Use of Fenfluramine and Phentermine," *New England Journal of Medicine* 337 (1997): 602–6; Gregory Curfman, "Diet Pills Redux," *New England Journal of Medicine* 337 (1997): 629–30; Alfred Fishman, "Aminorex to Fen/Phen: An Epidemic Foretold," *Circulation* 99 (1999): 156–61; Molly Sachdev et al., "Effect of Fenfluramine-Derivative Diet Pills on Cardiac Valves: A Meta-Analysis of Observational Studies," *American Heart Journal* 144 (2002): 1065–73; Randall Stafford and David Radley, "National Trends in Antiobesity Medication Use," *Archives of Internal Medicine* 163 (2003): 1046–50; Blanck, Khan, and Serdula, "Prescription Weight Loss Pill Use among Americans."

40. On sibutramine's potential antidepressant activity, see Carla A. Luque and Jose A. Rey, "The Discovery and Status of Sibutramine as an Anti-Obesity Drug," *European Journal of Pharmacology* 440 (2002): 119–28. On the continuing quest for more drugs related to amphetamine, see Brian Rothman and Michael Baumann, "Neurochemical Mechanisms of Phentermine and Fenfluramine: Therapeutic and Adverse Effects," *Drug Development Research* 51 (2000): 52–65.

41. Marian Burros, "The Mysteries and Dangers of Herbal Remedies," *New York Times,* June 16, 1993, C8; idem, Marian Burros, "With Some Dietary Supplements, What You Don't Know Can Hurt You," *New York Times,* July 14, 1993, C4; Warren Leary, "Federal Panel Suggests Restrictions on Herbal Stimulant," *New York Times,* August 29, 1996, D18; Timothy Gower, "Weight Loss the Herbal Way: No All Natural Silver Bullet," *New York Times,* June 13, 1999, WH13; Mary Duffy, "Side Effects Raise Flag on Dangers of Ephedra," *New York Times,* October 12, 1999, F7; Anon., "FDA Announces Plans to Prohibit Sales of Dietary Supplements Containing Ephedra," U.S. Food and Drug Administration, http://www.fda.gov/oc/initiatives/ephedra/december2003 (accessed December 15, 2006); Anon., "Sales of Supplements Containing Ephedrine Alkaloids (Ephedra) Prohibited," U.S. Food and Drug Administration, http://www.fda/gov/oc/initiatives/ephedra/february2004 (accessed December 15, 2006); Cynthia Bulik, "Abuse of Drugs Associated with Eating Disorders," *Journal of Substance Abuse* 4 (1992): 69–90.

42. Parry et al., "National Patterns of Psychotherapeutic Drug Use." This 5 percent includes people taking amphetamines prescribed for weight loss, but because depression or emotional distress is often seen as the cause of weight gain, the distinction is not sharp.

43. J. Mallerstein, "Depression as a Pivotal Affect," *American Journal of Psychotherapeutics* 22 (1968): 202–17; C. G. Watson, W. G. Klett, and T. W. Lorei, "Toward an Operational Definition of Anhedonia," *Psychological Reports* 26 (1970): 371–76; J. Schildkraut, "The Catecholamine Hypothesis of Affective Disorders," *American Journal of Psychiatry* 122 (1965): 509–52; Hagop Askisal and William McKinney, "Overview of Recent Research in Depression," *Archives of General Psychiatry* 32 (1975): 285–305.

44. Askisal and McKinney, "Overview of Recent Research in Depression"; Donald Klein, "Endogenomorphic Depression: A Conceptual and Terminological Revision," *Archives of General Psychiatry* 31 (1974): 447–54; Paul Meehl, "Hedonic Capacity: Some Conjectures," *Bulletin of the Menninger Clinic* 39 (1975): 295–307.

45. Askisal and McKinney, "Overview of Recent Research in Depression"; American Psychiatric Association, *Diagnostic and Statistical Manual*, 3rd ed. (Washington, D.C.: American Psychiatric Association, 1980), 213–14, 220–21. Elizabeth Cooksey and Phil Browne, in "Spinning on Its Axes: DSM and the Social Construction of Psychiatric Diagnosis," *International Journal of the Health Sciences* 28 (1998): 525–54, point out the *DSM*'s function in improving the professional status of psychiatrists compared to nonmedical rivals like psychologists, for which greater unity and cooperation appeared essential in the 1970s. Also see Edward Shorter, *A History of Psychiatry: From the Era of the Asylum to the Age of Prozac* (New York: Wiley, 1997), chap. 8.

46. David Healy, *The Antidepressant Era* (Cambridge, Mass.: Harvard University Press, 1996), 165–69 and passim.

47. Ibid. The chemists who invented Prozac describe themselves as moonlighting, doing work outside their official tasks. However, because serotonin plays a role in lowering blood pressure, a selective serotonin-booster might turn out to be a valuable heart medicine, a possibility commercially interesting enough to allow employees to investigate the topic. See D. T Wong et al., "Prozac (fluoxetine, Lilly 110140), the First Selective Serotonin Uptake Inhibitor and an Antidepressant Drug: Twenty Years Since Its First Publication," *Life Sciences* 57 (1995): 411–41.

48. David Healy, "The Three Faces of the Antidepressants: A Critical Commentary on the Clinical-Economic Context of Diagnosis," *Journal of Nervous & Mental Disease* 187 (1999): 174–80.

49. Healy, *The Antidepressant Era*. The finding that tricyclics work as well or better than SSRIs for at least some patients has proved robust, and, indeed, the exploration of which patient types respond better to tricyclics is an active research field; see G. Parker et al., "Assessing the Comparative Effectiveness of Antidepressant Therapies: A Prospective Clinical Practice Study," *Journal of Clinical Psychiatry* 62 (2001): 117–25; G. Parker, "Differential Effectiveness of Newer and Older Antidepressants Appears Mediated by an Age Effect on the Phenotypic Expression of Depression," *Acta Psychiatrica Scandinavica* 106 (2002): 168–70.

50. Kramer, Listening to Prozac, 1–12, 246–49, quote at 246.

51. Ibid., quote at 14.

52. Ibid., 210, 245.

53. Christopher Callahan and German Berrios, *Reinventing Depression: A History of the Treatment of Depression in Primary Care 1940–2004* (Oxford: Oxford University Press, 2005), esp. chaps. 8–9.

54. According to IMS retail prescription audit data, more than 100 million SSRI prescriptions were dispensed in the year 2003. See M. Marketos, "The Top 200 Brand Drugs in 2003," *Drug Topics* 148 (2004): 76; cited in Patricia G. Moorman et al., "Antidepressant Medication Use for and Risk of Ovarian Cancer," *Obstetrics and Gynecology* 105, no. 4 (April 2005): 725–30. According to David Healy (personal communication, October 2006) 20 million individuals is the best estimate of how many Americans consumed these prescriptions per year in recent years. According to Erica Goode, consumption rates were leveling out at 7 million Americans using SSRI antidepressants in 2001, clearly a minimal estimate, based on drug industry sources; see Goode, "Antidepressants Lift Clouds, but Lose 'Miracle Drug' Label," *New York Times,* June 29, 2002, http://www.essentialdrugs.org/edrug/archive/200206/msg00064.php (accessed January 20, 2006).

55. Even the figure of 8 million users, 2.6 percent of the national population, exceeds the proportion of Americans ever using amphetamines psychiatrically, by prescription. As we have seen, 5 percent of Americans over the age of twelve used amphetamines by prescription in the year 1969–70, or up to 8 million people (4 percent of the total population) and half that figure was supposedly accounted for by weight loss prescriptions, although there was much overlap (Parry et al., "National Patterns of Psychotherapeutic Drug Use"; also see chap. 6 above). The proportion of psychotropic drug prescribing attributable to primary care physicians has declined greatly since the 1960s and dipped below 50 percent in the mid-1990s. See H. A. Pincus et al., "National Trends in the Prescribing Trends in Psychotropic Medications: Primary Care, Psychiatry, and Other Medical Specialties," *JAMA* 279 (1998): 526–31. On the economics of treating depression with SSRIs in an American private insurance setting, see David Cutler, *Your Money or Your Life* (Oxford: Oxford University Press, 2004), chap. 4.

56. L. T. Wu and J. C. Anthony, "The Estimated Rate of Depressed Mood in U.S. Adults: Recent Evidence for a Peak in Later Life," *Journal of Affective Disorders* 60 (2000): 159–71. The National Institute of Mental Health has assessed the number of adult Americans suffering mood disorders in any year at 21 million or 9.5 percent of the population, three-quarters of which are major or minor depression (dysthymia) and the remainder bipolar disorders; see Anon., "The Numbers Count: Mental Disorders in America," National Institute of Mental Health, http://www.nimh.nih.gov/publicat/numbers.cfm# Dysthymic (accessed October 16, 2006).

57. Taking the prevalence of tricyclic and MAOI antidepressant consumption in the 1960s (1–2 percent of the population per year) as indicative of the medical profession's assessment of depression's prevalence, today's estimated annual prevalence of 10 percent reflects an increase no greater than tenfold. Taking Healy's view that depression was thought to affect fewer than a

hundred people per million per year in the 1960s, today's prevalence of 10 percent reflects a thousandfold increase (Healy, "The Three Faces of the Antidepressants"). Of course, MAOIs and especially tricyclics, like amphetamines, were also deliberately prescribed as placebos by physicians to patients they must not have considered clinically depressed. This must be true of SSRIs to at least as great a degree, as I argue further below. The concept that mood disorders were not recognized as common conditions by general practitioners before the 1990s is absolutely false, as amply shown in chapters 2–6 of this book.

58. Irving Kirsch and Guy Saperstein, "Listening to Prozac but Hearing Placebo: A Meta-Analysis of Antidepressant Medications," in *How Expectancies Shape Experience,* ed. I. Kirsch, 303–20 (Washington, D.C.: American Psychological Association, 1999). Irving Kirsch et al., "Initial Severity and Antidepressant Benefits: A Meta-Analysis of Data Submitted to the Food and Drug Administration," *PLoS Medicine* 5(2) (2008):e45, DOI:10.1371/journal.pmed.0050045. As for tests comparing tricyclics to placebos and Dexamyl, see E. H. Hare, C. Mc-Cance, and W. O. McCormick, "Impiramine and 'Drinamyl' in Depressive Illness: A Comparative Trial," *British Medical Journal* (28 March, 1964): 818–20; also see Overall et al., "Drug Therapy in Depressions," although this was an inpatient study population that included psychotic depressives and schizophrenics.

59. In the New York studies, only 13 percent of users of "diet pill"–type amphetamines, the great majority of whom were medical users, also used prescription-type psychiatric amphetamines. Epidemiological research on legal polydrug use today is needed. See Inciardi and Chambers, "The Epidemiology of Amphetamine Use in the General Population," and chap. 6 above.

60. Ecstasy's use for sociability and soul-searching bears resemblances to both the psychiatric and recreational use of amphetamine. But this complexity is consistent with the general argument, since, as an illicit drug, Ecstasy would not necessarily be expected to enhance conformity to social norms.

61. Jean Baudrillard, *The Consumer Society: Myths and Structures,* trans. Chris Turner (London: Sage, 1998), chap. 11, esp. 182–83.

62. Ivan Illich, *Limits to Medicine: Medical Nemesis, the Expropriation of Health* (London: Marion Boyars, 1976), 88; Nikolas Rose, *Inventing Our Selves: Psychology, Power, and Personhood* (Cambridge: Cambridge University Press, 1996).

Notes to the Conclusion

1. *Diet Pills (Amphetamines) Traffic, Abuse, and Regulation,* Hearings Before the Subcommittee to Investigate Juvenile Delinquency, Senate Committee on the Judiciary, 92nd Congress, 1st session, February 7, 1972, 88.

2. See Office of Applied Studies, Substance Abuse and Mental Health Services Administration, "National Survey on Drug Use and Health, Short Re-

port: Nonmedical Use of Prescription Pain Relievers," May 21, 2004, U.S. Department of Health and Human Services, http://oas.samhsa.gov/2k4/pain/ pain.htm (accessed September 23, 2006); for detailed findings on past year abuse of prescription drugs, 2004, see Office of Appled Studies, "National Survey on Drug Use and Health: Detailed Tables 2004," U.S. Department of Health and Human Services, http://oas.samhsa.gov/NSDUH/2k4nsduh/ 2k4tabs/Sect1peTabs1to66.htm#tab1.26b, (accessed September 23, 2006).

3. P. Kozlov et al., "HIV Incidence and Factors Associated with HIV Acquisition among Injection Drug Users in St. Petersburg, Russia," *AIDS* 20 (2006): 901–6

4. HIV/AIDS incidence in the U.S. was about 42,000, with more than 10,000 of these infections (almost 25 percent) acquired directly by injecting drug use, according to E. Schneider et al., "Epidemiology of HIV/AIDS— United States, 1981—2005," *Morbidity and Mortality Weekly Report* 55 (June 2, 2006): 589–92, http://www.cdc.gov/mmwr/preview/mmwrhtml/mm5521a2 .htm (accessed September 23, 2006), whereas in Australia HIV/AIDS incidence is 200–250 annually since 2000, and less than 5 percent are injecting drug users, according to Australian Institute of Health and Welfare, "Australia's Health 2004," http://www.aihw.gov.au/publications/aus/ah04/ah04- c00.rtf (accessed September 23, 2006), and lecture by Alex Wodak, University of Sydney School of Public Health, August 9, 2006.

5. Amphetamines were 1.4 percent of new prescriptions in 1968 compared to 2.9 percent in the U.S. See *National Prescription Audit, General Information Report,* 9th ed. (Gosselin, 1970), 12–14, where 2.9 percent is the sum of the two categories "psychostimulants" and "anti-obesity preparations—amphetamine"; for British data, see Istvan Bayer, "The Abuse of Psychotropic Drugs," *Bulletin on Narcotics* 2 (1973), United Nations Office on Drugs and Crime, http://www.unodc.org/unodc/es/bulletin/bulletin_1973-01-01_3_page003 .html#tnr101 (accessed January 30, 2006). This calculation of the British amphetamine prescription rates takes 280 million (5 scrips/person × 56 million people) as the total U.K. prescriptions for 1968, and 4 million as the number of amphetamine prescriptions, as per Derrick Dunlop, "The Use and Abuse of Psychotropic Drugs," *Proceedings of the Royal Society of Medicine* 63 (1970): 1279–82. The overall U.K. per capita prescription rate was closely comparable to that of the U.S. at the time. In the early 1960s, based on the Newcastle-area studies, amphetamine preparations accounted for about 3 percent of British prescriptions.

6. Jerry Avorn, Milton Chen, and Robert Hartley, "Scientific versus Commercial Sources of Influence on the Prescribing Behavior of Physicians," *American Journal of Medicine* 73 (1982): 4–8; P. R. Lichstein, R. C. Turner, and K. O'Brien, "Impact of Pharmaceutical Company Representatives on Internal Medicine Residency Programs," *Internal Medicine* 152 (1992): 1009–13; J. A. Hopper,

M. W. Speece, and J. L. Musial, "Effects of an Educational Intervention on Residents' Knowledge and Attitudes Toward Interactions with Pharmaceutical Representatives," *Journal of General Internal Medicine* 12 (1997): 639–42; M. A. Steinman, M. G. Shlipak, and S. L. McPhee, "Of Principles and Pens: Attitudes of Residents and House Staff toward Pharmaceutical Industry Promotions," *American Journal of Medicine* 110 (2001): 551–57; S. L. Coyle, "Physician-Industry Relations. Part 1: Individual Physicians," *Annals of Internal Medicine* 136 (2002): 396–402; R. S. Watkins and J. Kimberly, "What Residents Don't Know about Physician-Pharmaceutical Industry Interactions," *Academic Medicine* 79 (2004): 432–37; Richard Adair and Leah R. Holmgren, "Do Drug Samples Influence Resident Prescribing Behavior? A Randomized Trial," *American Journal of Medicine* 118, no. 8 (August 2005): 881–84. This is but a small sampling of a large and expanding literature that documents the powerful effects on prescribing of corporate marketing, sponsored medical education, and so forth.

7. T. Bodenheimer, "Clinical Investigators and the Pharmaceutical Industry," *New England Journal of Medicine* 342 (May 18, 2000): 1539–44; Lise L. Kjaergard and Bodil Als-Nielsen, "Association between Competing Interests and Authors' Conclusions: Epidemiological Study of Randomised Clinical Trials Published in the BMJ," *British Medical Journal* 325 (2002): 249–52; J. E. Bekelman, Y. Li, and C. P. Gross, "Scope and Impact of Financial Conflicts of Interest in Biomedical Research: A Systematic Review," *Journal of the American Medical Association* 289, no. 4 (January 22, 2003): 454–65; Joel Lexchin et al., "Pharmaceutical Industry Sponsorship and Research Outcome and Quality: Systematic Review," *British Medical Journal* 326 (2003): 1167–70; Mohit Bhandari et al., "Association between Industry Funding and Statistically Significant Pro-Industry Findings in Medical and Surgical Randomized Trials," *Canadian Medical Association Journal* 170 (2004): 477–80.

8. Sheila W. Smith, "Sidelining Safety: The FDA's Inadequate Response to the IOM," *New England Journal of Medicine* 357 (2007): 960–63. Recent efforts to protect the medical research literature from sponsorship bias includes strict guidelines on disclosure of sponsorship, and universal pre-registration of clinical trials so that the existence of unreported negative trials can be detected. International Committee of Medical Journal Editors, "Uniform Requirements for Manuscripts Submitted to Biomedical Journals," http://www.icmje.org/ (accessed October 15, 2005). Anon., "WHO Clinical Trials Initiative to Protect the Public," *Bulletin of the World Health Organization* 84 (2006): 10–11. I would further propose a lifetime ban on all authors proven to have failed knowingly in disclosure, from a set of coooperating major journals such as the ICMJE group, because it is essential for purposes of meta-analysis that sponsored trials can be treated separately.

9. For statistics on health outcomes and expenditures by country, see *Health at a Glance: OECD Indicators 2007* (Paris: Organisation for Economic Cooperation

and Development, 2007), 23, 87, 89, and passim. Also see CIA, *The World Fact-book*, Central Intelligence Agency, https://www.cia.gov/cia/publications/factbook (accessed September 28, 2006). For an accessible if inward-looking overview of the health economic problems of the United States, see David Cutler, *Your Money or Your Life* (Oxford: Oxford University Press, 2004); on pharmaceuticals as part of the problem, see John Abramson, *Overdosed America: The Broken Promise of American Medicine* (New York: HarperCollins, 2004).

List of Archival Sources

ANRP: Alfred Newton Richards papers, University of Pennsylvania Archives UPT50/R514.

BFSP: B. F. Skinner papers, Harvard University Archives HUG (FP) 60.20, Boston

GAP: Gordon Alles Papers, California Institute of Technology Archives, Pasadena (many of these documents are also found in the *SKF vs. Alles* records, below).

NAS: National Academy of Sciences (USA), Reports and Correspondence Files of the Advisory Committees to the Surgeons General of the War & Navy Departments and United States Public Health Service, Washington, D.C.

RAC: Rockefeller Archive Center, Tarrytown, New York.

SKF vs. Alles records: Records of *Smith, Kline & French, Inc., vs. the Estate of Gordon Alles,* Civil Action 67-280-IH (1967), U.S. District Court, Central California District, Federal District Courts, Civil Case Files, National Archives and Records Administration Pacific Region Archives (Laguna Niguel, California).

SKF vs. Clark & Clark records: Records of *Smith, Kline & French, Inc., vs. Clark & Clark, Inc.,* Case C-2311 (1943), U.S. District Court, New Jersey District, Federal District Courts, Civil Case Files, National Archives and Records Administration Central Plains Region Archives (Lee's Summit, Missouri).

UCSF-PH: Department of Pharmacology and Experimental Therapeutics records, PH S/M, University of California, San Francisco Archives.

UKNA: United Kingdom National Archives, Public Record Office, Kew.

USNA: National Archives of the United States, College Park, Maryland.

Index

Abel, John Jacob 7, 13
Abuse of amphetamines, 138–141, 171,
175–176, 208, 210, 236–237, 248, 250;
British, 31, 88, 137, 172–173, 203, 258,
318n62, 327n52; in military, 85, 89–91,
100, 190–191; in 1940–1950s counterculture, 91–100, 103; in 1960s counterculture, 171–175, 179, 181–189; among
students, 30–31, 41, 47, 50, 54, 87, 236,
253, 319n8. *See also* Ecstasy; Methamphetamine
Acetylcholine, 11, 38–39, 151
Addiction, 175, 189–190, 192, 210, 255; to
amphetamines, 31, 46–50, 55, 99, 124,
132, 137–138, 140–143, 178–179, 197–
204, 214, 218, 224, 231, 236–237, 257,
303n52, 317n62, 324n45; definition of,
48–50, 140–143, 170, 197, 199, 203–204
Adrenaline: or epinephrine and norepinephrine, natural functions, 10–12, 25–
27, 38–39, 57, 62, 151, 160, 202, 241, 246,
262n2, 273nn24, 26; as a pharmaceutical,
7–12, 14, 16, 20, 27
Aggression: amphetamines and, 29, 53, 64–
65, 68, 70–71, 82, 87, 139, 173, 185, 187,
192, 195, 225
Alles, Gordon, 13–15, 221, 226–227; and
collaboration with Smith, Kline &
French, 22–24, 51–53, 102–103, 106,
125–126; and invention and patenting
of amphetamine, 6–7, 15–22, 108–112,
115–119, 130, 144
Aminorex, 240
Amphetamine psychosis, 80, 98, 138–141,
143, 165, 167, 169, 173, 185, 188, 195, 203,
218, 225, 231, 239, 241–242, 255
Anhedonia, 33–35, 38–39, 41–42, 106, 121,
124–125, 131, 158–160, 180–181, 246, 248,
251–253, 307n16, 325n46
Antibiotics, 1–3, 47, 113, 128, 145, 151, 160
Antidepressants, 136, 162–165, 177, 210,
244–253, 278n52, 305n1, 309n26, 341n49,

342n57; amphetamines as, 3, 36–42, 50–
52, 109–110, 114–115, 131, 136, 142–143,
150, 158–161, 163–164, 180–181, 214,
217–218, 226, 231, 236, 244–245, 248–251,
258, 295n4, 308n21; mechanism of action,
38–39, 151–152, 158–159, 246, 273n26;
monoamine oxidase inhibitors (MAOIs),
160–164, 202, 244, 247; selective serotonin reuptake inhibitors (SSRIs), 1–2, 202,
225–226, 246–251, 300n39, 341n47,
342n54; screening and discovery, 149–
158, 246–247, 305n4, 325n46; tricyclic,
155, 157–164, 244, 246–249, 307n12,
308n21, 342n57. *See also* Benzedrine Sulfate; Dexamyl; Dexedrine
Antipsychotics, 1–2, 154, 157, 176, 203.
See also Chlorpromazine
Anxiety, 35, 36, 40, 41, 51, 56–57, 63–64,
82–83, 124, 133, 136, 145–147, 149, 153–
154, 165, 167, 172, 175; and depression,
33, 51, 120–121, 131, 164, 300n39
Asthma, 10, 14, 16–18, 20–21, 28
Attention Deficit Disorder, 29–30, 164–166,
214, 216, 220, 231–237, 244, 248, 250–252,
255–256, 258, 270n9, 334n19, 335n20

Barbiturates, 31, 34, 56–57, 112, 113, 122–
123, 196, 198, 291n26, 293n4, 313n53;
abuse of, 100–101, 130, 190, 208–210,
328n60; combined with amphetamines,
51, 90, 100, 121, 124–126, 136, 161, 166,
174, 194, 297n18, 309n23. *See also*
Dexamyl
Barger, George, 12, 14, 112
Bartlett, F. C., 63
Beatles, 104
Beatniks, 94–99, 171, 183–184
Bebop, 91–95
Behaviorism, 152–157, 200–201, 235, 245
Benzedrex, 105, 119; Inhaler, 102–105
Benzedrine Inhaler, 22, 43–44, 46, 87–105,
139, 183

348

About the Author

NICOLAS RASMUSSEN is the author of *Picture Control: The Electron Microscope and the Transformation of Biology in America, 1940–1960* (Stanford: Stanford University Press, 1997). He has taught history of life sciences and medicine for fifteen years, ten at the University of New South Wales, and also at the University of Sydney, Princeton University, the University of California at Berkeley and UCLA. He has had broad practical experience in the life sciences and, briefly, in the drug industry. He holds advanced degrees in the History and Philosophy of Science, the Biological Sciences, and Public Health.

Printed in the United States
By Bookmasters